High-Resolution CT of the Chest

Comprehensive Atlas

THIRD EDITION

■ **ERIC J. STERN, M.D.**

Professor of Radiology
Adjunct Professor of Medicine
Adjunct Professor of Medical Education and Bioinformatics
Vice-Chair for Academic Affairs
University of Washington
Seattle, Washington

■ **STEPHEN J. SWENSEN, M.D., M.M.M., FACR**

Professor of Radiology
Mayo Clinic
Rochester, Minnesota

■ **JEFFREY P. KANNE, M.D.**

Associate Professor
Vice Chairman of Quality and Safety
Department of Radiology
University of Wisconsin - Madison
Madison, Wisconsin

Wolters Kluwer | Lippincott Williams & Wilkins
Health
Philadelphia · Baltimore · New York · London
Buenos Aires · Hong Kong · Sydney · Tokyo

Acquisitions Editor: Brian Brown
Product Manager: Ryan Shaw
Vendor Manager: Bridgett Dougherty
Senior Manufacturing Manager: Benjamin Rivera
Senior Marketing Manager: Angela Panetta
Design Coordinator: Teresa Mallon
Production Service: Aptara, Inc.

Library of Congress Cataloging-in-Publication Data
Stern, Eric J.
  High-resolution CT of the chest : comprehensive atlas / Eric J. Stern, Stephen J. Swensen, Jeffrey P. Kanne. – 3rd ed.
     p. ; cm.
  Includes bibliographical references and index.
  ISBN 978-0-7817-9190-8 (alk. paper)
  1. Chest—Tomography—Atlases.   I. Swensen, Stephen J.   II. Kanne, Jeffrey P.   III. Title.
  [DNLM: 1. Respiratory Tract Diseases—radiography—Atlases.   2. Radiography, Thoracic—Atlases.   3. Respiratory System—pathology—Atlases.   4. Tomography, X-Ray Computed—Atlases. WF 17 S839h 2009]
  RC941.S85 2009
  617.5′40757—dc22

                                                                        2009023437

Care has been taken to confirm the accuracy of the information presented and to describe generally accepted practices. However, the authors, editors, and publisher are not responsible for errors or omissions or for any consequences from application of the information in this book and make no warranty, expressed or implied, with respect to the currency, completeness, or accuracy of the contents of the publication. Application of the information in a particular situation remains the professional responsibility of the practitioner.

The authors, editors, and publisher have exerted every effort to ensure that drug selection and dosage set forth in this text are in accordance with current recommendations and practice at the time of publication. However, in view of ongoing research, changes in government regulations, and the constant flow of information relating to drug therapy and drug reactions, the reader is urged to check the package insert for each drug for any change in indications and dosage and for added warnings and precautions. This is particularly important when the recommended agent is a new or infrequently employed drug.

Some drugs and medical devices presented in the publication have Food and Drug Administration (FDA) clearance for limited use in restricted research settings. It is the responsibility of the health care providers to ascertain the FDA status of each drug or device planned for use in their clinical practice.

To purchase additional copies of this book, call our customer service department at (800) 638-3030 or fax orders to (301) 223-2320. International customers should call (301) 223-2300.

Visit Lippincott Williams & Wilkins on the Internet at: LWW.com. Lippincott Williams & Wilkins customer service representatives are available from 8:30 am to 6 pm, EST.

10 9 8 7 6 5 4 3 2

To Karen, and our beautiful life together.

-*EJS*

To my three favorite people: Lynn, Scott and Callie.

-*SJS*

To Elizabeth, Max, Alan, and Liza for all of their love, support, and patience.

-*JPK*

Foreword to Third Edition

As co-author of the textbook *High-Resolution CT of the Lung*, it is with great pleasure that I write the foreword to the atlas on the same subject that I see as its companion and that is now in its 3rd edition.

The aim of a reference textbook on high-resolution CT of the chest is to provide a thorough review of the literature and to illustrate the most common and characteristic features of diseases that affect the airways and pulmonary parenchyma. The aim of this atlas is to provide a pictorial essay of the spectrum of abnormalities that may be seen in any given disease entity. The textbook and the atlas therefore are complementary.

The atlas has been updated and the text and images have been greatly improved in this edition, thanks to the recognized expertise of the two original authors, Drs. Eric Stern and Stephen Swensen, and to the addition of a new star in chest imaging, Dr. Jeffrey Kanne, who was one of the most talented and enthusiastic Chest Imaging Fellows that I have had the pleasure to have in my program. Congratulations to the authors on the publication of this excellent atlas of high-resolution CT.

Nestor L. Müller, M.D., Ph.D.

Contents

Contents

Introduction to High-Resolution Computed Tomography

High-resolution computed tomography (HRCT) has contributed significantly to the radiologic assessment of intrathoracic and pulmonary diseases since its refinement in the mid-1980s. The foremost reason is that HRCT scans detect and allow characterization of many disease processes, which with conventional chest radiography are occult, nonspecific, or equivocal. Computed tomography (CT) scanning is still the most common cross-sectional imaging examination for evaluation of the chest. In our practices, dedicated HRCT scans are performed in a minority of cases; however, it should be readily appreciated that most modern multidetector-row CT scanners, and their capability for volumetric scanning, quickly produce many thin sections, essentially equivalent to the HRCT techniques of the past, but now with easy generation of reformations in coronal or sagittal imaging planes, expanding our appreciation for the extent and distribution of various conditions and abnormalities. In many ways, all state-of-the-art thin section chest imaging, with or without contrast enhancement, is high-resolution chest imaging, making an understanding of the various presentations of lung abnormalities all the more important.

Technique

Dedicated HRCT is a technique that can be performed on any late-generation CT scanner. It differs from conventional CT only by optimizing technical parameters for spatial resolution by using the narrowest beam collimation possible <1.5 mm, and often down to 0.6 mm in diameter and a high spatial frequency reconstruction algorithm (e.g., bone, sharp). HRCT should not be used in the densitometric analysis of lung nodules because the high spatial frequency reconstruction algorithms may lead to erroneous diagnosis of calcification.

HRCT is usually performed using volumetric helical imaging of the entire thorax. Radiation dosage can be lowered considerably with negligible reduction in diagnostic accuracy. We suggest routine use of a single window/level combination [window level of approximately −750 Hounsfield units (HU) and a width of approximately 1,500 HU] but also recommend tailoring the window/level combination to accentuate certain disease processes. For instance, to increase confidence in detecting interstitial lung disease, we suggest using a window with higher contrast (window/level of approximately –750 HU and a width of approximately 1,000 to 1,200 HU). For accentuating more subtle differences in lung density, such as in emphysema or constrictive bronchiolitis, a lower window/level (–800 to –900 HU) and narrower width (500 to 1,000 HU) increase the contrast between abnormal and normal lung tissue, always keeping in mind that such a window can also make the normal interstitium appear abnormally prominent. Wider window widths of 1,500 to 2,000 HU reduce contrast between the lung and air-containing spaces but are useful for examining pleuroparenchymal abnormalities.

HRCT scanning is usually performed with the patient supine. In this position, a zone of increased lung attenuation in the dependent regions of the posterior lung bases can be seen. This is most often attributable to microatelectasis and other gravity-related changes. This appearance and distribution are very similar to the ground-glass attenuation associated with many of the etiologies of pulmonary fibrosis (e.g., usual interstitial pneumonia (UIP), scleroderma, and asbestosis). To definitively state whether these changes are a result of normal "dependent" lung attenuation or pulmonary fibrosis/inflammation, the patient should be rescanned after a deep inspiration and then, if necessary, in the prone position, to "rule out interstitial lung disease" in the clinical context. With normal lung parenchyma, the normal dependent lung density clears.

HRCT scanning has been also traditionally performed at suspended full inspiration. However, HRCT scanning performed at suspended full expiration shows the physiologic consequence of small airways (bronchiolar) diseases—air trapping. Lung regions that retain air during exhalation remain more lucent and show less decrease in volume than do lung regions supplied by normal airways. The distribution of air trapping is often lobular or multilobular and depends on the level and severity of the airway obstruction. When the level of airway obstruction is at or near the lobular level, a mosaic pattern of normal lung and hyperlucent lung can result. Lung regions that retain air show a decrease in the caliber and number of pulmonary vessels relative to normal lung. The inciting pathologic processes can be permanent, as are seen in patients with constrictive bronchiolitis, or reversible, as are seen in patients with asthma. In some instances, air trapping can be occult on routine suspended full-inspiration CT scanning, becoming evident only on CT scans obtained at suspended full expiration. Air trapping has been shown in patients with asthma, constrictive bronchiolitis of all etiologies, including the postinfectious Swyer-James syndrome, cystic fibrosis, and sarcoidosis. Expiratory CT scanning provides anatomic and physiologic information that is complementary to conventional suspended full-inspiration CT scanning and pulmonary function testing. Depending on the clinical scenario, the extent and distribution of air trapping are useful in indicating or directing further diagnostic workup, such as transbronchial, thoracoscopic, or surgical lung biopsy.

Regardless of the specific HRCT protocols that you chose for your practice, it is strongly suggested that your practice adopts a common set to optimize comparison and efficiency and to reduce errors.

Anatomy

HRCT scans can show lung anatomy and morphology not evident on conventional CT scans or conventional radiographs. Because abnormalities are easily detected and characterized at the level of the secondary pulmonary lobule, it is important to have an understanding of the secondary lobule's anatomy—the intralobular core structures (the intralobular artery and airway) and the interlobular septa (containing the lobular venous and lymphatic drainage).

The acinus, the respiratory unit of the lung, is that portion of lung supplied by a terminal bronchiole and includes the gas-exchange structures (usually three to eight respiratory bronchioles, with subtending alveolar ducts, and alveoli). Three to five acini form the secondary pulmonary lobule, or more simply, the pulmonary lobule. The acinus system of description is preferable in some circumstances for theoretical and functional reasons, whereas the lobular system is preferable in the situations in which macroscopic tissue abnormalities are the essence. The pulmonary acinus is not normally visible on HRCT (except in some disease states), whereas pulmonary lobular structures are well visualized by HRCT. It is the lobular terminology that is important in defining many lung diseases, and the one we use throughout this book. Other intrathoracic structures are better characterized by HRCT, such as the lobar fissures and accessory fissures, and the central and peripheral airways.

Specific General Indications

Below are some specific, but certainly not all-inclusive, indications for dedicated thin section chest imaging.

HRCT scans can identify small nodules not evident on chest radiographs. Small rounded opacities on HRCT, especially poorly defined nodules, do not have to be "nodules" per se. They can be inflammatory or fibrotic regions of lung, around small bronchovascular bundles, that appear only as "nodules" (e.g., with hypersensitivity pneumonitis). The lumen of small airways may be obliterated, thereby appearing as nodules (e.g., with panbronchiolitis and cystic fibrosis).

Especially in the early stages of lung damage, HRCT is more sensitive and accurate than chest radiographs or pulmonary function tests in defining the presence and extent of pulmonary emphysema and cystic lung diseases in symptomatic patients. In cystic lung diseases, HRCT separates out the superimposition of multiple thin walls of lung cysts responsible for the "interstitial" pattern observed at chest radiography, accurately displaying the extent and distribution of cystic change of the lung.

HRCT is also more sensitive than chest radiography or conventional CT for detecting lung and pleural abnormalities in asbestos-exposed individuals. HRCT is helpful in eliminating false-positive chest radiographic diagnoses of asbestos-related pleural disease caused by subpleural fat and false-positive diagnoses of asbestosis in patients with extensive pleural plaques or superimposed emphysema.

CT and HRCT have been shown to be very useful in the evaluation of focal lung disease. HRCT is more sensitive than CT and chest radiography in the detection of fat and calcium in lung nodules. HRCT often allows a confident, specific benign diagnosis to be made, such as granuloma, hamartoma, rounded atelectasis, arteriovenous malformation, and bronchopulmonary sequestration, thus obviating invasive diagnostic procedures and saving the patient expense and morbidity. In general, focal lung disease is best initially localized with conventional CT, usually of the entire thorax, to determine whether a lung lesion is solitary. Thin section CT scans can then be selectively obtained depending on the CT appearance and clinical situation. One-mm collimation using the standard (not high spatial frequency) algorithm should be used for lung nodule analysis.

HRCT scanning is useful in examining the lungs in immunocompetent and immunocompromised patients who have fever or respiratory symptoms but normal or nonspecific chest radiographs, again by detecting, characterizing, and localizing disease. For example, HRCT scanning can help assess the severity of disease in patients with bronchiectasis and cystic fibrosis or identify active granulomatous disease in patients with prior mycobacterial infection.

Common Descriptive HRCT Disease Patterns

Several colorful descriptive terms have been popularized in the radiology literature, becoming HRCT "buzz" words. These terms, originally coined to describe a particular disease process, are sometimes used inappropriately to imply a pathognomonic finding when, in fact, the terms are much less specific than once thought and are now associated with a number of other disorders. These HRCT buzz words include *crazy paving*, *mosaic perfusion* or *mosaic pattern*, *ground-glass opacity* (GGO), and *tree-in-bud* (TIB) and are described in greater detail below.

Crazy Paving

Crazy paving is a colorful, descriptive term for the HRCT scan findings of apparent thickened interlobular septa and intralobular structures, forming typical polygonal shapes with no architectural distortion. The diseased lung can be quite well demarcated from surrounding normal lung tissue, creating a "geographic" pattern, especially with pulmonary alveolar proteinosis.

Crazy paving was originally described as a pathognomonic finding of pulmonary alveolar proteinosis. The finding is still strongly suggestive of pulmonary alveolar proteinosis but only in the appropriate clinical setting. However, this HRCT scan pattern has also been described with such diverse disease processes as *Pneumocystis* pneumonia, sarcoidosis, bronchioloalveolar carcinoma, acute respiratory distress syndrome, pulmonary hemorrhage, and lipoid pneumonia.

Mosaic Pattern of Lung Attenuation

The original descriptive term *mosaic perfusion* refers to a CT finding of chronic pulmonary thromboembolic disease resulting from regions of hyperemic (higher attenuation) lung adjacent to oligemic (lower attenuation) regions of lung. The oligemic lung shows a decrease in the caliber and number of pulmonary vessels relative to normal or hyperemic lung. Similar findings are described for primary pulmonary hypertension. Acute pulmonary thromboembolism has been shown experimentally to not produce a mosaic pattern of lung attenuation, discrediting the concept of Westermark's sign.

However, since the original description of mosaic perfusion, areas of variable lung attenuation in a lobular or multilobular distribution similar to that of chronic pulmonary thromboembolism have been described in two other distinct disease categories: (i) small airways disease and (ii) infiltrative disease. Diseases from each of these categories can cause similar patterns, and since these etiologies are not all directly related to perfusion per se, the general term mosaic lung attenuation is preferred.

Areas of variable lung attenuation in a lobular or multilobular distribution are almost never a normal finding, except as a normal gravitational gradient of lung density. This mosaic pattern of lung attenuation presents a challenge to the radiologist when deciding which are the abnormal regions of lung, those of low attenuation, high attenuation, or both. It is often possible to distinguish among these categories by using the following additional CT scan findings, although admittedly, there are cases that defy a satisfactory interpretation.

A patchy infiltrative process within the interstitium of the lung or partial filling of the air spaces by fluid, cells, or fibrosis can occur, such that the CT attenuation of the affected lung increases relative to that of normal parenchyma. This patchy distribution can appear as a typical mosaic pattern. The vessel caliber and number are not appreciably different between the normal and abnormal regions of lung. Diseases that can produce such a CT pattern of mosaic lung attenuation include, for example, *Pneumocytis* pneumonia, chronic eosinophilic pneumonia, hypersensitivity pneumonia, or bacterial pneumonia.

In small airways disease and primary pulmonary vascular disease, the pulmonary vessels within the lucent regions of lung are small, relative to the vessels in the more opaque lung. This discrepancy in vessel size is likely caused, at least in part, by local hypoxic reflex vasoconstriction in small airways disease, whereas the difference in vessel size in primary vascular disease is caused by the underlying hypoperfusion. In proliferative diseases, the vessels are more uniform in size throughout the different regions of lung attenuation.

Paired inspiratory/expiratory CT scans are useful for confirming the presence of air trapping. Although air trapping is most often the result of small airway disease, it can also result from reflexive hypoxic bronchoconstriction secondary to primary oligemia. The presence of bronchiectasis as a marker of airway insult should strongly suggest that air trapping, when present, is the result of small airways disease rather than a chronic vascular disease.

Tree-in-Bud

Bronchiolitis and bronchiolectasis are nonspecific inflammatory processes of the small airways caused by many different insults. The TIB pattern is a direct HRCT scan finding of bronchiolar disease, originally and appropriately used as a descriptor for the CT scan findings of endobronchial infectious spread of *Mycobacterium tuberculosis*. This pattern is analogous to the larger airway "finger-in-glove" appearance of bronchial impaction but on a much smaller scale. The *TIB pattern* has become a popular descriptive term for many inflammatory bronchiolar disease processes, all with similar appearances, and as such is not a pathognomonic finding for tuberculosis.

The list of diseases associated with the bronchioles potentially producing a TIB pattern at CT scanning is extensive. The more common disease processes can be grouped as follows: (i) infection, (ii) immunologic disorders, (iii) congenital disorders, (iv) aspiration, and (v) idiopathic condition. Indirect CT scan signs of bronchiolar disease include air trapping, especially with expiratory CT scanning, and subsegmental atelectasis.

Ground-Glass Opacity

Ground-glass opacity describes a finding on HRCT of the lungs in which there is a hazy increased attenuation of lung, with preservation of bronchial and vascular margins, caused by partial filling of air spaces, interstitial thickening, partial collapse of alveoli, normal expiration, or increased capillary blood volume. This finding is not to be confused with consolidation, in which bronchovascular margins are obscured, and may be associated with an air bronchogram. GGO can represent interstitial or alveolar processes, findings beyond the resolution of the HRCT technique. The original descriptions of GGO on HRCT scanning suggested that it represented acute alveolitis. Over the years, GGO has become a nonspecific finding but in certain clinical circumstances can suggest a specific diagnosis, indicate a potentially treatable disease, or guide a bronchoscopist or surgeon to an appropriate area for biopsy. GGO is a frequent finding on HRCT, with a lengthy differential diagnosis. It is very important to correlate the HRCT scan finding of GGO with the clinical presentation to narrow the lengthy differential diagnosis. The following generalized disease processes can all result in a ground-glass pattern as the sole, dominant, or accompanying HRCT scan manifestation: infectious and noninfectious inflammation, simple edema without inflammatory cells, infiltration with tumor cells or granulomatous tissue, and blood within or outside vessels. These generalized "lung insults" can result from a myriad of more specific injuries or disease processes.

There are even some nondisease states, normal conditions, and technical factors in which one can find GGO (e.g., narrow window widths and levels that can erroneously create the appearance of GGO). Thick (5- to 10-mm) collimation may cause a false appearance of GGO that is shown to be volume averaging of planar structures with thin sections (i.e., fissures, discoid scarring). Lung attenuation normally increases with exhalation and is often misinterpreted as disease, especially when heterogeneous. In such instances, these areas or higher lung attenuation may in fact represent the "normal" areas of lung in patients with small airways disease and air trapping.

Conclusion

HRCT is a powerful technique for evaluation of the lung parenchyma and airways. It is established as a useful and cost-effective means to reach a definitive diagnosis and obviate further intervention or direct indicated intervention so that biopsy is optimized or unnecessary altogether.

2

Airway and Lung Anatomy

NORMAL AIRWAY AND LUNG ANATOMY
Normal tracheal anatomy
Normal bronchi
Normal interlobular septa
Normal lobar fissures
Accessory fissures
Incomplete fissures
Partially complete fissures
Normal pulmonary artery and vein anatomy

PATHOLOGY ACCENTUATING NORMAL ANATOMY
Lobular air trapping
Acinar air trapping
Pulmonary interstitial emphysema
Interlobular septal thickening
Lymphangitic carcinomatosis
Intralobular and interlobular septal anatomy: crazy paving
Pulmonary alveolar proteinosis
Intralobular and interlobular septal anatomy
Pulmonary interstitial emphysema

NORMAL AIRWAY AND LUNG ANATOMY
Normal tracheal anatomy

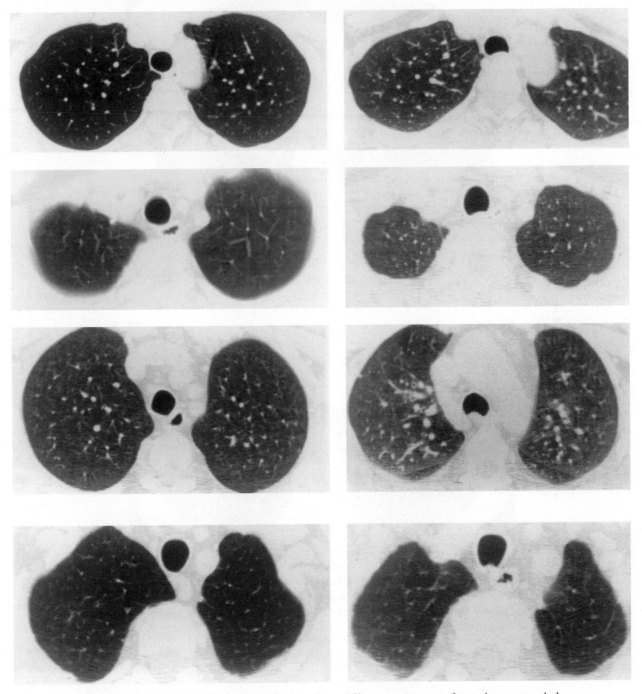

FIGURE 2-1 CT scans through the trachea in four different patients performed at suspended full inspiration and expiration show slight differences in the tracheal contours among patients. The trachea is usually round or nearly round at inspiration. The normal tracheal diameter should be between 16 and 25 mm, depending on gender and body habitus, and is smaller in women and smaller individuals. The coronal/sagittal diameter ratio is approximately 1.0. At expiration, the posterior membrane moves anteriorly, giving the trachea an inverted-U shape. The cross-sectional area of the trachea should not decrease more than 60% at end expiration. Note apparent "ground-glass opacity" in expiratory images.

Normal bronchi

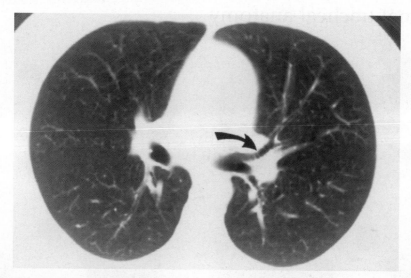

FIGURE 2-2 HRCT scan shows the bronchial cartilage rings (*arrow*) in the left upper lobe bronchus. This is a normal finding.

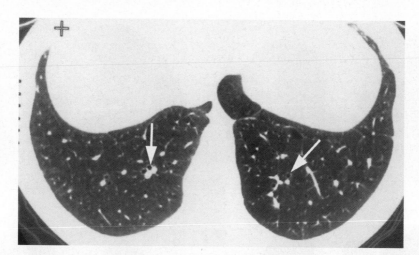

FIGURE 2-3 HRCT scan shows normal subsegmental bronchial airways in both lower lobes (*arrows*). Compare the size of the airway with its accompanying artery in the bronchovascular bundles; they should be of equal or nearly equal size. Note the barely perceptible thickness of the normal airway wall. At the lung periphery, the airway walls are not normally seen at all.

Normal bronchi *(continued)*

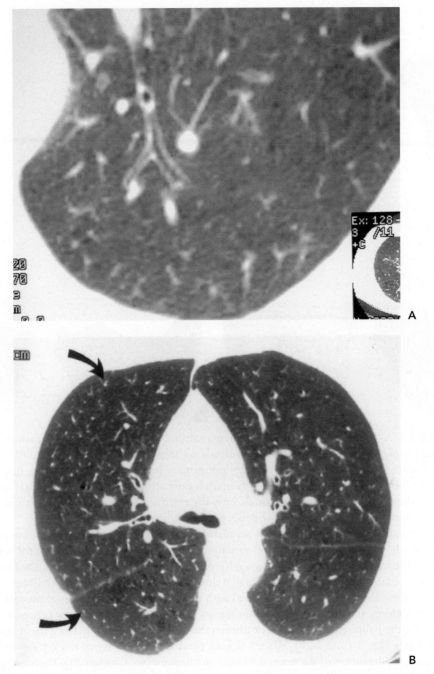

FIGURE 2-4 A: With optimal scanning technique, HRCT can routinely image airways to approximately their eighth-generation branches. Normal airways are, therefore, not detectable in the peripheral half of the lung. Note the size and caliber of the normally visualized airways in relation to the accompanying arteries. **B:** Pulmonary arteries may be imaged out to approximately 16th-generation branches *(arrows)*. This allows imaging of lobular bronchiolar arteries to within 5 to 10 mm of the pleura, often with a typical "V" shape, separated by 1 to 2 cm. Note that the accompanying intralobular bronchiole is not visualized at this level.

Normal interlobular septa

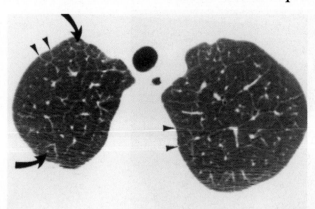

A

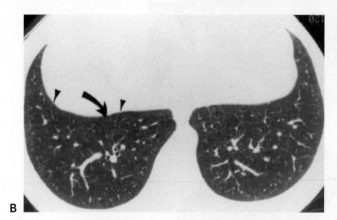

B

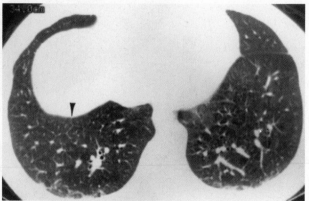

C

FIGURE 2-5 A–C: HRCT scans can show lung anatomy and morphology that cannot be obtained using conventional CT or conventional radiographs. Because abnormalities are easily detected at the level of the secondary pulmonary lobule, it is important to have an understanding of normal secondary pulmonary lobule structures and their normal appearance. Of the centrilobular core structures, only the centrilobular artery can be visualized (*arrows*); the centrilobular bronchiole is never seen in healthy individuals.

The secondary pulmonary lobules are separated by interlobular septa that are not normally visible on HRCT, except as an occasional very thin line at the extreme periphery of the lung, usually at the lung apices or bases (*arrowheads*), often in gravity-dependent areas. The interlobular septa contain venules and lymphatics that drain the secondary pulmonary lobules. Normally, these thin septa are not associated with any architectural distortion of the lobule or any other features, such as nodules or ground-glass opacity. Certain pathologic processes that can involve the lymphatics accentuate or thicken the interlobular septa, making them visible by HRCT (see Figs. 2-19 to 2-27). When a fibrotic process results in septal thickening, there will usually be distortion of the normal lobular architecture (see Chapter 10). There are usually other associated intralobular and perilobular abnormalities, such as nodules or ground-glass opacities.

Note the normal gravity-dependent density in **C**, not evident in the prone position in **B**.

Normal lobar fissures

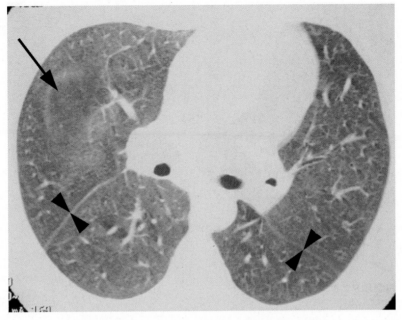

FIGURE 2-6 HRCT scan shows the normal interlobar fissures as thin, sharply defined white lines in the expected positions of the fissures, which depend on the level of the slice (*arrowheads*). The right minor fissure may not be seen well with cross-sectional imaging and may appear as an area of relative hypovascularity (*arrow*).

Accessory fissures

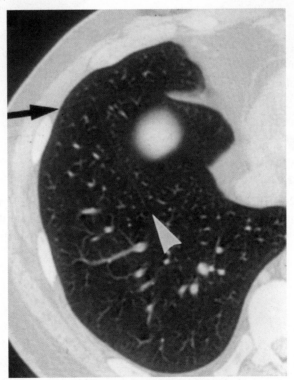

FIGURE 2-7 HRCT scan shows right major (*arrow*) and inferior accessory (*arrowhead*) fissures. The inferior accessory fissure separates the medial basal segment from the other basilar segments. Accessory fissures are present to some degree in 5% to 30% of the population. They do not imply an alteration in the underlying bronchial or lobular pattern of the lung.

Accessory fissures *(continued)*

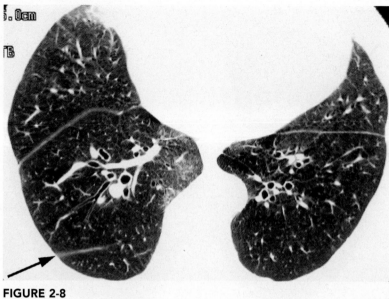

FIGURE 2-8

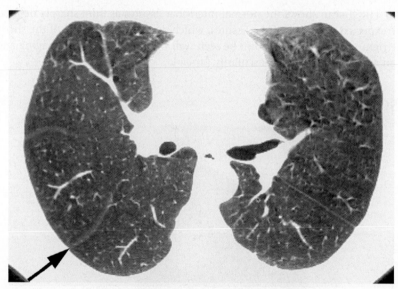

FIGURE 2-9

FIGURES 2-8 and 2-9 HRCT scans show two examples of the superior accessory fissure, in these cases, separating the superior segment of the right lower lobe from the basal segments (*arrows*). Note that in these cases the accessory fissures are incomplete. This is a common scenario.

Incomplete fissures

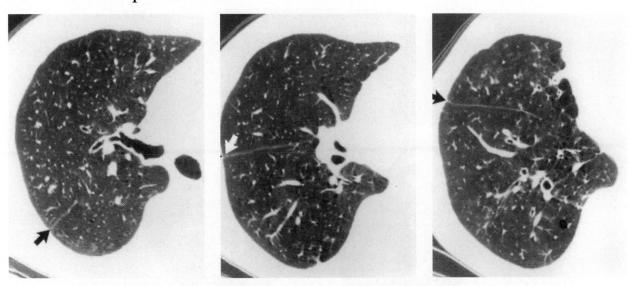

A–C

FIGURE 2-10 A–C: HRCT scans show an incomplete right major (*arrows*) fissure as a discontinuous linear opacity that remains in contact with the chest wall. Bronchovascular structures cross through the two fused lobes. This is a common finding that may be seen in as many as 80% of individuals and should not be misinterpreted as a linear scar or atelectasis. Recognition of an incomplete interlobar fissure is occasionally important in understanding the spread of pulmonary disease or in explaining various patterns of collapse or lack thereof from obstructed airways.

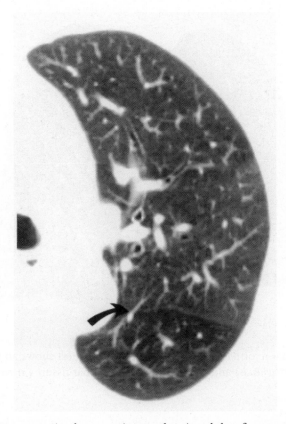

FIGURE 2-11 HRCT scan again shows an incomplete interlobar fissure as a discontinuous linear opacity that remains in contact with the chest wall. Note the small pulmonary artery crossing through the fused portion of the lung (*arrow*).

Incomplete fissures *(continued)*

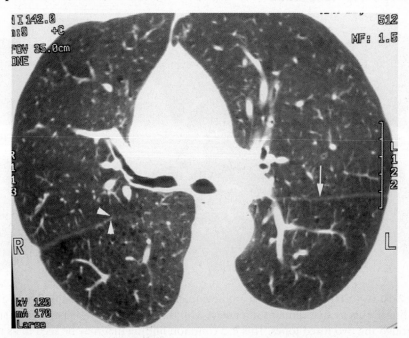

FIGURE 2-12 HRCT scan shows an incomplete right interlobar fissure (*arrowheads*) and a complete left interlobar fissure (*arrow*). Asymmetry of the fissures is a common normal finding.

Partially complete fissures

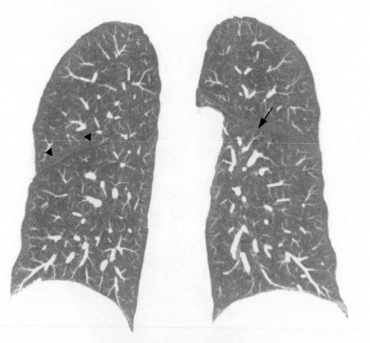

FIGURE 2-13 Coronal reformat CT through the posterior chest shows an incomplete right interlobar fissure (*arrowheads*) and a complete left interlobar fissure (*arrow*).

Normal pulmonary artery and vein anatomy

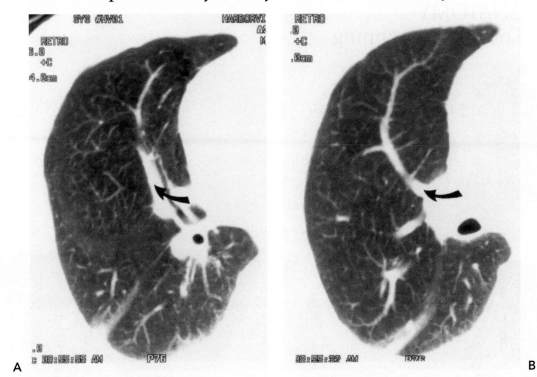

FIGURE 2-14 A,B: Consecutive 3-mm CT scans through the right hilum show the middle lobe pulmonary artery and bronchus (*arrow*) **(A)** traveling together in the bronchovascular bundle; they show a dichotomous branching pattern, the branches arising at acute angles. The middle lobe vein (*arrow*) **(B)**, like all pulmonary veins, has a monopodial branching pattern; the branches arise at approximately 90-degree angles, with no accompanying airway.

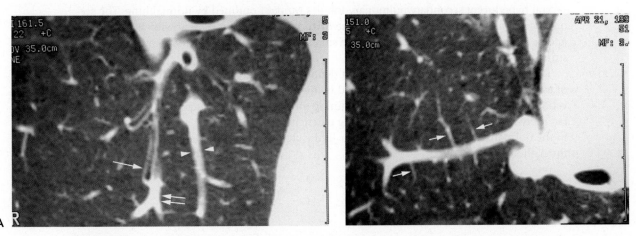

FIGURE 2-15 A,B: HRCT scans show the normal relationship of the pulmonary arteries and airways to the pulmonary veins. Note the intimate relationship of the artery (*double arrow*) and airway (*arrow*), forming the bronchovascular bundle that is surrounded by connective tissue, including lymphatics **(A)**. The pulmonary veins (*arrowheads*) are quite distinct, anatomically, from the artery and airway. In **B**, again note the monopodial branching pattern (*arrows*) of the vein, without an accompanying airway.

PATHOLOGY ACCENTUATING NORMAL ANATOMY
Lobular air trapping

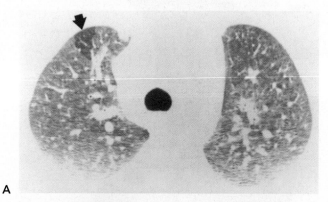

A

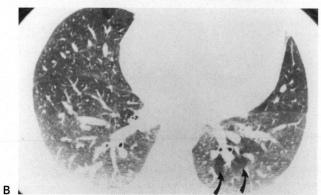

B

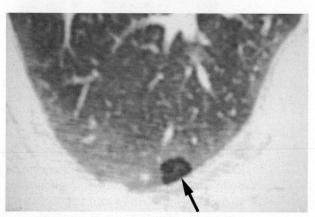

C

FIGURE 2-16 A–C: In these cases, HRCT scans obtained at suspended end expiration show several hyperlucent secondary pulmonary lobules (*arrows*) outlined by normal lung. The secondary pulmonary lobules are seen because of air trapping in this patient with asthma (**A,B**) and as an incidental finding in **C**. Note the small white dots—the centrilobular core structures—at the center of the lucencies.

The secondary pulmonary lobule is best defined at the lung periphery and can be thought of as anatomically that unit of lung divided by the interlobular septa (containing the lobular venous and lymphatic drainage) and containing intralobular core structures (the intralobular artery and airway) and intralobular lung parenchyma. Because they are not well defined in the normal state, except as shown earlier in the chapter, they are often better delineated in the pathologic state.

Acinar air trapping

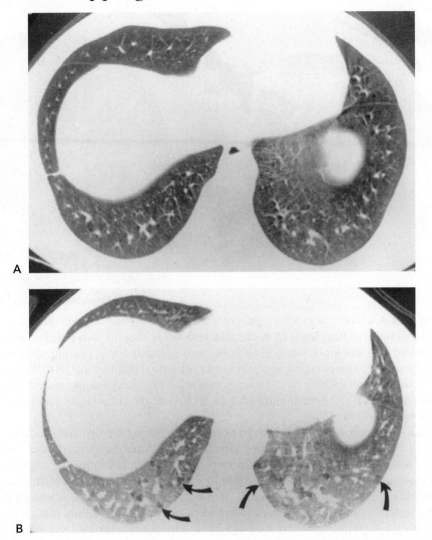

FIGURE 2-17 A,B: HRCT scan from a patient with acquired immunodeficiency syndrome and chronic cough, obtained at suspended end inspiration (**A**), is normal. HRCT scan obtained at suspended end expiration (**B**), at the same level as in **A**, shows multiple acinar-sized hyper-lucencies (*arrows*) outlined by normal lung in this patient with presumptive bronchiolitis. Again, note the small white dots—the centrilobular core structures—at the center of the lucencies. Recall that there are approximately 3 to 12 acini per secondary pulmonary lobule that, when pathologic, can appear in a cluster or rosette pattern around the centrilobular core structure.

Pulmonary interstitial emphysema

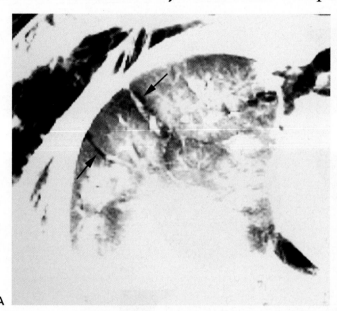 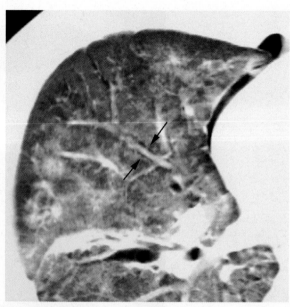

A   B

FIGURE 2-18 A,B: HRCT scan from a patient with acute respiratory distress syndrome (ARDS) that required high levels of mechanical ventilatory support with positive end-expiratory pressure who developed severe barotrauma with pneumothorax, pneumomediastinum, severe subcutaneous emphysema, and pulmonary interstitial emphysema (PIE). In **A**, note the air within the interlobular septa (*arrows*), indicating PIE, as well as the associated subcutaneous emphysema and pneumomediastinum. In **B**, note the air around a pulmonary vein (*arrows*), again indicating PIE.

PIE is a commonly recognized entity in neonates but is rarely recognized in adults. PIE results from dissection of air from ruptured alveoli into the pulmonary interstitium. Virtually any phenomenon that increases intrapulmonary pressure or lung volume can result in PIE.

On most occasions, PIE is suspected clinically. The sequelae of PIE include decreased ventilation and perfusion caused by an overall decrease in lung space, as well as being a precursor for potentially life-threatening pneumothorax or pneumomediastinum. PIE has been reported as a transient phenomenon, although in our experience it can be a stable finding over a several-week period.

Interlobular septal thickening

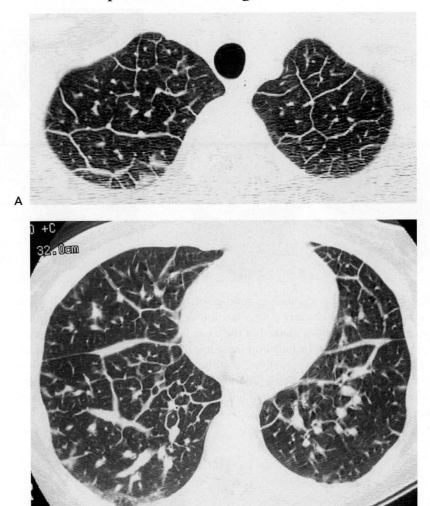

FIGURE 2-19 **A,B:** HRCT scans from the upper and lower lungs of a 32-year-old woman who had recently received massive fluid resuscitation show marked distention of innumerable normal interlobular septa as the excess fluid is drained via the lymphatics. Note how these distended septa outline and nicely show the size and shape of the secondary pulmonary lobules.

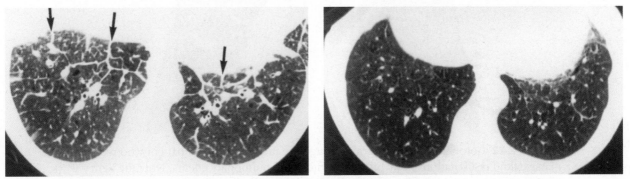

FIGURE 2-20 **A,B:** HRCT scans performed at the same anatomic level before and after medical therapy for cardiogenic pulmonary edema show resolution (**B**) of the thickened interlobular septa (*arrows*) in **A**. In this patient, distention of lymphatic channels and interstitial edema secondary to elevated left ventricular end-diastolic pressure result in thickened interlobular septa. These structures represent the Kerley B lines seen on chest radiographs. This case illustrates the nonspecific nature of visible, thickened septa.

Interlobular septal thickening *(continued)*

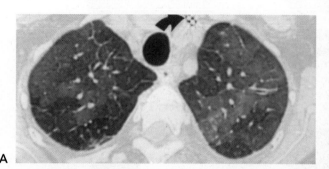
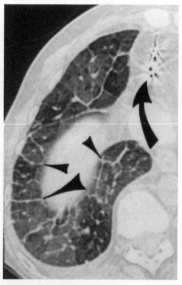

A   B

FIGURE 2-21 A,B: HRCT scans show ground-glass opacification throughout the lungs with patchy sparing of many secondary pulmonary lobules. There is moderate smooth thickening of the interlobular septa, most marked in the bases (*arrowheads*). Also present were small bilateral pleural effusions, not included on these images. Note star artifacts from transvenous cardiac pacemaker (*curved arrows*). These HRCT findings are characteristic of cardiogenic pulmonary edema, related to primary elevation of left atrial pressure (such as with mitral stenosis or mitral regurgitation) or to elevated left ventricular end-diastolic pressure (such as with dilated or restrictive cardiomyopathy).

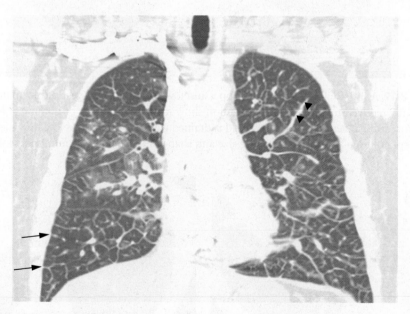

FIGURE 2-22 Coronal reformat CT scan through the mid chest from a patient who received massive fluid resuscitation shows bilaterally interstitial pulmonary edema. Note the Kerley B lines (*arrows*) representing edema within the interlobular septa and Kerley A lines (*arrowheads*).

Interlobular septal thickening *(continued)*

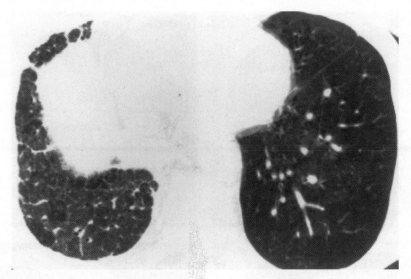

FIGURE 2-23 HRCT scan from this patient who underwent right lung transplantation for pulmonary emphysema shows smooth thickening of ipsilateral peripheral interlobular septa caused by pulmonary lymphatic disruption.

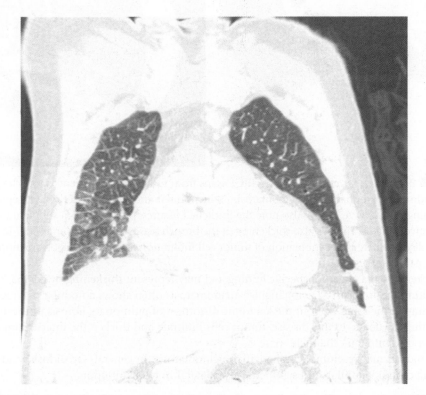

FIGURE 2-24 Coronal reformat CT scan through the anterior chest from a patient with right hilar lung cancer and unilateral obstruction of central lymphatics shows unilateral interstitial pulmonary edema. Note distended/thickened centrilobular septa, also known as Kerley B lines.

Lymphangitic carcinomatosis

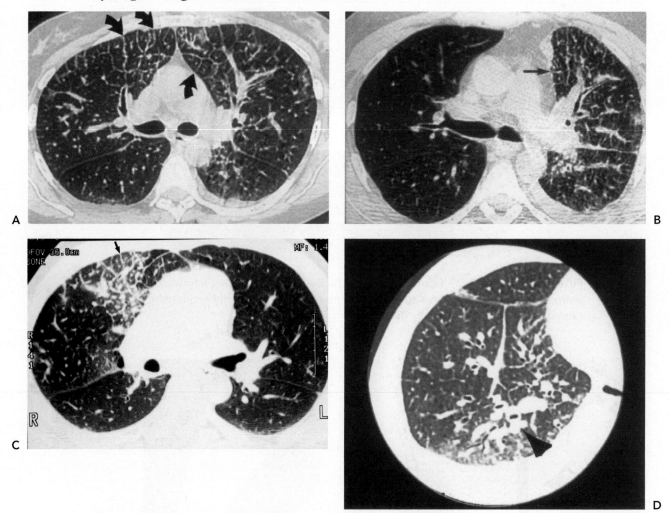

FIGURE 2-25 A–D: (*arrows in* **A, B, C**) HRCT scans from four different patients show characteristic findings of lymphangitic carcinomatosis. Note nodular and smooth interlobular septal thickening (*arrows in* **A, B, C**). Also note the thickened fissures, probably from subpleural lymphatic involvement. There is also thickening of the bronchovascular bundle (*arrowhead in* **D**). In this disease, there is a combination of tumor cell infiltration and lymphatic obstruction in the interstitial space.

Thickened septa are a nonspecific finding and may represent thickening by edema, cellular infiltration, or fibrosis. Lymphangitic carcinomatosis often shows a nodular or irregular thickening of the septa without the anatomic distortion of pulmonary fibrosis or the smooth thickening of edema. In this disease, tumor cells infiltrate and thicken the interstitium and obstruct the lymphatic channels.

Sarcoidosis may resemble lymphangitic carcinomatosis. In general, sarcoidosis tends to be more central, perihilar, and symmetrically bilateral in its distribution.

Lymphangitic carcinomatosis *(continued)*

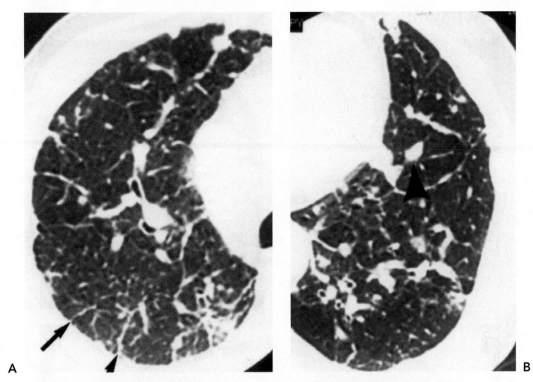

A   B

FIGURE 2-26 A,B: HRCT scans show two different appearances of lymphangitic carcinomatosis in the same patient. The distribution of disease in the left lung has a prominent axial (central) distribution (*arrowhead*), with thickened bronchovascular bundles. There is a more peripheral distribution (septal lines) in the right lung (*arrows*).

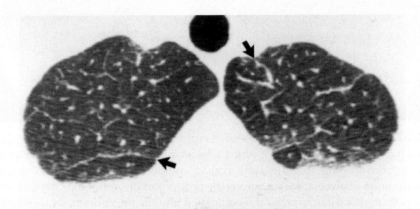

FIGURE 2-27 HRCT scan shows minimal, somewhat beaded, interlobular septal thickening (*arrows*) in early lymphangitic carcinomatosis.

Intralobular and interlobular septal anatomy: crazy paving

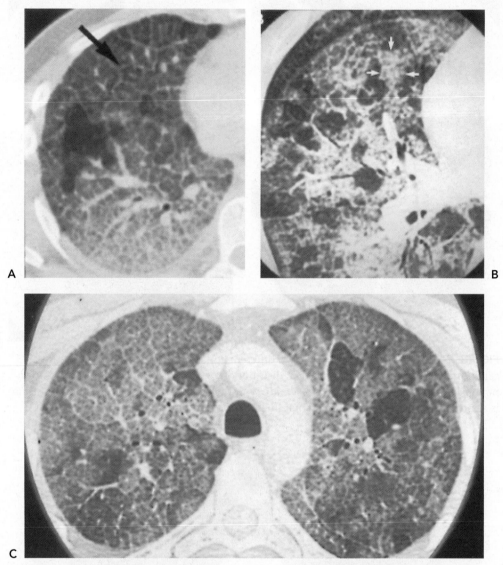

FIGURE 2-28 **A–C:** HRCT scans from three patients with alveolar proteinosis. Note the thickened interlobular septa, many of which have a typical polygonal shape (*black arrow*).

Alveolar proteinosis has interstitial and airspace components (*white arrows*). The ground-glass opacification of alveolar spaces reflects the presence of phospholipid/proteinaceous material in them. The same material is incorporated into the interstitium, with consequent thickening of the interlobular septa, an HRCT finding not appreciable on chest radiographs. Crazy paving was originally thought to be a pathognomonic finding of pulmonary alveolar proteinosis. The finding is still strongly suggestive of pulmonary alveolar proteinosis in the appropriate clinical setting. In isolation, however, this HRCT scan pattern has also been described in such diverse disease processes as sarcoidosis, pulmonary hemorrhage, *Pneumocystis jiroveci* pneumonia, mucinous bronchioloalveolar carcinoma, ARDS, and lipoid pneumonia, all of which can have a similar appearance.

Crazy paving is a colorful, descriptive term for the HRCT scan findings of apparent thickened interlobular septa and intralobular structures, forming typical polygonal shapes, with no architectural distortion. The diseased lung is usually quite well demarcated from surrounding normal lung tissue, creating a "geographic" pattern. The apparent interlobular septal thickening in alveolar proteinosis may be actually peripheral acinar accumulation of phospholipid adjacent to the septa but not actually involving them directly.

Intralobular and interlobular septal anatomy: crazy paving *(continued)*

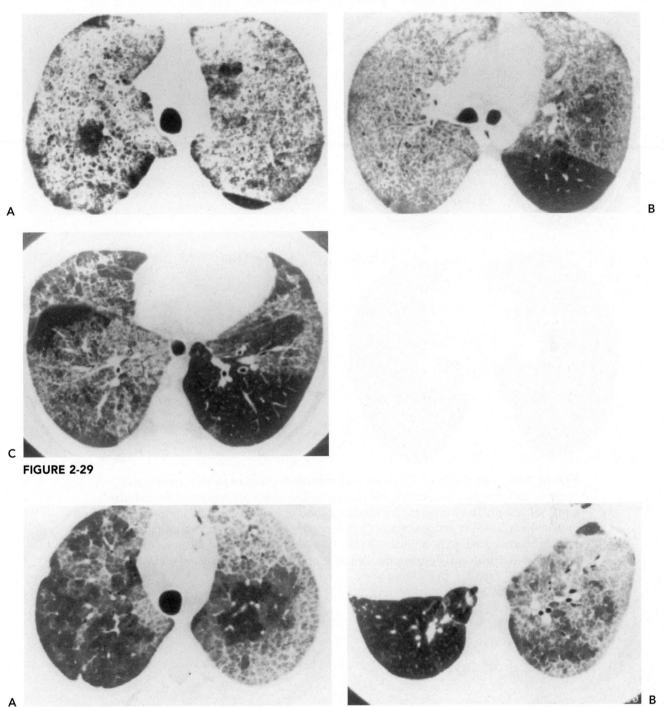

FIGURE 2-29

FIGURE 2-30

FIGURES 2-29 A–C and 2-30 A,B: HRCT scans from multiple levels in two different patients with pulmonary alveolar proteinosis show the patchy distribution of disease that may occur with this disease. Note the patchy distribution of the disease between the upper and lower regions of the lungs, often completely and unpredictably sparing large portions of the lung.

Pulmonary alveolar proteinosis

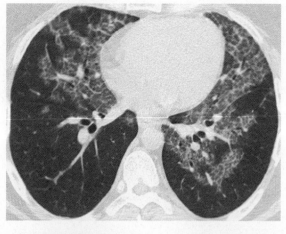

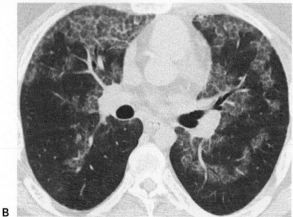

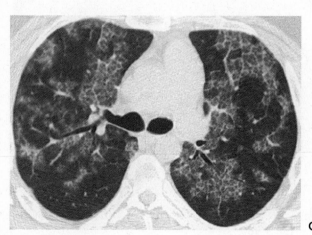

A

B

C

FIGURE 2-31 High-resolution CT shows characteristic findings of alveolar proteinosis. Note multifocal regions of ground-glass opacity within which are regions of interlobular septal thickening. There is no architectural distortion or honeycombing. Pulmonary alveolar proteinosis is caused by accumulation of a phospholipoprotein derived from surfactant. The lung architecture tends to be normal and without associated fibrotic or inflammatory changes. Note the well-demarcated nonanatomic demarcation between abnormal and normal lung.

Pulmonary alveolar proteinosis *(continued)*

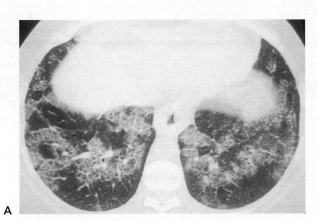

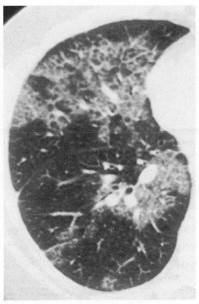

A   B

FIGURE 2-32 A: HRCT scan through lung base from a 54-year-old woman with exogenous lipoid pneumonia and mild dyspnea shows patchy areas of increased lung attenuation and thickened interlobular and intralobular septa in lower lobes. In **B,** HRCT scan through the middle lobe shows a prominent geographic ground-glass attenuation with superimposed reticular pattern, a typical "crazy-paving" pattern. The appearance is identical to that of alveolar proteinosis. (Reprinted with permission from Franquet T, Giménez A, Bordes R, et al. The crazy-paving pattern in exogenous lipoid pneumonia: CT-pathologic correlation. *AJR Am J Roentgenol* 1998;170:315–317.)

Exogenous lipoid pneumonia is an uncommon pulmonary disorder resulting from chronic aspiration or inhalation of mineral oil or a related material into the distal lung. Predisposing factors, such as neuromuscular disorders or structural abnormalities of the pharynx and esophagus, are frequently associated with this condition. Exogenous lipoid pneumonia may also be related to excessive use of oil-based nose drops, mainly at bedtime. Radiologically, exogenous lipoid pneumonia is characterized by the presence of bilateral lower lobe consolidations, mixed alveolar and interstitial opacities, and ill-defined masslike infiltrates. CT scanning is considered the imaging technique of choice for its diagnosis. When ill-defined masslike infiltrates are present, the resulting typical CT appearance is that of a low-density masslike consolidation with negative Hounsfield units, indicating the presence of lipid deposits.

The crazy-paving pattern on thin-section CT has been described as a characteristic appearance of alveolar proteinosis. However, this pattern may be mimicked by a number of processes other than alveolar proteinosis, such as sarcoidosis, pulmonary hemorrhage, *P. jiroveci* pneumonia, mucinous bronchioloalveolar carcinoma, pulmonary venoocclusive disease, and ARDS.

Pulmonary alveolar proteinosis *(continued)*

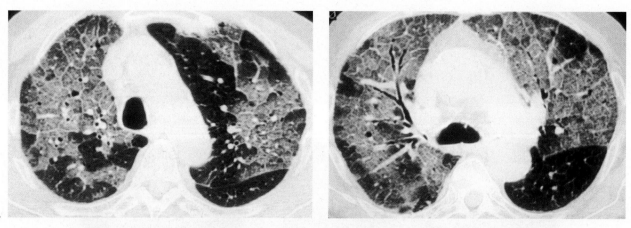

A   B

FIGURE 2-33 A,B: HRCT scan through the upper lungs from a 45-year-old woman who developed diffuse pulmonary hemorrhage after autologous bone marrow transplant for breast carcinoma shows extensive ground-glass opacity with a superimposed reticular pattern representing thickening of the intralobular and interlobular septa, a crazy-paving pattern. Note the patchy distribution of the process, affecting some lung regions, whereas others appear spared. Again, we emphasize the nonspecific nature of this pattern, as it can be seen with a number of processes, such as alveolar proteinosis, sarcoidosis, pulmonary hemorrhage, *P. jiroveci* pneumonia, mucinous bronchioloalveolar carcinoma, lipoid pneumonia, and ARDS.

Intralobular and interlobular septal anatomy

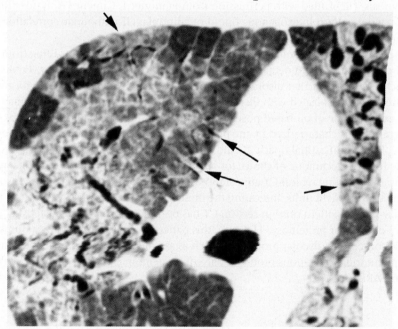

FIGURE 2-34 HRCT scan from a 27-year-old man with ARDS who developed severe barotrauma and PIE. Note the air within the interlobular septa *(arrows)* indicating PIE. This patient also exhibits intralobular and interlobular septal thickening, often called *crazy paving*. As stated earlier, the crazy-paving pattern can be seen in a number of other processes, such as alveolar proteinosis, sarcoidosis, pulmonary hemorrhage, *P. jiroveci* pneumonia, and mucinous bronchioloalveolar carcinoma.

Pulmonary interstitial emphysema

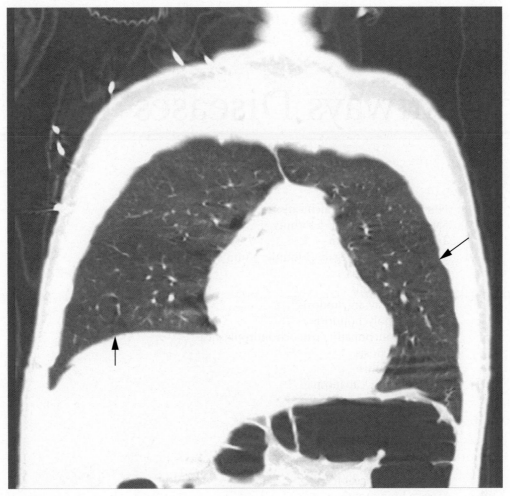

FIGURE 2-35 Coronal reformat CT scan through the anterior chest from a patient with PIE secondary to an asthma exacerbation shows air within the interlobular septa (*arrows*).

3

Large Airways Diseases

Normal airway wall calcifications
Saber sheath tracheal deformity
Tracheal diverticulum
Tracheobronchomegaly (Mounier-Kuhn syndrome)
Tracheal bronchus
Cardiac bronchus
Central airway amyloidosis
Relapsing polychondritis
Tracheobronchopathia osteochondroplastica
Tracheal stenosis
Crohn tracheitis
Adenoid cystic carcinoma
Leiomyoma
Chondrosarcoma
Main bronchus metastasis
Thyroid goiter
Bronchopleural fistula
Tracheoesophageal fistula
Erosive broncholith
Right middle lobe syndrome
Fibrosing mediastinitis
Postpneumonectomy syndrome
Posttraumatic bronchial stenosis
Endobronchial renal cell metastasis
Metastatic cancer to the airways
Mucoid impaction
Atypical carcinoid tumor with mucoid impaction
Mucoid impaction secondary to lung cancer
Bronchial atresia

Normal airway wall calcifications

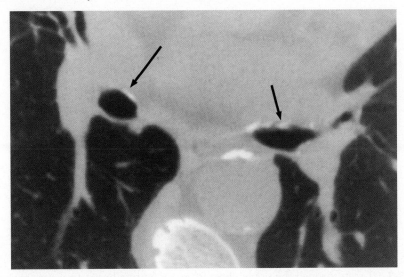

FIGURE 3-1 HRCT scan shows smooth, thin calcification of the walls of the main bronchi (*arrows*), with no intraluminal encroachment. This is usually an incidental finding, especially with advancing age.

Saber sheath tracheal deformity

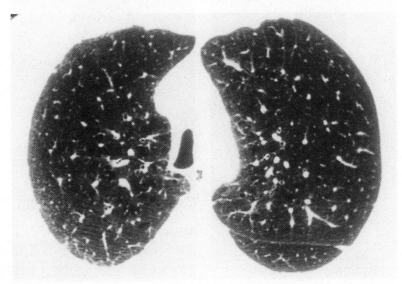

FIGURE 3-2 HRCT scan shows a typical severe saber sheath tracheal deformity commonly found in conjunction with chronic bronchitis and chronic obstructive pulmonary disease. Because this abnormality reflects the influence of chronically increased intrathoracic pressures, probably from chronic coughing, the characteristic deformity involves only the intrathoracic trachea. The trachea is usually round or elliptical in cross section (Fig. 2-1); however, in saber sheath deformity the sagittal dimension is often twice the coronal dimension or greater.

Other disease processes that can decrease the caliber of the trachea include tracheomalacia, saber sheath deformity, amyloidosis (primary and secondary types), relapsing polychondritis, tracheobronchopathia osteochondroplastica (TBO), and complete cartilage rings (also called *napkin ring anomaly* or *congenital tracheal stenosis*).

Saber sheath tracheal deformity *(continued)*

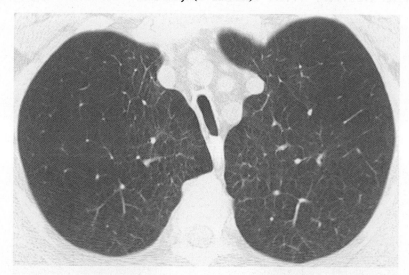

FIGURE 3-3 CT scan through the upper chest from a longtime heavy cigarette smoker shows a typical saber sheath tracheal deformity and extensive centrilobular pulmonary emphysema.

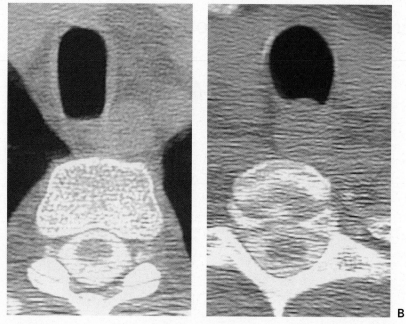

A   B

FIGURE 3-4 CT scan through the intrathoracic trachea from a 55-year-old man with pulmonary emphysema and chronic obstructive pulmonary disease shows the typical cross-sectional appearance of the saber sheath tracheal deformity. The coronal diameter of the trachea is less than two thirds of the sagittal diameter. Compare this shape with the normal round shape of the trachea (**B**), as seen at an extrathoracic level in the neck from the same patient.

Saber sheath tracheal deformity *(continued)*

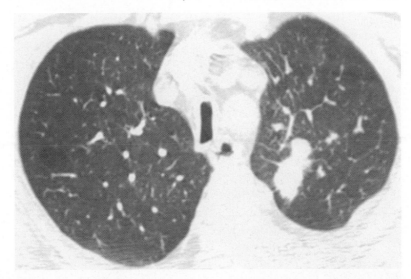

FIGURE 3-5 CT scan through upper chest from a longtime cigarette smoker shows a typical saber sheath tracheal deformity and left upper lobe lung cancer. Mild bilateral upper lobe centrilobular pulmonary emphysema.

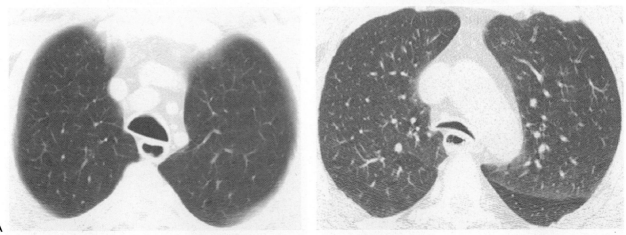

A   B

FIGURE 3-6 Paired inspiratory and expiratory CT scans through the upper chest from a patient with a lunate tracheal deformity. Note the typical semilunar shaped and the expiratory collapse in the coronal plane. A lunate trachea is characterized by a coronal/sagittal diameter ratio greater than 1 (normal is ~1), which is the opposite of the saber sheath tracheal deformity, and is frequently associated with tracheomalacia and associated lung parenchymal air trapping on expiratory views.

Tracheal diverticulum

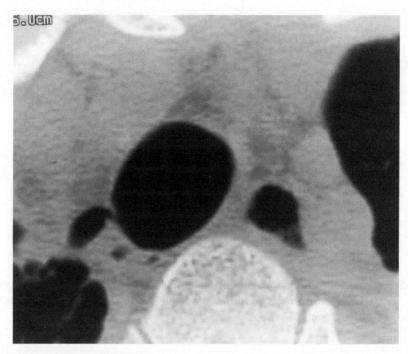

FIGURE 3-7

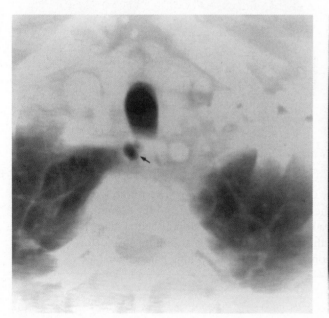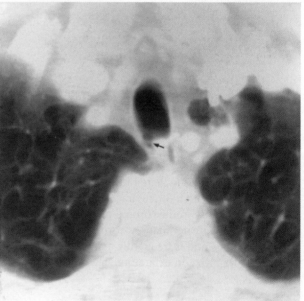

FIGURE 3-8

FIGURES 3-7 and 3-8 CT scans show two patients with tracheal diverticula extending posterolaterally from the posterior membrane. These diverticula may extend cephalad or caudad as illustrated in Figure 3-8 (*arrow*). These may occur with tracheobronchomegaly (TBM) or may be incidental, as in these two patients.

Tracheal diverticulum *(continued)*

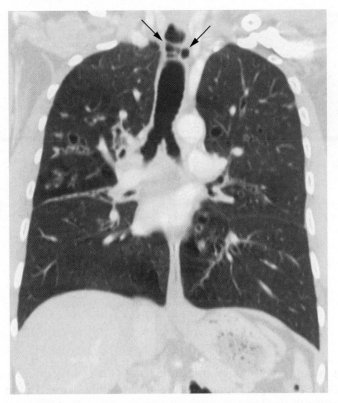

FIGURE 3-9 Coronal reformat CT scan at the level of the trachea shows several bilateral tracheal diverticula extending from the posterolateral tracheal wall, at the thoracic inlet (*arrows*).

Tracheal diverticulum *(continued)*

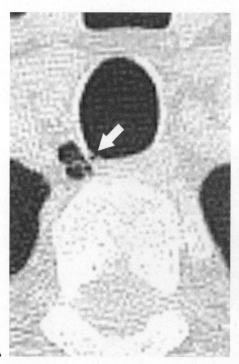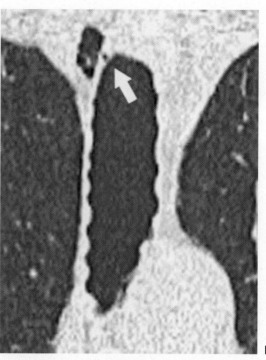

A   B

FIGURE 3-10 A,B: Coned-down transverse and coronal HRCT images show a small right paratracheal air collection representing a tracheal diverticulum. There is a tiny connection (*arrows*) between the tracheal lumen and the diverticulum. Tracheal diverticula are usually incidental findings and most commonly occur on the right posterolateral to the trachea at the junction between the cartilaginous and membranous portions of the tracheal wall. A connection to the trachea may or may not be identified. They can range in size from a few millimeters to several centimeters. They occur more commonly in patients with chronic obstructive pulmonary disease and may be multiple.

Tracheobronchomegaly (Mounier-Kuhn syndrome)

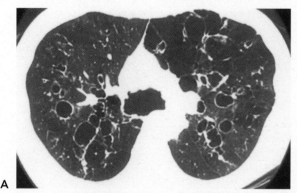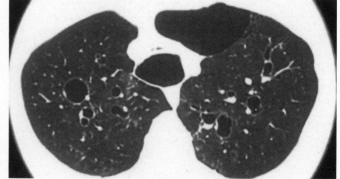

A   B

FIGURE 3-11 A,B: HRCT scans show typical findings of TBM. Note marked tracheal enlargement (more than 30 mm in this patient; normal is less than 25 mm) and extensive central bronchiectasis bilaterally. The typical CT features of TBM are dilatation of the trachea and mainstem bronchi, tracheal diverticulosis, bronchiectasis, and chronic pulmonary parenchymal disease.

Tracheal disorders can be categorized as diffuse or focal abnormalities. Although some of these tracheal abnormalities are fairly common, most are very uncommon.

The trachea (and usually the main bronchi) may be diffusely increased in caliber and includes such diseases as TBM and the very rare congenital tracheobronchomalacia (Williams-Campbell syndrome).

Tracheobronchomegaly (Mounier-Kuhn syndrome) *(continued)*

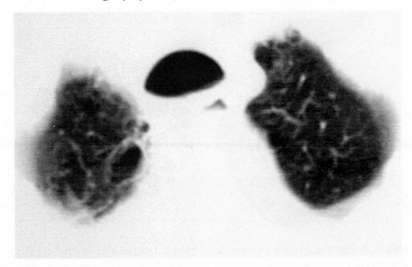

FIGURE 3-12 CT scan through the upper intrathoracic trachea from a patient with TBM (Mounier-Kuhn syndrome) shows marked enlargement of the trachea, especially the coronal diameter. There was associated mild central bronchiectasis (not shown).

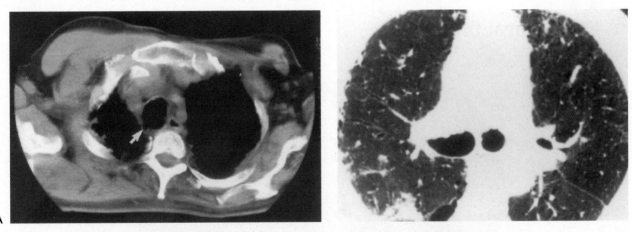

A   B

FIGURE 3-13 A,B: HRCT scan from a patient with TBM shows an associated tracheal diverticulum (*arrow* in **A**). The bronchus intermedius is dilated to the size of a normal trachea. Note the mild peripheral bronchiectasis and chronic parenchymal scarring in **B**.

Tracheobronchomegaly (Mounier-Kuhn syndrome) *(continued)*

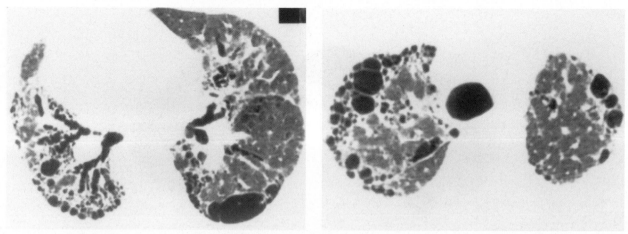

A   B

FIGURE 3-14 **A,B:** HRCT scans show severe cystic bronchiectasis and parenchymal scarring **(A)** associated with TBM (32-mm tracheal diameter in **B**). TBM is a rare disorder, likely congenital in origin. The diagnosis is made radiologically: Although it may be suggested on chest radiographs, CT has been used to confirm the diagnosis. Note the differences in severity of the tracheal dilatation and associated bronchiectasis and lung scarring in these four cases (Figs. 3-11 to 3-14).

Tracheal bronchus

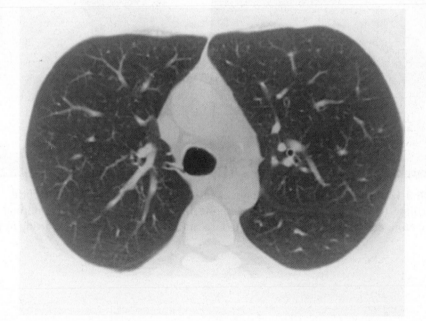

FIGURE 3-15 HRCT scan shows an anomalous bronchus to the right lung that arose just above the right mainstem bronchus. The tracheal bronchus, also called a *bronchus suis*, is a rare congenital abnormality in which a bronchus originates directly from the tracheal wall. This may represent one of two conditions, a true supernumerary bronchus occurring in addition to the usual three upper lobe segmental bronchi or an apical segmental bronchus displaced from the right upper lobe bronchus. A true supernumerary bronchus gives rise to a true tracheal lobe. In humans, such lobes are usually asymptomatic but can give rise to recurrent infections; postobstructive

(continued)

Tracheal bronchus *(continued)*

FIGURE 3-15 *(continued)*
pneumonias; bronchiectasis; troubled endotracheal intubation, either by intubation of the ectopic bronchus or by intraoperative hypoxemia caused by tube obstruction of the tracheal bronchus with collapsing of the right upper lobe; and technical problems in case of double-lung transplantation using donor lungs with tracheal bronchus. The tracheal bronchus does not usually necessitate specific treatment unless surgical excision of the involved segment is indicated for localized bronchiectasis, hemorrhage, or cancer.

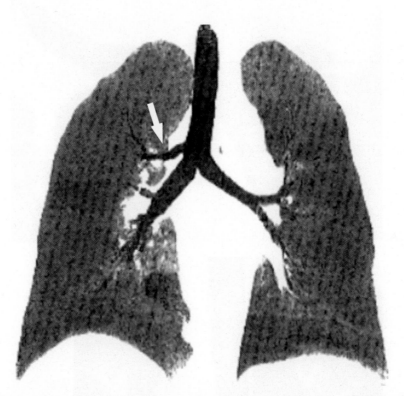

FIGURE 3-16 Coronal minimum intensity projection shows right upper lobe bronchus arising from the distal trachea (*arrow*). A tracheal bronchus occurs in 0.5% to 3% of individuals and usually arises from the lateral tracheal wall near the carina. Right tracheal bronchi are far more common than those on the left. They most commonly occur on the right, often simply ectopically placed, and may supply the entire right upper lobe (pig bronchus or *bronchus suis*), the apical segment, or be a true supranumerary upper lobe bronchus.

Cardiac bronchus

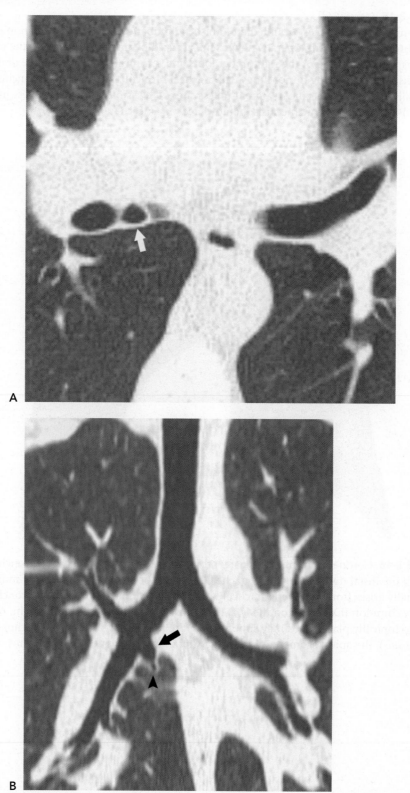

FIGURE 3-17 A,B: Transverse and coronal HRCT images show a cardiac bronchus (*arrow*) arising medially from the bronchus intermedius and coursing medially. Cardiac bronchi occur in 0.07% to 0.5% of the population. Most commonly they are blind ending but occasionally supply a few secondary pulmonary lobules as in this case (*arrowhead*).

Central airway amyloidosis

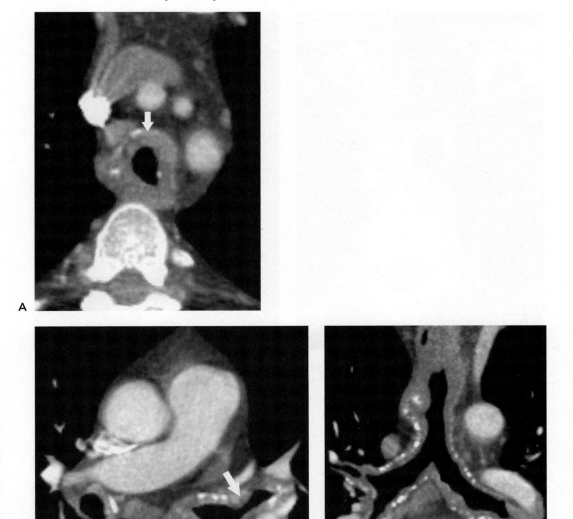

FIGURE 3-18 A: Transverse contrast-enhanced CT image shows circumferential tracheal wall thickening (*arrow*). **B:** The bronchial walls are also involved, and there is mild stenosis of the left upper lobe bronchus (*arrow*). **C:** Coronal reformation show diffuse thickening of tracheal and bronchial walls and numerous foci of dystrophic calcification. In amyloidosis, deposition of a protein-polysaccharide complex occurs in the submucosa and muscular layers of the airways. This forms irregular masses that are circumferential and encroach on the airway lumen, narrowing it. This may be a focal or diffuse process and occurs as a primary or secondary abnormality.

Relapsing polychondritis

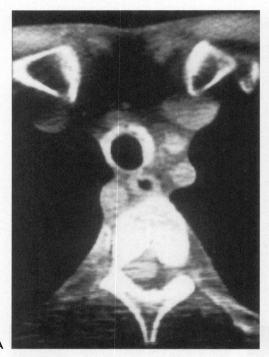
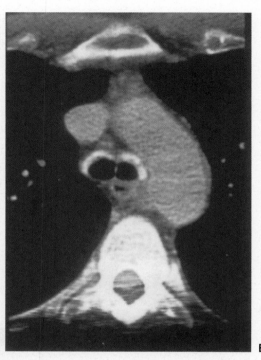

FIGURE 3-19 A,B: CT scans from a patient with relapsing polychondritis show thickening of the tracheal and mainstem bronchial walls with diffuse calcification that spares the posterior membrane. Differential diagnostic considerations include tracheobronchopathia osteochondroplastica.

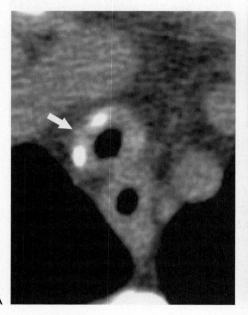
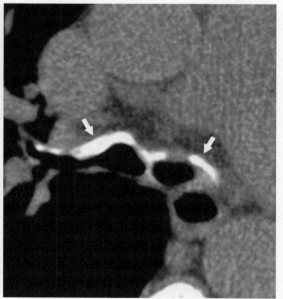

FIGURE 3-20 Transverse CT images show thickening and calcification of the tracheal and bronchial walls. Typically only the cartilagenous portions of the tracheobronchial tree are involved, the posterior membrane is spared. Recurrent inflammation may lead to tracheobronchomalacia, best depicted on expiratory CT.

Relapsing polychondritis *(continued)*

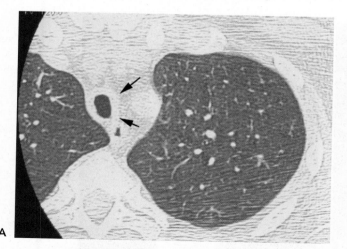

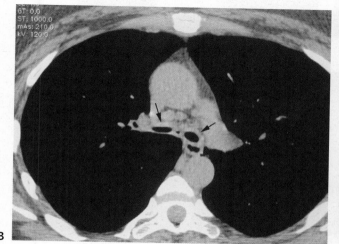

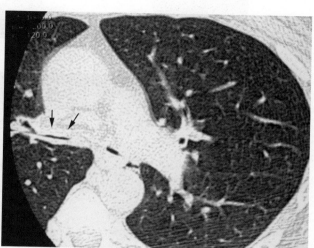

FIGURE 3-21 **A–C:** CT scans from a patient with relapsing polychondritis show diffuse narrowing and thickening of the tracheal and mainstem bronchial walls (*arrows*), especially the right mainstem bronchus, with sparing of the posterior membrane (case courtesy of L. Deal, Madigan Army Medical Center, Tacoma, WA).

Relapsing polychondritis is an unusual idiopathic inflammatory systemic disease that affects the cartilage at many sites, including the ears, nose, joints, and tracheobronchial cartilages. Relapsing polychondritis causes a diffuse or focal fixed narrowing of the airway that is shown well by CT. The CT findings included diffuse, smooth tracheobronchial wall thickening with narrowing and deformity of the lumen, as in this case. These findings may decrease or return to normal after steroid therapy. There may be dense calcium deposition within the thickened tracheal cartilages, as in Figure 3-19.

Tracheobronchopathia osteochondroplastica

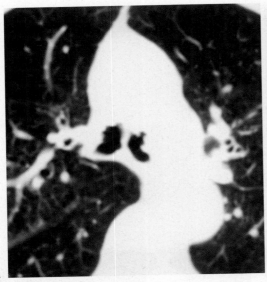
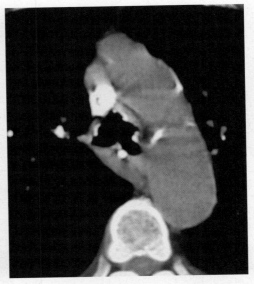

A   B

FIGURE 3-22

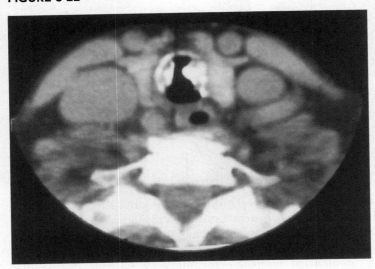

FIGURE 3-23

FIGURES 3-22 A,B and 3-23 CT scans from two different patients show the characteristic findings of tracheobronchopathia osteochondroplastica, calcified tracheal cartilaginous ring with nodular calcific protuberances that narrow the lumen. TBO is an unusual idiopathic condition of unknown origin in which nodules of mature bone, bone marrow, and cartilage form and protrude into the lumen of the airway, usually the trachea but with subglottic sparing. The pathogenesis of TBO remains unclear; hypotheses include exostosis and enchondrosis of cartilaginous rings and submucosal connective tissue metaplasia. It is most common in men older than 50 years and is usually asymptomatic but can present with symptoms related to airway obstruction, such as expiratory wheezing and recurrent pneumonia. The incidence is reported as one in 200 in autopsy series; 90% of cases are diagnosed at autopsy as an incidental finding, although some cases may present during life with hemoptysis, usually caused by mucosal erosion. Most cases are diagnosed incidentally during intubation or endoscopy. The differential diagnosis for nodular tracheal lesions includes TBO, tracheal amyloidosis, endobronchial sarcoidosis, and tracheal papillomatosis. The CT appearance is similar to amyloidosis except there is sparing of the posterior membrane; this process affects primarily the cartilage rings. Bronchoscopic evaluation or CT scanning usually confirms the diagnosis of TBO. The course of TBO is generally indolent and does not represent a malignant process.

Tracheal stenosis

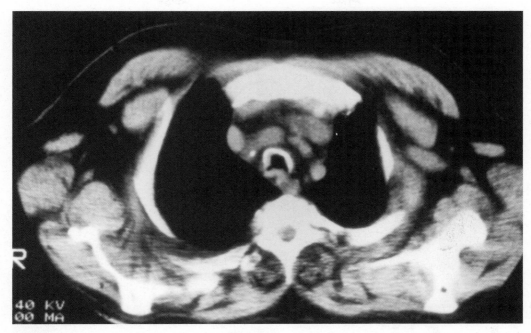

FIGURE 3-24

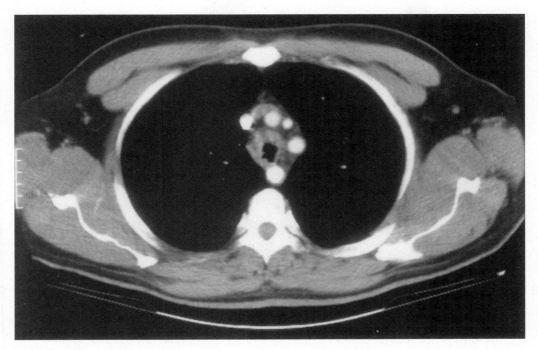

FIGURE 3-25

FIGURES 3-24 and 3-25 In Figure 3-24, the CT scan shows circumferential narrowing of the midtrachea caused by inflammatory granulomata. In Figure 3-25, the CT scan shows, in addition to narrowing, diffuse thickening of the tracheal wall. The tracheal narrowing in these two patients was caused by Wegener's granulomatosis. Other etiologies that yield similar CT findings include trauma, tuberculosis, fungal infection, and laryngeal papillomatosis. CT is useful in ruling out extrinsic compression of the trachea by a mass or vascular anomaly.

Tracheal stenosis *(continued)*

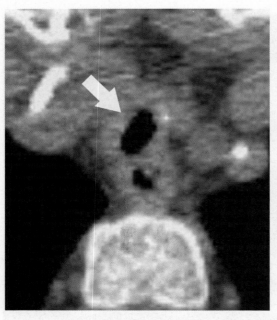

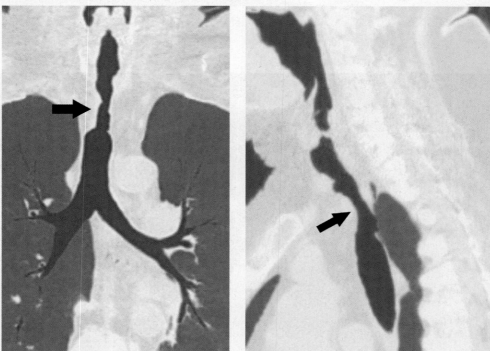

FIGURE 3-26 Focal subglottic tracheal stenosis in patient who had prolonged tracheal intubation. **A:** Transverse CT image shows concentric tracheal wall thickening and stenosis (*arrow*). **B,C:** Coronal oblique and sagittal oblique minimum intensity projections demonstrate the typical "hour-glass" configuration of tracheal stenosis resulting from prolonged endotracheal intubation.

Crohn tracheitis

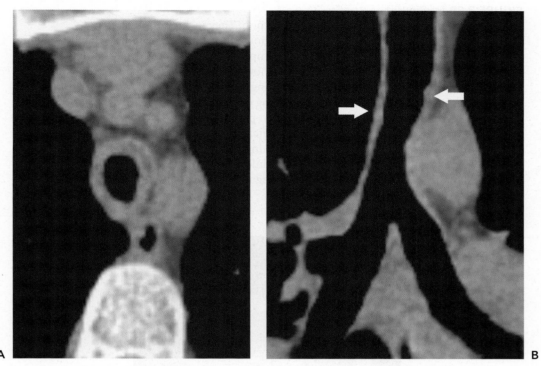

FIGURE 3-27 **A:** Transverse noncontrast CT image shows concentric tracheal wall thickening. **B:** Coronal reconstruction shows only short segment involvement of the trachea (*arrows*). Large airway involvement in inflammatory bowel disease is uncommon. Tracheobronchitis may develop years after the initial diagnosis and even after total colectomy for ulcerative colitis. Tracheal or bronchial stenosis may develop and bronchiectasis may occur.

Adenoid cystic carcinoma

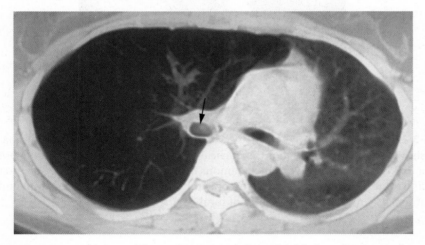

FIGURE 3-28 CT scan shows a right mainstem endobronchial lesion that was subsequently shown to be an adenoid cystic carcinoma, also called a *cylindroma* (*arrow*). This expiratory CT shows significant shift of the mediastinum to the left because of air trapping by the right lung with normal left lung deflation.

(continued)

Adenoid cystic carcinoma *(continued)*

FIGURE 3-28 *(continued)*

Benign neoplasms of the trachea are uncommon. They include chondromatous hamartoma, squamous cell papilloma, hemangioma, granular cell myoblastoma, leiomyoma, and other mesenchymal tumors. It should be emphasized that the CT appearance of these lesions is usually nonspecific. CT scanning best shows the extent of the intraluminal and extraluminal components of the tumor, usually distinguishing primary airway tumors from invasion of other primary tumors, as well as allowing detection of other lesions.

Squamous cell papillomas arise from human papilloma virus infection disseminated from the larynx to the trachea; they are most often seen in children and are usually multiple. The papilloma virus may also spread into the lung parenchyma—especially after instrumentation—where it causes multiple cavitating nodules, usually in a dependent distribution. Rarely, squamous cell papillomas undergo malignant transformation.

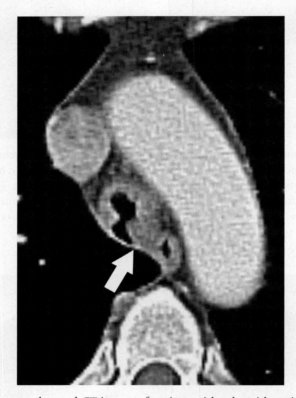

FIGURE 3-29 Contrast-enhanced CT image of patient with adenoid cystic carcinoma of the trachea shows nodular thickening of the tracheal wall *(arrow)*, with sparing of the posterior membrane. While less aggressive than squamous cell carcinomas, adenoid cystic carcinomas can be difficult to cure surgically as microscopic tumor growth often extends longitudinally in the submucosa, resulting in high rates of local recurrence.

Adenoid cystic carcinoma *(continued)*

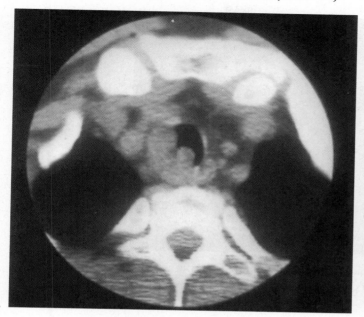
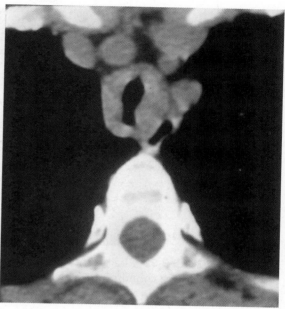

FIGURE 3-30 A,B: CT scan in **A** shows a lobulated mass arising from the right posterior and lateral aspect of the trachea and in **B** shows circumferential thickening of the wall of the trachea, both typical of infiltrative neoplasms in these examples of adenoid cystic carcinoma. Differential diagnostic considerations would include squamous cell carcinoma, papilloma, chondrosarcoma, mucoepidermoid carcinoma, carcinoid, and metastasis.

Leiomyoma

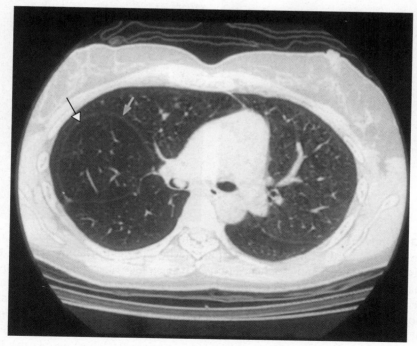

FIGURE 3-31 HRCT scan shows an endobronchial lesion nearly completely filling the bronchus intermedius just below the origin of the right upper lobe bronchus. Note hyperlucent and hyperexpanded right lung caused by air trapping. The diagnosis was benign leiomyoma. Note the normal HRCT appearance of the minor fissure (*arrow*).

Chondrosarcoma

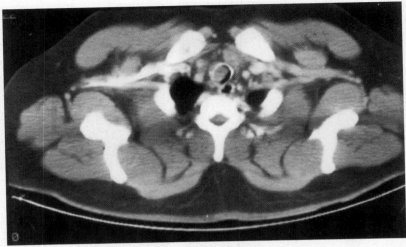

FIGURE 3-32 CT scan shows a 1.5-cm tracheal nodule extending from the right lateral wall. This was a chondrosarcoma arising from one of the tracheal cartilage rings.

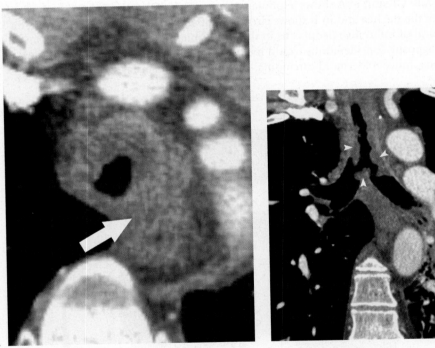

A   B

FIGURE 3-33 Advanced tracheal squamous cell carcinoma in a former smoker. **A:** Coned-down contrast-enhanced CT image shows diffuse tracheal mural thickening. Loss of the fat plane between the trachea and esophagus (*arrow*) is suggestive of esophageal wall invasion. **B:** Coronal reconstruction shows multiple tumor nodules (*arrowheads*) in the tracheal wall and lumen. Left lower lobe pneumonia (*arrow*) has developed as a consequence of airway obstruction. Squamous cell carcinoma is the most common primary malignant neoplasm of the trachea followed by adenoid cystic carcinoma. Primary malignant neoplasms are unusual, although slightly more frequent than benign primary tracheal neoplasms. Primary malignant neoplasms of the trachea are often caused by squamous cell carcinoma, or adenoid cystic carcinoma (the most common of the mixed salivary gland tumors

(continued)

Chondrosarcoma *(continued)*

FIGURE 3-33 *(continued)*

or cylindromas). Carcinomas account for 60% to 90% of primary malignant tracheal neoplasms. Less common are chondrosarcoma, fibrous sarcoma, carcinoid, and other rare mesenchymal tumors.

Tracheal squamous cell carcinoma represents just 0.1% of all primary malignancies. Malignant tumors above and below the trachea (laryngeal and bronchial) are 75 to 180 times more common. Tracheal squamous cell carcinomas arise most often in the caudad third of the trachea. These tumors are often sessile and eccentric, although 10% may be circumferential in contrast to benign tumors.

Chest radiographs have limited ability to detect tracheal tumors. CT, on the other hand, clearly shows the abnormal soft tissue mass, usually arising from the posterior or lateral wall, as in this case. Also, up to 40% of tracheal squamous cell carcinomas may have mediastinal invasion, well seen on CT images.

Main bronchus metastasis

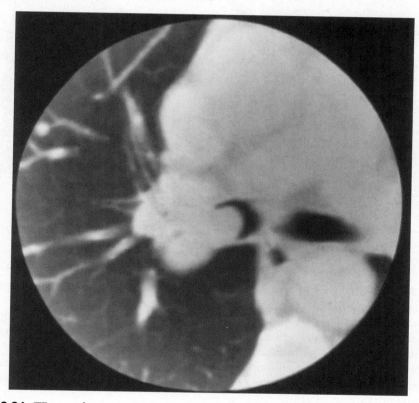

FIGURE 3-34 CT scan shows an 8-mm lesion arising from the lateral aspect of the right mainstem bronchus. It nearly occludes the airway. There was mild air trapping on expiratory views. Diagnosis was uterine leiomyosarcoma metastasis.

Main bronchus metastasis *(continued)*

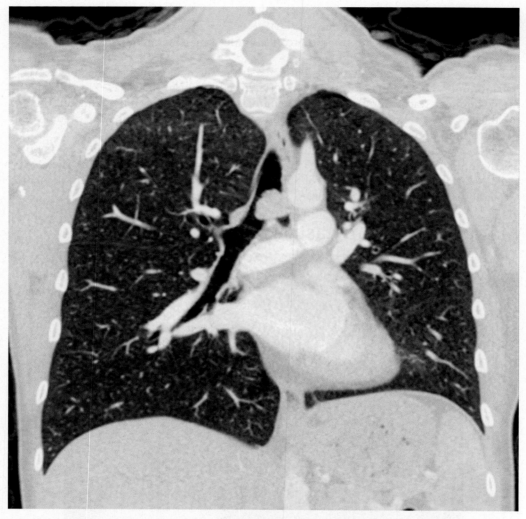

FIGURE 3-35 Coronal CT scan from a 32-year-old woman with melanoma shows a large metastasis at the origin of the left mainstem bronchus, nearly including the airway.

Metastases to the trachea are unusual, although more common than primary malignancies. They are seen in approximately 2% of patients dying from solid tumors and 5% of patients with multiple metastases. The common primary neoplastic sites to metastasize to the trachea and bronchi are breast, colon, genitourinary system (including testes), melanoma, and Kaposi's sarcoma. For focal masses, the radiographic and CT features can be indistinguishable from central primary neoplasms.

Thyroid goiter

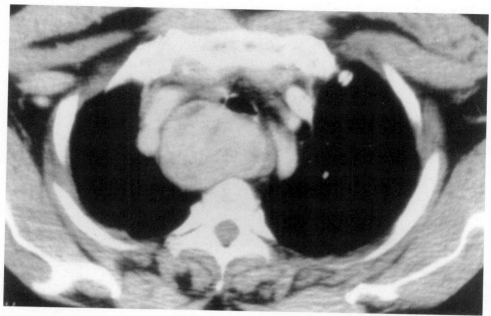

FIGURE 3-36

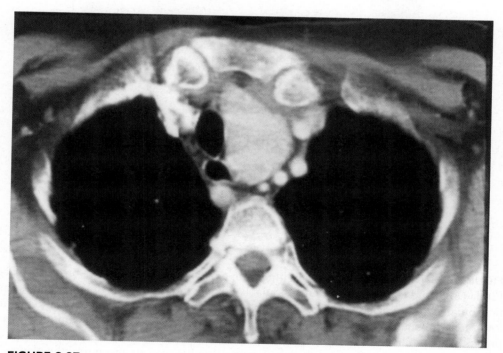

FIGURE 3-37

FIGURES 3-36 and 3-37 CT scans from two different patients with superior mediastinal masses both show a large hypervascular mass displacing the trachea and the great arterial vasculature. Cephalad images showed both masses connected to the thyroid. Findings are compatible with benign goiter, as was the surgical diagnosis. Because of their natural iodine content, thyroid goiters are often of relatively high attenuation before intravenous contrast material administration. To make a diagnosis of goiter with CT, one must show that it is connected to the cervical thyroid gland. There are often punctuate regions of calcification and low attenuation nodules within goiters.

Bronchopleural fistula

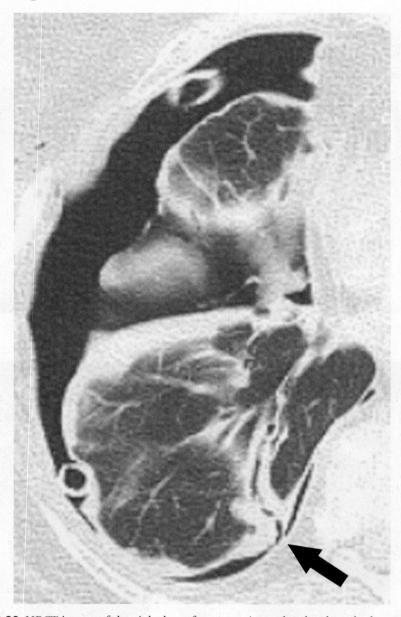

FIGURE 3-38 HRCT image of the right lung from a patient who developed a bronchopleural fistula (BPF) and empyema from pneumonia. Following thoracopscopic drainage and decortication, there was a persistent pneumothorax. Note the direct connection between the right lower lobe subsegmental bronchus and the pleural space (*arrow*). A small pneumothorax is present despite tube thoracostomy. Bronchopleural fistulae can develop when a neoplastic or inflammatory process leads to an abnormal connection between an airway and the pleura. Radiation, infection (especially tuberculosis and other necrotizing pneumonias), pulmonary laceration, and neoplasm can all result in BPF formation.

Bronchopleural fistula (*continued*)

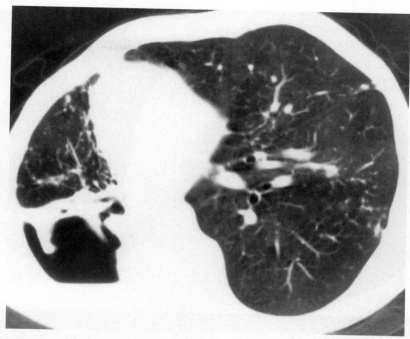

FIGURE 3-39 CT scan shows a dilatated and tortuous airway leading into a large air-fluid collection in the pleural space, indicative of a BPF. A BPF is a process, not a specific disease, in which there is a direct communication between the pleural cavity and the bronchial tree (a true BPF) or lung parenchyma (really a parenchymal-pleural fistula). BPFs remain a serious complication of a variety of lung diseases or injuries and, therefore, can prolong hospital admissions, often necessitate operative procedures, significantly increase patient morbidity, and can have a high mortality. Large airway BPFs—involving segmental airways or larger—usually occur after blunt or penetrating trauma and after surgical resection of lung parenchyma at the suture line across the subtending airway. These types of BPFs are diagnosed clinically and by bronchoscopy. However, small peripheral airway BPFs, although often apparent clinically, manifest by prolonged thoracostomy tube air leak, recalcitrant pneumothorax, or massive subcutaneous emphysema, and are not usually identified by bronchoscopy or chest radiography. CT scanning of the chest is useful not only in directly visualizing and localizing the BPF(s) but also in identifying the probable underlying etiology, number, and size of BPFs and thus is helpful in treatment planning.

In most clinical populations, the most common causes of BPF are pulmonary infections and surgical procedures, with chest trauma and idiopathic causes being less common. Infectious etiologies include necrotizing pneumonias, septic pulmonary emboli, infected pulmonary infarction, and tuberculosis. Specific traumatic and iatrogenic injuries that can cause a BPF include blunt and penetrating lung injuries (e.g., stab wounds and gunshot wounds), complication of pneumonectomy, thoracentesis, pleural drains, and ventilatory support with positive-end expiratory pressure. BPFs can also occur secondary to malignancy or its therapy, especially those malignancies that have a pleural-parenchymal component.

CT scanning is the imaging modality of choice for visualizing and characterizing BPFs. Peripheral BPFs are most evident when there are chronic inflammatory changes that lead to bronchiectasis/bronchiolectasis; airways are not normally visualized at the lung periphery.

Tracheoesophageal fistula

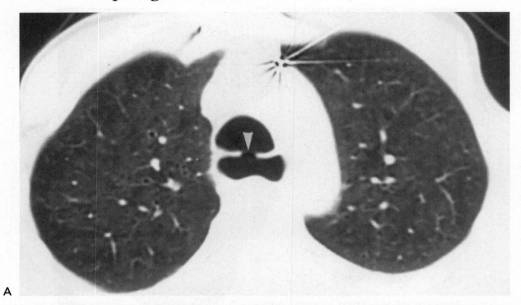

A

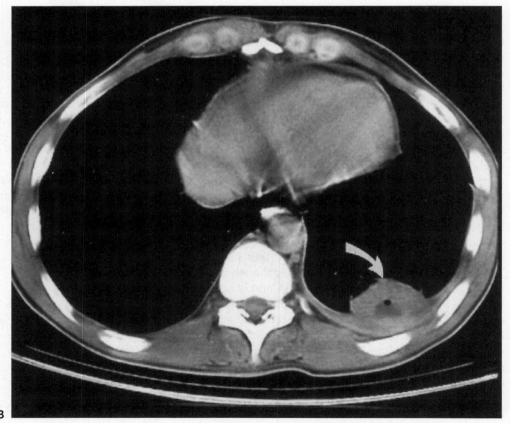

B

FIGURE 3-40 A,B: CT scan of the upper thorax shows a tracheoesophageal fistula (*arrowhead*). This tracheoesophageal fistula predisposed the patient to aspiration that resulted in the left lower lobe lung abscess (*curved arrow*). Tracheoesophageal fistulae may result from endoscopy, surgery, lye ingestion, mediastinitis, radiation, neoplasm, trauma, and so forth.

Erosive broncholith

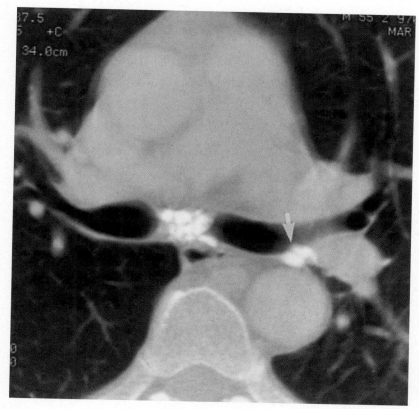

FIGURE 3-41 CT scan shows large, calcified subcarinal and left hilar nodes secondary to histoplasmosis. In this case, the left hilar nodes were eroding through the airway (*arrow*), producing a broncholith that caused hemoptysis.

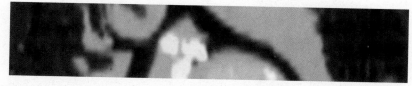

FIGURE 3-42 Coronal reconstruction of volumetric scans through the left mainstem bronchus shows a fistula from the left mainstem bronchus to calcified subcoronal nodes. This patient presented with a history of lithoptysis and this CT examination confirmed the presumed diagnosis of broncholithiasis.

Right middle lobe syndrome

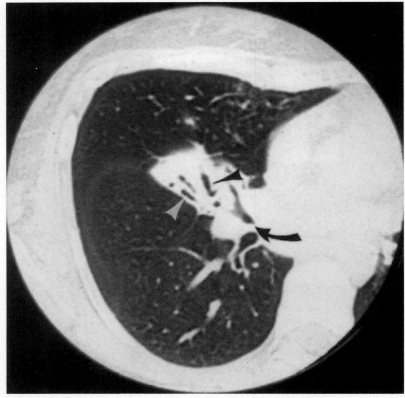

FIGURE 3-43

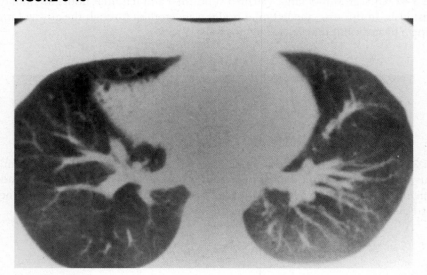

FIGURE 3-44

FIGURES 3-43 and 3-44 HRCT scans from two patients with right middle lobe syndrome show complete collapse of the middle lobe. There is ectasia of the visualized bronchi (*arrowheads*). On the right, note that the middle lobe bronchus is patent (*curved arrow*). Both patients had a history of recurrent middle lobe infections. Bronchoscopy in each showed no obstructing lesion.

Right middle lobe syndrome is characterized by a spectrum of diseases from recurrent atelectasis and pneumonia to bronchiectasis. In 60% of cases, the cause is benign inflammation (i.e., tuberculous adenopathy or bronchostenosis). However, retained foreign body or tumor may also cause this syndrome and must be excluded. Some authors speculate that right middle lobe syndrome is related to relative isolation of the middle lobe, where lack of collateral ventilation impairs mucus clearance.

Right middle lobe syndrome *(continued)*

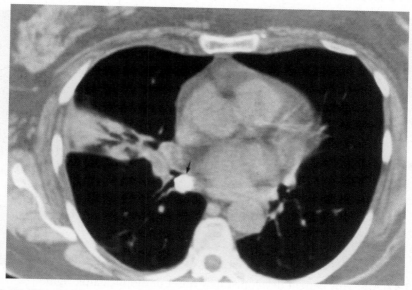

FIGURE 3-45 CT scan shows a large calcified lymph node eroding into the bronchus intermedius (*arrow*), with resultant parenchymal opacification (chronic) in the right middle lobe. In this patient, right middle lobe syndrome is secondary to prior histoplasmosis infection, now with erosive broncholith.

Fibrosing mediastinitis

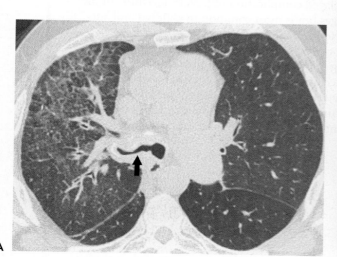

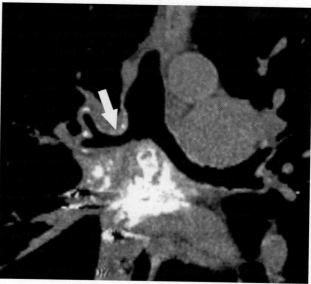

A

B

FIGURE 3-46 A: HRCT image from a patient with fibrosing mediastinitis resulting from histoplasmosis shows marked narrowing of the right main and upper lobe bronchus (*arrow*). Interlobular septal thickening in the right upper lobe and thickening of the bronchovascular bundles are from stenosis or occlusion of the right superior pulmonary vein. **B:** Coned-down coronal reformation (mediastinal window settings) shows a large partially calcified subcarinal mass and right bronchial stenosis (*arrow*). Differential diagnostic considerations would include lymphoma and bronchogenic carcinoma. Fibrosing mediastinitits is rare disorder most commonly caused by infection with *Histoplasma capsulatum*. Other causes include other fungal infections, sarcoidosis, Behçet's disease, radiation, and treated neoplasm (especially nodular sclerosing Hodgkin lymphoma). An idiopathic form exists, and there is an association with other fibrosing diseases such as retroperitoneal fibrosis, Riedel's thyroiditis, and orbital pseudotumor.

Postpneumonectomy syndrome

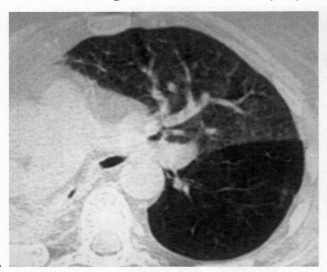
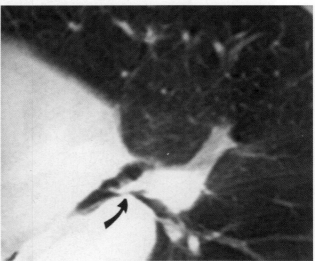

A

B

FIGURE 3-47 A,B: This patient developed new onset of dyspnea after right pneumonectomy. The chest radiograph showed only normal postoperative findings of pneumonectomy. Expiratory CT scan **(A)** shows air trapping in the left lower lobe. The left upper lobe deflated normally. Also note the marked relative oligemia of the left lower lobe compared with the upper lobe. HRCT scan **(B)** shows marked narrowing of the left lower lobe bronchus, where it is tethered over the descending aorta (*arrow*). Findings are compatible with postpneumonectomy syndrome and are secondary to stretching and extrinsic pressure on the lower lobe bronchus. Surgery to reposition the mediastinum more centrally with prosthetic filling of the right thorax was helpful in alleviating the left lower lobe bronchial obstruction in this patient.

Postpneumonectomy syndrome is a rare, delayed complication of pneumonectomy of the right lung (less than 0.5%) that occurs in all ages but is most common in children and adolescents. During the first year after pneumonectomy, there is marked right posterior deviation of the mediastinum, with counterclockwise rotation of the heart and great vessels and displacement of the hyperinflated left lung into the right anterior hemithorax. After the mediastinal shift, some patients develop marked airway obstruction, leading to severe dyspnea, stridor, and recurrent episodes of pneumonia. The realignment of intrathoracic structures results in compression of the left main bronchus, distal trachea, or left lower lobe bronchus between the left pulmonary artery anteriorly and the aorta or thoracic spine posteriorly.

Postpneumonectomy syndrome (*continued*)

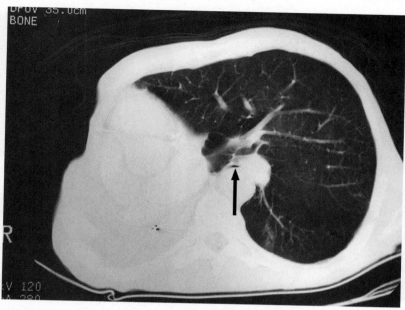

FIGURE 3-48 HRCT scan at the level of the left main bronchus from a 63-year-old man with a right pneumonectomy for bronchogenic carcinoma 2 years before and several episodes of recurrent left lower lobe pneumonia. Chest CT scan performed to evaluate for recurrent tumor shows a hyperinflated left lung and narrowing of the left lower lobe bronchus (*arrow*) squeezed between the descending thoracic aorta and the left pulmonary artery. Also note a small focal opacity in the posterior left lower lobe as evidence of prior pneumonia.

Posttraumatic bronchial stenosis

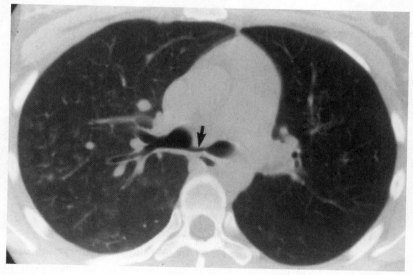

FIGURE 3-49 CT scan shows the results of a traumatic rupture of the left main bronchus many years before, now with severe stenosis of the bronchus (*arrow*). Note the resulting air trapping in the left lower lobe. Ventilation-perfusion study revealed 1% of total ventilation and 12% of total perfusion in the left lung. Incidental bronchoalveolar lavage fluid in the right lung produced patchy ground-glass opacification.

Posttraumatic bronchial stenosis *(continued)*

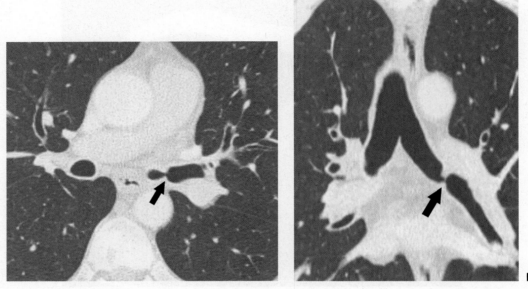

FIGURE 3-50 A,B: Transverse and coronal HRCT images show focal stenosis of the distal left main bronchus (arrows). The patient had suffered an occult bronchial injury several years ago in a motor vehicle accident. Most blunt traumatic injuries to the airways occur within 2 cm of the carina.

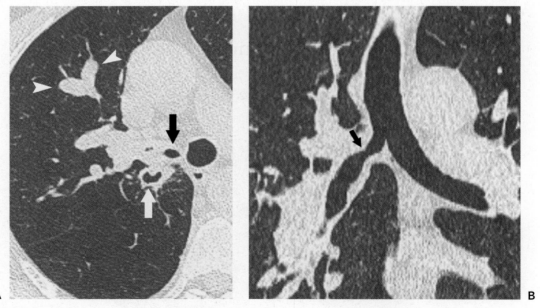

FIGURE 3-51 A,B: Transverse and coronal HRCT images show wall thickening and focal narrowing of the right main bronchus (*black arrows*) from *Mycobacterium tuberculosis* infection. The right upper lobe posterior segmental bronchus is ectatic with a thick wall (*white arrow*), and the anterior subsegmental bronchi are dilated and filled with secretions (*arrowheads*). Bronchial strictures from tuberculosis can be focal or involve multiple airway segments.

Endobronchial renal cell metastasis

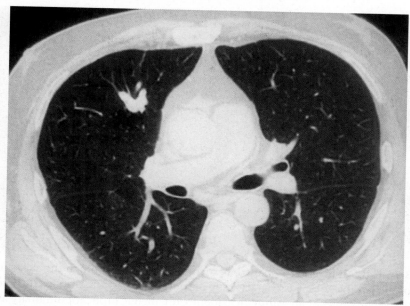

FIGURE 3-52 HRCT scan shows a branched tubular structure in the anterior segment of the right upper lobe. This finding would be compatible with a mucoid impaction; however, endobronchial metastasis can have an identical appearance. This patient had a renal cell carcinoma and this focal lung lesion was shown to be an endobronchial metastasis.

Metastatic cancer to the airways

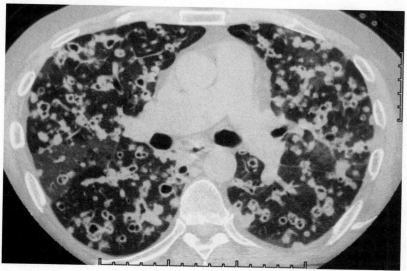

FIGURE 3-53 HRCT scan from a patient with a gastrointestinal primary adenocarcinoma metastatic to the airways shows that the bronchi are diffusely dilatated and thick walled. Solid nodular densities represent impacted bronchi. The airways were essentially carpeted with tumor, diagnosed by bronchoscopic biopsy of central mucosa. There is disseminated endobronchial metastatic cancer, presumably spreading through a lepidic mechanism. The bronchiectasis is assumed to be consequent to the tumor infiltration. Note a mosaic pattern of lung attenuation as a manifestation of obstructed small airways by tumor.

Mucoid impaction

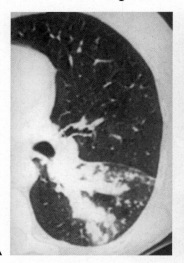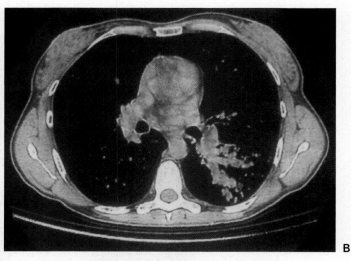

A   B

FIGURE 3-54 A,B: An inverted V-shaped, branching tubular structure in the superior segment of the left lower lobe is characteristic of mucoid impaction on this HRCT scan (lung and soft tissue windows) of an asthmatic patient with allergic bronchopulmonary aspergillosis. Central bronchiectasis and mucoid impaction are common findings in patients with this malady.

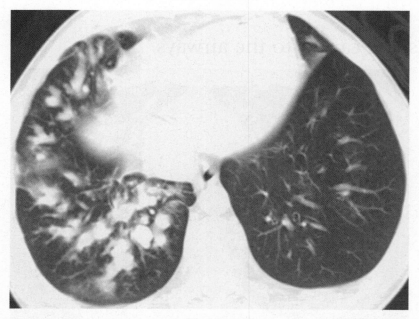

FIGURE 3-55 CT scan through the lower chest from a patient with cystic fibrosis who underwent a left-sided, single lung transplant shows extensive "finger-in-glove" deformities throughout the right lung, resulting from mucus/debris–filled bronchiectatic airways.

Atypical carinoid tumor with mucoid impaction

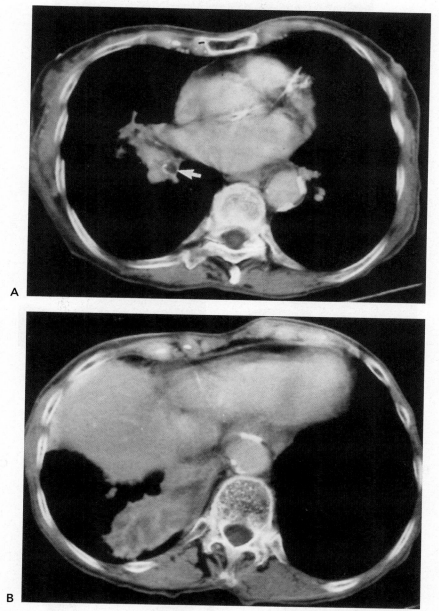

FIGURE 3-56 A,B: CT scan from a patient with an atypical carcinoid tumor in the bronchus intermedius (*arrow*) shows mucoid impaction. Note the relatively low attenuation of mucus in the branching bronchi compared with the surrounding enhancing lung parenchyma.

Mucoid impaction secondary to lung cancer

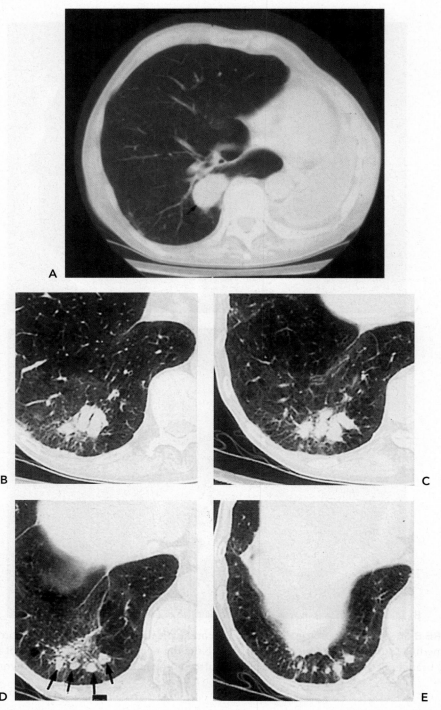

FIGURE 3-57 A–E: Serial contiguous HRCT scans show a 3-cm mass in the posterior basal segment of the right lower lobe (*arrow*). Note branched tubular structures inferior to this mass. Findings were caused by an obstructing squamous cell carcinoma with distal mucoid impaction in subsegmental bronchi (*arrows*); parenchymal aeration was maintained by collateral air drift. Mucoid impaction may be caused by an obstructing lesion, such as endobronchial tumor, bronchostenosis, broncholithiasis, and so forth. Other considerations include asthma, allergic bronchopulmonary aspergillosis, dysmotile cilia syndrome, tuberculosis with resultant bronchiectasis, and postoperative pulmonary status.

Bronchial atresia

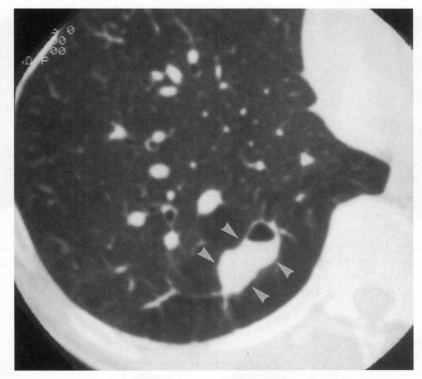

FIGURE 3-58 HRCT scan shows typical findings of bronchial atresia. There is a dilatated bronchus that contains mucus and a small amount of air in the posterior basal segment of the right lower lobe (*arrowheads*). Note marked hyperlucency of lung surrounding the mucus-filled atretic bronchus. All of the subsegmental parenchyma distal to this point was hyperinflated as well.

Congenital bronchial atresia is a developmental anomaly caused by atresia of a segmental or lobar bronchus. The resulting blind-end bronchus has no connection to the rest of the tracheobronchial tree. Mucus secretion in the obstructed segment leads to a dilatated, mucus-filled bronchus—a bronchocele. Bronchoceles can also be seen in obstructing neoplasms of the bronchus, such as carcinoid tumor and bronchogenic carcinoma, and in nonobstructive disorders, such as allergic bronchopulmonary aspergillosis, bronchocentric granulomatosis, and cystic fibrosis. Chest CT scanning better shows the characteristic branching pattern of a bronchocele over serial slices and adjacent hyperinflated lung parenchyma. The most common sites of involvement include segmental bronchi in the left upper (apicoposterior), left lower, and right upper lobes. Patients typically require no treatment. Rarely, surgical intervention may be warranted in the setting of recurrent lung infections or if there is impaired ventilation of the adjacent lung from progressive hyperinflation.

Bronchial atresia *(continued)*

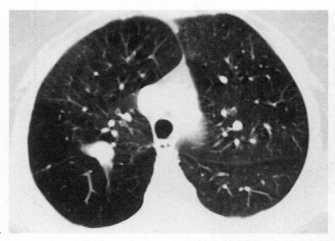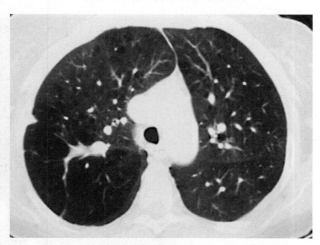

A · B

FIGURE 3-59 A,B: CT scan through the right upper lobe from this 64-year-old asymptomatic woman shows a smoothly marginated mass with a characteristic Y-shape branching pattern of a bronchocele over serial slices. Also note the adjacent hyperinflated lung parenchyma (case courtesy of W. Caras, Tacoma, WA).

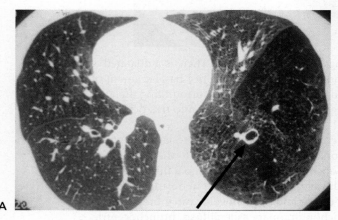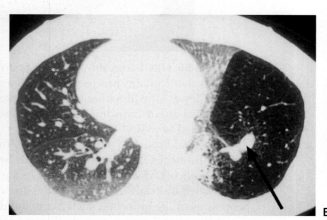

A · B

FIGURE 3-60 A,B: Paired inspiratory-expiratory HRCT scans from a patient with bronchial atresia show a tubular opacity in the left lower lobe representing a mucus-filled bronchocele (*arrow in* **B**). Expiratory CT scans show air trapping. The presence of air is clearly seen within the bronchial lumen more proximal to the bronchocele (*arrow in* **A**). Note the shift of the midline to the right as a result of the hyperinflated left lower lobe.

4

Bronchiectasis

Bronchiectasis
Varicose bronchiectasis
Saccular bronchiectasis
Williams-Campbell syndrome
Cystic bronchiectasis
Mild central bronchiectasis secondary to allergic
   bronchopulmonary aspergillosis
Allergic bronchopulmonary aspergillosis
Cystic fibrosis
Bronchocentric granulomatosis
Bronchiectasis secondary to chronic granulomatous
   disease of childhood
Combined variable immunodeficiency
Traction bronchiectasis
Reversible bronchiectasis
Diffuse panbronchiolitis
Primary ciliary dyskinesia

Bronchiectasis

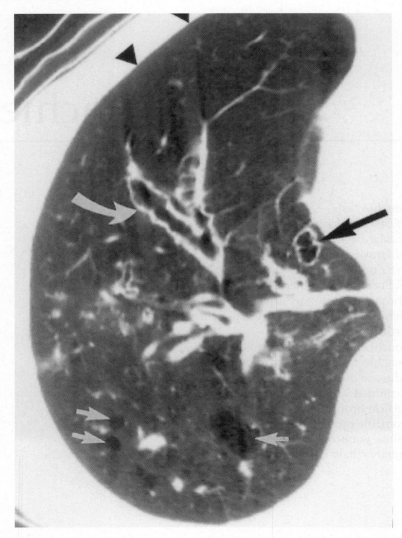

FIGURE 4-1 HRCT scan shows the difference between emphysematous spaces (*small arrows*), bronchiectatic airways in the cross section (*straight arrow*) and longitudinal planes (*curved arrow*), and air trapping (*arrowheads*).

Bronchiectasis is a chronic, usually inflammatory, often suppurative process that leads to *irreversibly* dilatated airways. Depending on severity, the HRCT signs of bronchiectasis include bronchial wall thickening caused by peribronchial inflammation and fibrosis; dilatated, non-tapering bronchi in the periphery of the lung; air-fluid levels in distended bronchi; and a linear array or cluster of cystlike spaces. Distended bronchi are easily distinguished from bulla, which generally have no definable wall thickness and no accompanying vessels.

Although bronchiectasis has been classically categorized into cylindrical, varicose, and saccular (cystic) types, the spectrum of disease may prevent neat classification in patients with varying severity among different regions of the lung. Because these categories have little clinical use, they are used infrequently in current practice.

Cylindrical bronchiectasis is the least severe form. Varicose bronchiectasis has alternating dilatation and constriction, yielding a beaded, varicoid appearance. Saccular and cystic bronchiectasis are the most severe forms; in them, the airways are markedly dilatated. In patients with bronchiectasis, there is frequently concomitant severe parenchymal destruction and obliteration of the distal airways (obliterative bronchiolitis).

Bronchiectasis *(continued)*

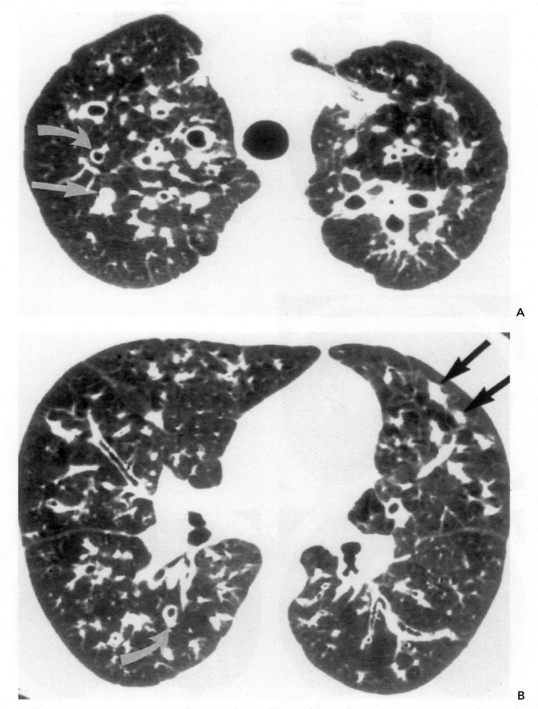

A

B

FIGURE 4-2 A,B: HRCT scans show multiple dilatated bronchiectatic airways (*curved arrows*) that form the classic "signet-ring" sign with their accompanying pulmonary artery (*straight arrows*).

Bronchiectasis *(continued)*

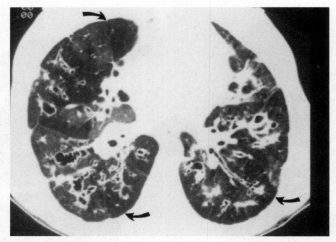

FIGURE 4-3

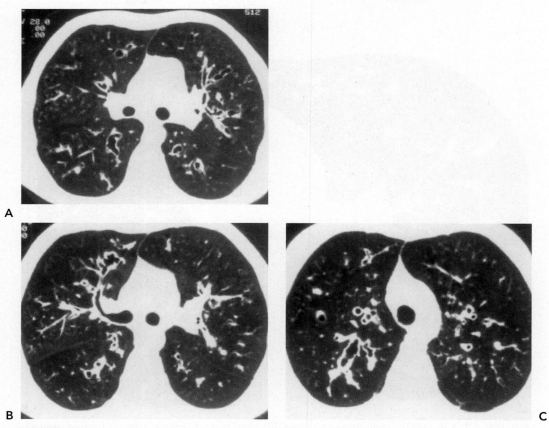

FIGURE 4-4

FIGURES 4-3 and 4-4 A–C: HRCT scans show multiple irregularly shaped bronchiectatic airways in two patients with cystic fibrosis. Bronchiectatic airways can attain different, often bizarre shapes even in the same patient, reflecting an often chronic and ongoing inflammatory airways disease. Note a mosaic pattern of lung attenuation (*arrows*). Hyperlucent regions are caused by air trapping, either from mucus plugging or associated obliterative bronchiolitis.

Varicose bronchiectasis

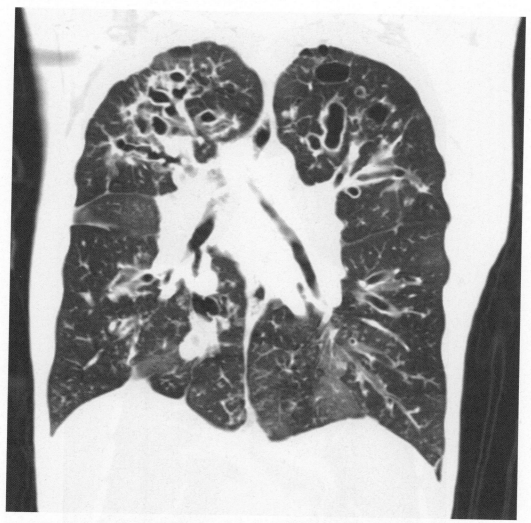

FIGURE 4-5 Coronal reformat CT scan from a 23-year-old man with cystic fibrosis shows typical bilateral upper lobe predominant bronchiectasis. Note the associated patchy air trapping in the lower lobes of lung attenuation.

Varicose bronchiectasis *(continued)*

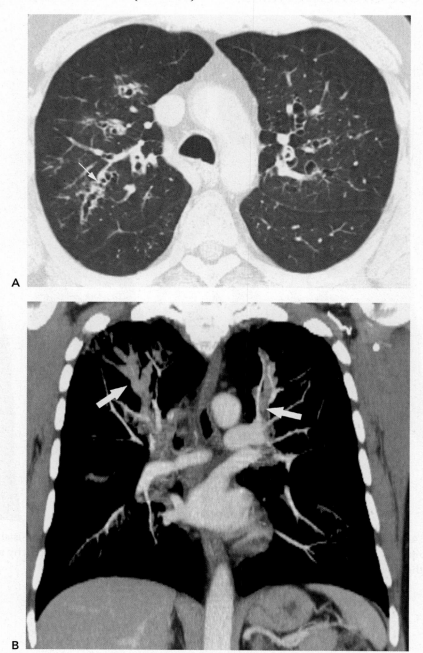

FIGURE 4-6 ABPA 2. **A:** HRCT image from this patient with allergic bronchopulmonary aspergillosis (ABPA) shows bilateral central varicoid bronchiectasis with bronchial wall thickening. Note string of pearls or varicose appearance of abnormally tapering and dilatated bronchus (*arrow*). There are three classifications of bronchiectasis in increasing order of severity: cylindrical, varicose, and saccular, also called *cystic*. Low attenuation areas in the lungs represent regional air trapping. **B:** Coronal maximum intensity projection (MIP) shows dilated upper lobe bronchi filled with high attenuation material (*arrows*).

Saccular bronchiectasis

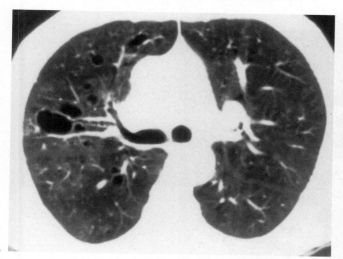
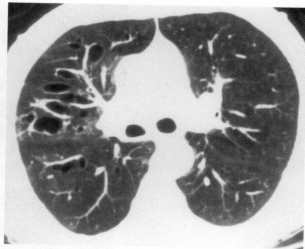

A

B

FIGURE 4-7 A,B: HRCT scans show marked dilatation and airway wall thickening of multiple small- to moderate-sized airways in the right lung. Although the central bronchi are normal, the presence of marked dilatation and thickened walls in small and moderate airways indicates saccular bronchiectasis peripherally.

Williams-Campbell syndrome

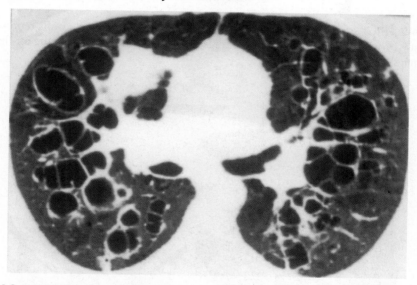

FIGURE 4-8 HRCT scan from this patient with Williams-Campbell syndrome shows extensive changes of saccular bronchiectasis. Williams-Campbell syndrome is congenital bronchomalacia caused by absence of annular cartilage distal to the first division of the peripheral bronchi. There is characteristically advanced bronchiectasis. Expiratory views may show ballooning of the distal airways (case courtesy of Steve Primack, Oregon Health Sciences University, Portland, OR).

Cystic bronchiectasis

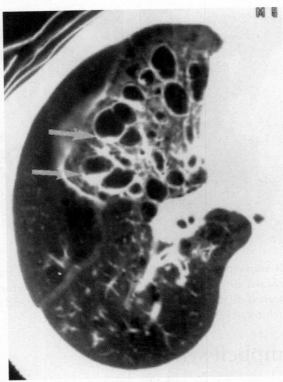

FIGURE 4-9 HRCT scan shows multiple rounded lucencies with discrete walls representing severe cystic bronchiectasis almost entirely replacing the middle lobe. Note the air-fluid levels (*arrows*).

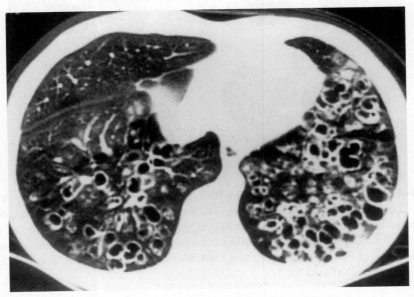

FIGURE 4-10 HRCT scan from this patient who suffered an episode of severe pneumonia in childhood shows extensive cystic bronchiectasis. Note multiple air-fluid levels within the airways. When severe, bronchiectasis can appear very similar to cystic lung diseases. Cystic bronchiectatic airways can be usually followed over serial slices and shown to be contiguous with one another. Remember, the cross section of a tubular structure will appear round and cystic.

Cystic bronchiectasis *(continued)*

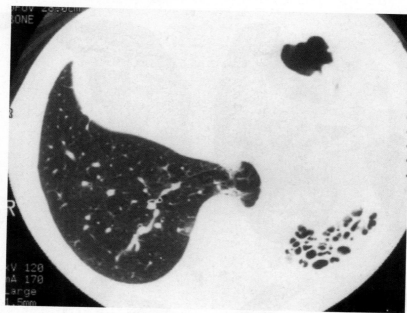

FIGURE 4-11 HRCT scan shows unilateral bronchiectasis in this patient whose left lung parenchyma was destroyed by tuberculosis. Ipsilateral severe bronchiectasis is the consequence of that infection. Bronchiectasis of this severity does not necessarily imply remote or long-standing infection. Postprimary tuberculosis may cause this amount of lung destruction in as little as 6 to 12 months.

Cystic bronchiectasis *(continued)*

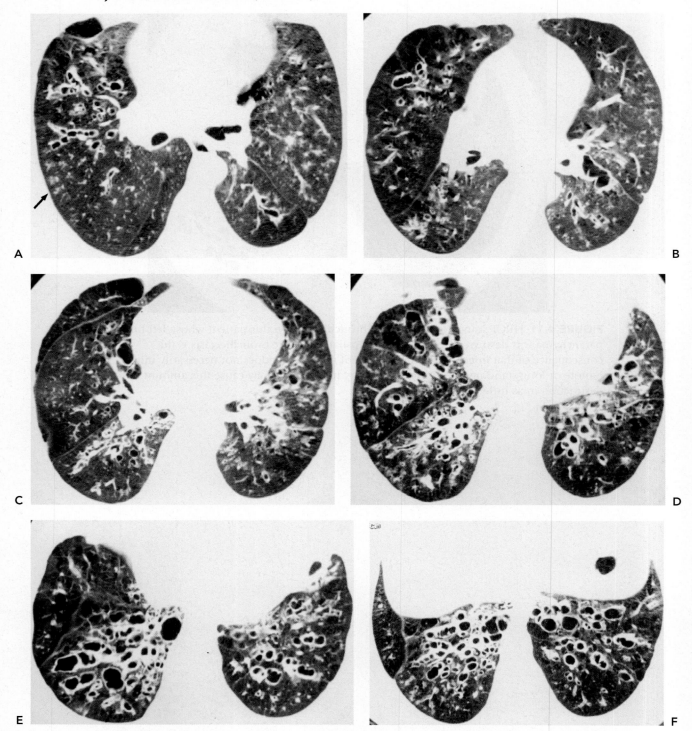

FIGURE 4-12 A–F: Six selected HRCT scans through the mid and lower lungs from a man with a long history of productive cough show the extent of the cystic bronchiectasis. Mentally stack the images in your mind's eye to see the tubular nature of the "cysts." Note that the smaller mucus-filled airways in **A** have a more nodular "tree-in-bud" appearance (*arrow*). Also note the heterogeneity of the extent of airway involvement and size of airway dilatation on all the images.

Cystic bronchiectasis *(continued)*

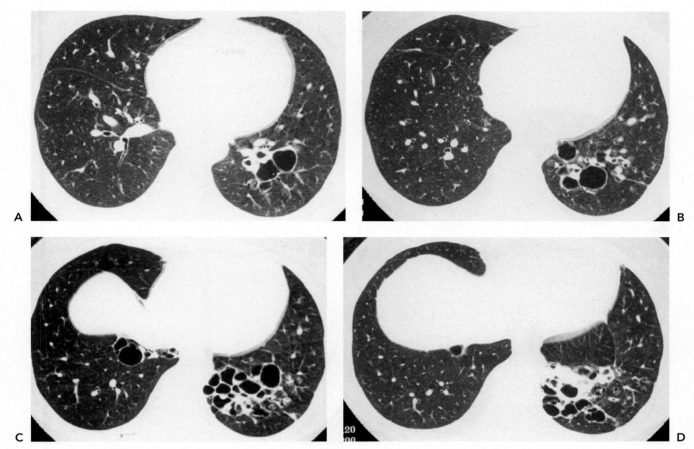

FIGURE 4-13 A–D: Four selected HRCT scans through the lower lobes show focal cystic bronchiectasis involving several basilar subsegmental airways of the left lower lobe and, to a much lesser extent, of the right lower lobe. Again, mentally stack the images in your mind's eye to see the tubular nature of the "cysts." Note just how focal bronchiectasis can be.

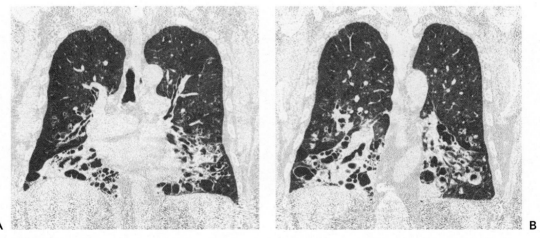

FIGURE 4-14 A–B: Coronal reformat CT scans through the mid chest from a patient with a lifelong history of bronchiectasis, of unknown etiology, show extensive and destructive cystic bronchiectasis throughout both lower lobes. There is also less severe bronchiectasis in the upper lungs, as well as features of mild air trapping in the upper lobes.

Cystic bronchiectasis *(continued)*

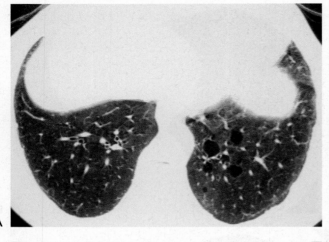

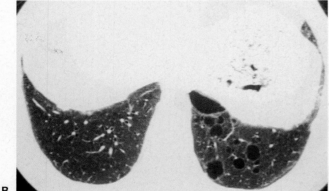

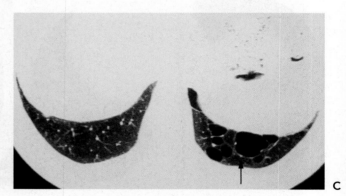

FIGURE 4-15 **A–C:** Three selected HRCT scans through the lower lobes show focal cystic bronchiectasis, again involving several basilar subsegmental airways of the left lower lobe. In this case, note the very thin, balloonlike walls of the bronchiectatic airways, all of which have a small white dot representing the accompanying pulmonary arteriole somewhere at the edge of the "cyst" (*arrow* in **C**).

Cystic bronchiectasis *(continued)*

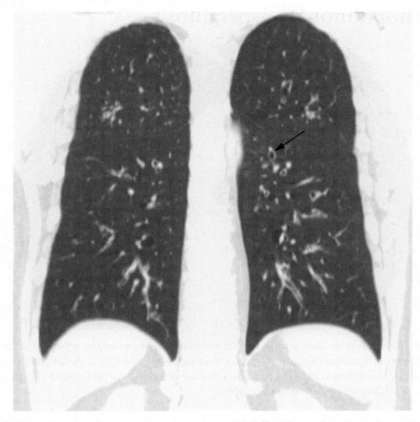

FIGURE 4-16 Coronal reformat CT scan shows mild diffuse bronchiectasis. Cross-sectional views through bronchiectatic airways result in the "signet-ring" sign; note the typical signet ring appearance (*arrow*).

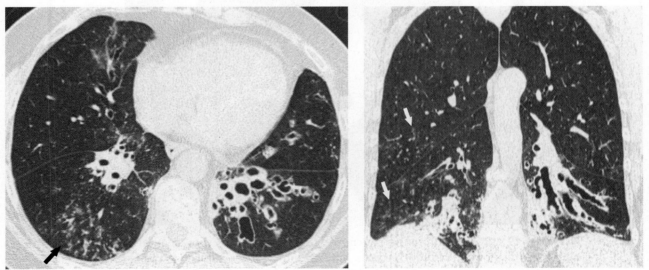

FIGURE 4-17 Transverse and coronal HRCT images show extensive basal predominant bronchiectasis with a varicoid morphology in the left lower lobe and more cylindrical bronchiectasis in the right middle and lower lobes. The bronchial walls are thickened and some retained secretions are present. Multiple poorly defined centrilobular nodules in the right lung (*arrows*) represent impacted smaller bronchi.

Mild central bronchiectasis secondary to allergic bronchopulmonary aspergillosis

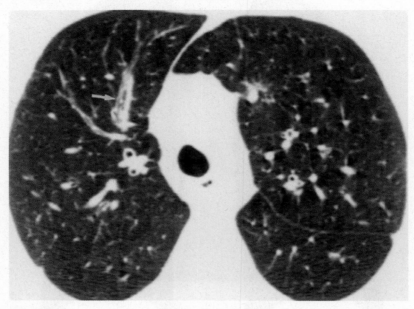

FIGURE 4-18 HRCT scan shows mild central bronchiectasis (*arrow*) in a patient with asthma. This combination of clinical and CT findings suggest ABPA, a destructive inflammatory disease of the airways. Patients with this disease usually have an immediate cutaneous reaction to a challenge by *Aspergillus fumigatus*.

Allergic bronchopulmonary aspergillosis

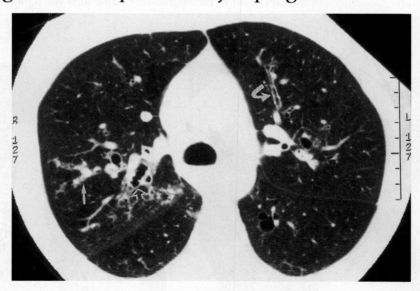

FIGURE 4-19 HRCT scan from this patient with asthma and ABPA shows typical central multilobar distribution of bronchiectasis. Both cylindrical (*curved arrow*) and varicose (*open arrow*) bronchiectases are present. Tenacious secretions impregnated with fungal hyphae opacify some dilatated bronchi, recognized as opaque branching structures (*arrow*). Also note thick and thin dilatated airway walls.

Allergic bronchopulmonary aspergillosis *(continued)*

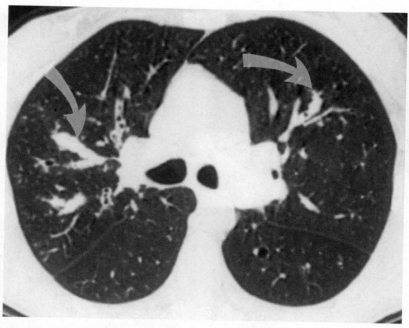

FIGURE 4-20 HRCT scan from a patient with ABPA shows bilateral bronchiectatic airways with mucoid impactions (*arrows*). ABPA is not an infection but a hyperimmune response to *Aspergillus* species. It results in excessive mucus production, impaction, and bronchiectasis. These patients usually have asthma and have elevated serum immunoglobulin E levels.

Cystic fibrosis

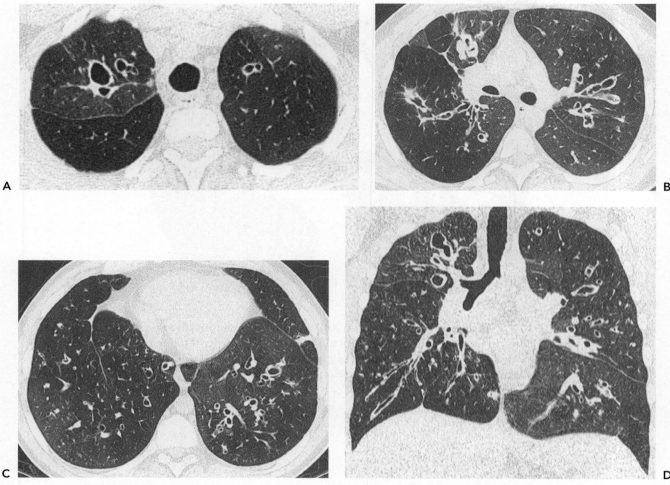

FIGURE 4-21 Transverse and coronal HRCT images show diffuse central bronchiectasis with a mid and upper lung predominance. Associated bronchial wall thickening and scattered foci of bronchial mucoid impaction are present. Additionally, the lungs are heterogeneous with hypoattenuating areas representing air trapping, the manifestation of the underlying small airways disease of cystic fibrosis.

Bronchocentric granulomatosis

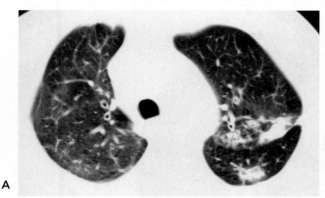

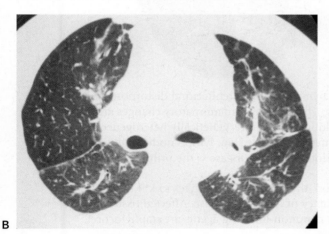

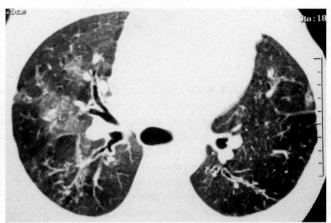

FIGURE 4-22 A–C: Three HRCT scans through the upper mid and lower lungs from a middle-aged woman with bronchocentric granulomatosis (BCG). Note the nonspecific multifocal areas of mild bronchiectasis, lung parenchymal architectural distortion, and non-specific areas of ground-glass opacity.

BCG can be categorized as one of five distinct clinical syndromes of pulmonary angiitis and granulomatosis: Wegener's granulomatosis, lymphomatoid granulomatosis, necrotizing sarcoid granulomatosis, BCG, and allergic angiitis and granulomatosis (Churg-Strauss syndrome). Some authors have classified BCG as part of the spectrum of ABPA. There are two different clinical subgroups of BCG: those with asthma and those without.

The HRCT manifestations of BCG are nonspecific and reflect the limited ways in which bronchi can respond to injury. Multifocal areas of bronchiectasis and lung scarring are seen, the essential requirement for its development being a sustained or intense inflammatory insult of the bronchial wall.

Bronchiectasis secondary to chronic granulomatous disease of childhood

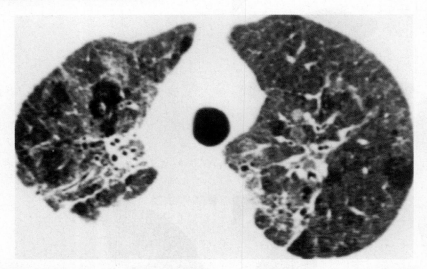

FIGURE 4-23 HRCT scan shows bilateral parenchymal scarring, architectural distortion, and bronchiectasis, which are worse in the right lung. These chronic inflammatory changes are caused by chronic granulomatous disease of childhood. This rare, genetically heterogeneous, heritable disorder is characterized by repeated infections of the skin, lymph nodes, and viscera. The lung is the most common site of infection, and lung disease is the primary cause of death in more than 50% of affected children.

In chronic granulomatous disease of childhood, the ability of phagocytes to kill ingested microorganisms is severely hampered by a deficiency of NADPH oxidase. Affected tissues respond with a granulomatous reaction. The most common infecting agents are staphylococci, gram-negative organisms, *Candida*, and *Aspergillus*.

Combined variable immunodeficiency

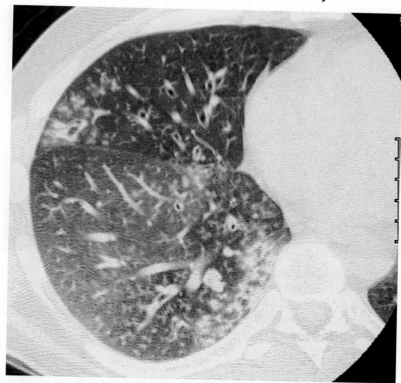

FIGURE 4-24 Targeted right-lung HRCT scan from a 39-year-old man complaining of 10 years of cough shows mild, patchy bronchiectasis involving the middle and lower lobes. The patient was subsequently discovered to have combined variable immunodeficiency. Note the associated mild air trapping in the regions of lung with bronchiectasis.

 Bronchiectasis is a common, nonspecific result of an inflammatory insult to the airways. The most common causes of bronchiectasis are necrotizing bacterial or viral infections in childhood. Other causes include cystic fibrosis, ABPA, immotile cilia syndromes, and immunoglobulinopathies, as in this case (case courtesy of Bruce Davidson M.D., Seattle, WA).

Traction bronchiectasis

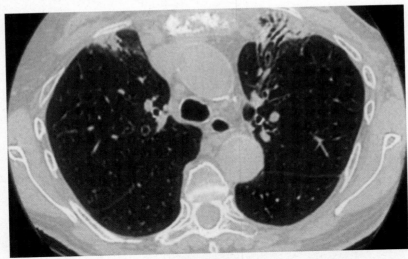

FIGURE 4-25 HRCT scan shows a fibrotic infiltrative process in the anterior aspects of the lungs, with consequent traction bronchiectasis. This patient had metastatic tumor to the sternum for which she received radiation therapy. Note that the distribution of fibrosis does not conform to any normal segmental or lobar lung anatomy; rather, it reflects the radiation port, often presenting in a geometric, nonanatomic appearance.

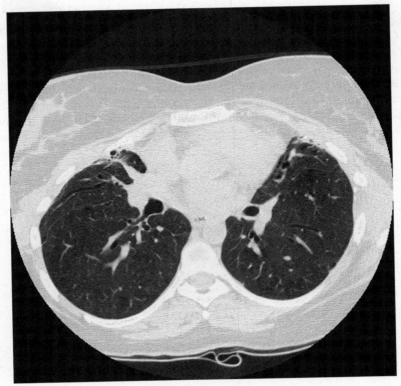

FIGURE 4-26 Thin section CT scan through the lower chest from this patient who suffered a prolonged episode of acute respiratory distress syndrome shows extensive residual scarring with volume loss in the anterior portions of the lung and associated traction bronchiectasis. Long-term survivors of ARDS often show this striking anterior distribution of lung fibrosis, which is thought to result from prolonged exposure to high partial pressures of oxygen, with resulting oxygen toxicity.

Traction bronchiectasis *(continued)*

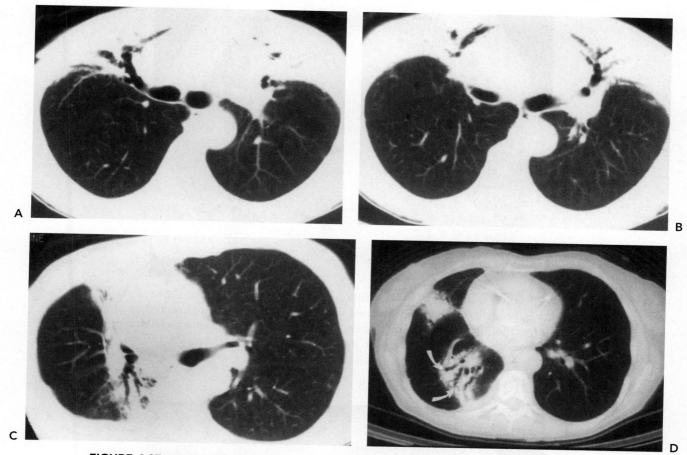

FIGURE 4-27 A–C: HRCT scan appearances of bronchiectasis secondary to radiation fibrosis and cicatrization in three patients. Note the straight, nonanatomic lateral border that marginates the area of abnormality, corresponding to the radiation port. The bronchiectasis that develops is caused by cicatrization and consequent traction reflecting the diffuse fibrotic nature of late-stage radiation pneumonitis (*arrows*). It is not caused by intrinsic disease of the airways. Findings of radiation pneumonitis usually are apparent on CT within 16 weeks after radiotherapy; however, they can be detected as early as 4 weeks after completion of radiotherapy. There can be progression of injury for several months, but by 6 to 9 months after radiation therapy has been completed, the injury stabilizes and healing with subsequent scarring begins.

Traction bronchiectasis (*continued*)

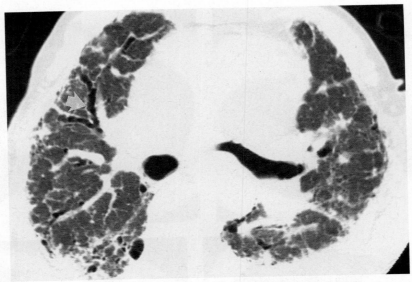

FIGURE 4-28 HRCT scan from a patient with idiopathic pulmonary fibrosis shows traction bronchiectasis. Bronchial dilatation associated with pulmonary fibrosis is produced by high retractive forces resulting from increased parenchymal elastic recoil and extremely high negative pleural pressure. Note the characteristic corkscrew appearance of the airway (*arrow*).

Reversible bronchiectasis

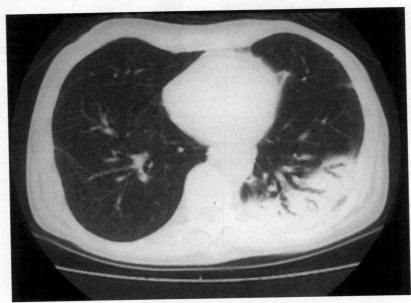

FIGURE 4-29 CT scan from patient with acute aspiration pneumonia of the left lower lobe shows bronchial dilatation within the region of disease. Subsequent HRCT examination showed that the airways had returned to normal caliber.

In pneumonia or atelectasis, the airways may dilate transiently. This "reversible bronchiectasis" is probably related to alterations in airway compliance and parenchymal stresses. Because dilatated airways can be present in patients who have recently had a suppurative pneumonia, one should consider delaying an HRCT examination for the accurate diagnosis of bronchiectasis at least 3 to 6 months after the resolution of the infection to avoid a false diagnosis of bronchiectasis.

Diffuse panbronchiolitis

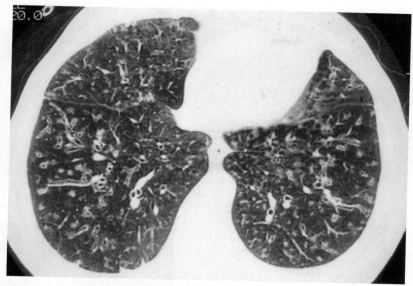

FIGURE 4-30 HRCT scan through the lower lung from a 63-year-old man with diffuse pan-bronchiolitis (DPB) shows diffuse ill-defined and branching bronchiolar structures throughout both lungs in this non-Asiatic patient. Lung attenuation is inhomogeneous, resulting in a mosaic pattern of lung attenuation.

DPB is a chronic idiopathic disease of bronchi and bronchioles, primarily affecting those of Asian origin, characterized by chronic airflow limitation and diffuse airway inflammation. Clinically, the patients have chronic sinusitis and chronic and recurrent infections of the airways. In the advanced stage, patients typically produce large amounts of purulent sputum and have chronic superinfection with *Pseudomonas* species. The usual cause of death in such patients is respiratory failure or *P. aeruginosa* pneumonia. HLA-Bw 54 is found in 60% to 70% of cases.

The HRCT scan features of DPB include diffuse ectasia of bronchi and bronchioles, which are usually filled with intrabronchial fibrosis or secretion, yielding numerous small nodular and linear opacities centrally located in secondary pulmonary lobules. A mosaic pattern of lung attenuation in peripheral areas can also be seen and is caused by air trapping. Similar HRCT scan features of DPB can be seen in patients with multifocal cylindrical bronchiectasis and dyskinetic cilia syndromes.

Diffuse panbronchiolitis *(continued)*

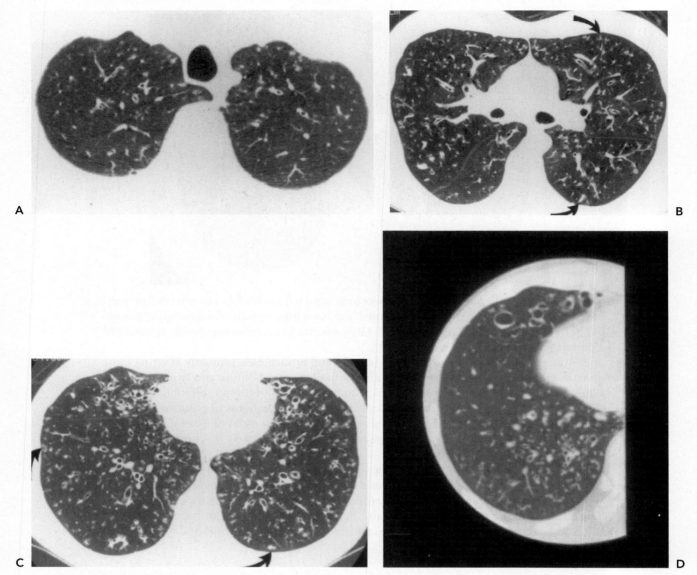

A

B

C

D

FIGURE 4-31 A–D: HRCT scans from two patients with DPB **(A–C)** and **(D)** show diffuse ectasia of bronchi and bronchioles and numerous small, round nodular and linear opacities centrally located in secondary pulmonary lobules *(arrows)*. The small nodular and linear opacities represent dilatated bronchioles filled with intrabronchial secretion. Note the decreased lung attenuation in peripheral areas due to air trapping caused by peripheral bronchiolar narrowing. In **D**, there are several dilatated airways with air-fluid levels.

Diffuse panbronchiolitis (*continued*)

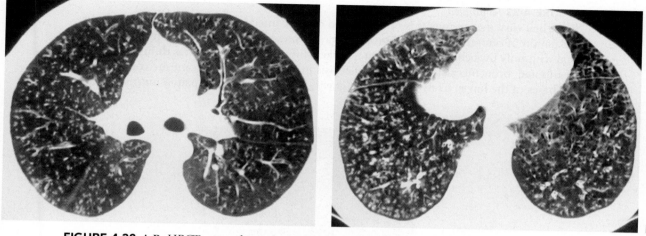

FIGURE 4-32 A,B: HRCT scans through the mid and lower lungs from this patient with DPB again show the typical features of this disease: diffuse ectasia of bronchi and bronchioles and numerous small, round nodular and linear opacities centrally located in secondary pulmonary lobules. Note that the cluster of lobular nodular opacities appear as small "rosettes" (case courtesy of Julie Takasugi, University of Washington, Seattle, WA).

Primary ciliary dyskinesia

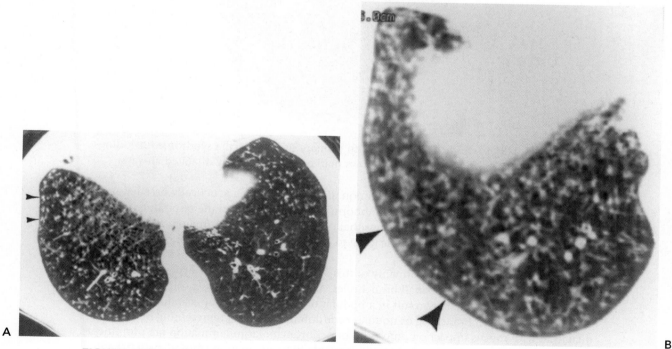

FIGURE 4-33 A,B: HRCT scans show numerous dilatated and mucus-filled bronchioles with thick walls that have the appearance of small ill-defined nodules (*arrowheads*). This patient had situs inversus and carried the diagnosis of Kartagener's syndrome. The presence of bronchiolectasis supports this diagnosis.

Primary ciliary dyskinesia results in chronic infection of the airways and sinuses, infertility in males, and a high incidence of abnormal thoracic, cardiac, and/or abdominal situs. When situs inversus is present, the syndrome is called *Kartagener's*. In patients with abnormal cilia,

(*continued*)

Primary ciliary dyskinesia (continued)

FIGURE 4-33 (continued)
bronchial clearance of mucus is impaired and chronic infection with bronchiectasis results. Dilatation of central or segmental bronchi may be present, or those airways may appear normal with only bronchiolectasis evident. Unlike panbronchiolitis, which is diffusely distributed, bronchiectasis and bronchiolectasis in amotile cilia syndrome are confined to the bases of the lungs, likely as a result of gravity exacerbating the impaired mucus clearance.

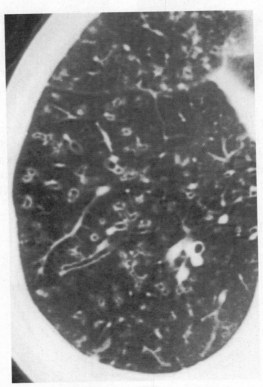

FIGURE 4-34 HRCT scan from a patient with primary dyskinetic cilia syndrome, including situs inversus (Kartagener's syndrome), shows markedly and diffusely dilatated airways, some obviously branching.

Primary ciliary dyskinesia is an uncommon disease caused by a genetically based abnormality of ciliary structure and function. Abnormal ciliary function in the respiratory tract results in recurrent and persistent infections that cause an intense inflammatory response in the bronchial and bronchiolar walls, leading to bronchiectasis and bronchiolectasis formation.

The earliest radiographic abnormality of this syndrome in children is hyperinflation caused by mucus plugging of small bronchioles. As the disease progresses, obstruction and plugging of small airways may result in a nodular or reticulonodular appearance on chest radiographs. On HRCT, branching or nodular centrilobular opacities representing bronchiolar dilatation with mucus impaction, infection, or peribronchiolar inflammation are prominent features of this disease. Geographic areas of variable lung attenuation (mosaic pattern) are also seen in patients with this syndrome.

Primary ciliary dyskinesia *(continued)*

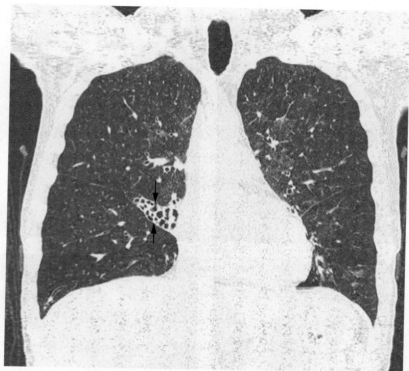

FIGURE 4-35 Coronal reformat CT scan through the midchest from a patient with immotile cila syndrome shows extensive bronchiectasis (*arrows*) in the right middle lobe and less so in the lingula.

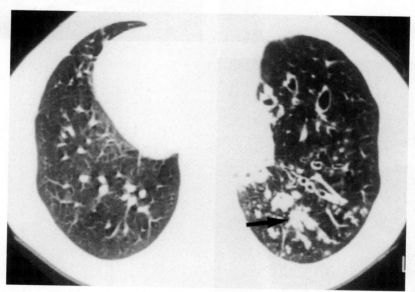

FIGURE 4-36 HRCT scan shows bronchiectasis and dextrocardia in this patient with Kartagener's syndrome. Asymmetry of the bronchiectasis does not exclude this diagnosis. Figures 4-33, 4-34 and 4-36 show the spectrum of bronchiectasis that occurs in Kartagener's syndrome. Note the thin-walled patent bronchiectatic airways anteriorly in the "left middle lobe" and the mucus-filled airways in the left lower lobe (*arrow*). The lung periphery is more lucent on the left when compared with the right lung, likely caused by air trapping.

Primary ciliary dyskinesia *(continued)*

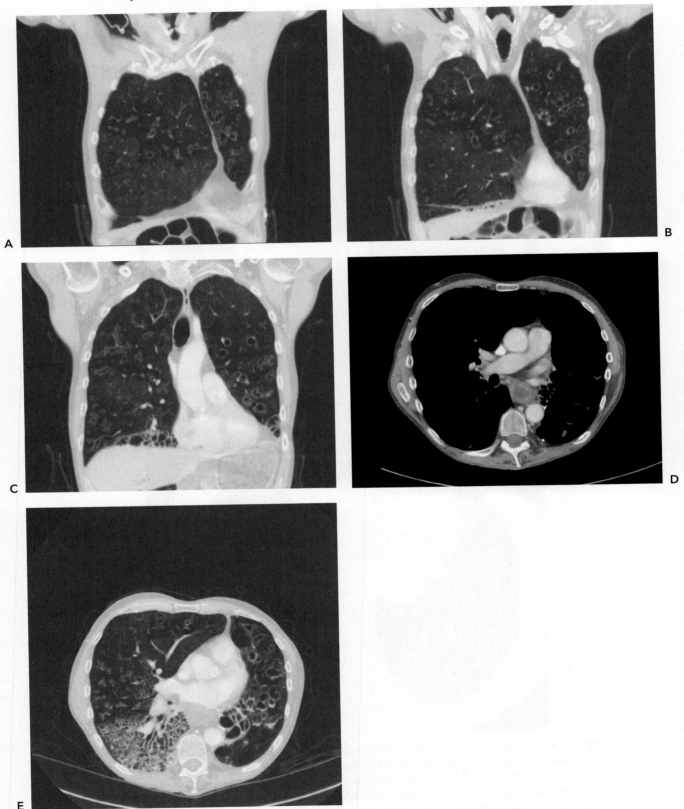

FIGURE 4-37 High-resolution axial and coronal reformat CT scan from patient with primary ciliary dyskinesia (immotile cilia syndrome) shows diffuse changes of cylindrical and cystic

(continued)

Primary ciliary dyskinesia *(continued)*

FIGURE 4-37 *(continued)*
bronchiectasis. Note the regional hypoattenuated lung secondary to small airways obstructive disease and air trapping. Primary ciliary dyskinesia is a rare genetic disorder of dysfunctional cilia associated with situs inversus. The demarcation between the hyperlucent lung is along the lines of interlobular septa that define the secondary pulmonary lobule. Note the markedly thickened esophageal wall from chronic reflux esophagitis. There may be a higher rate of esophagitis due to gastroesophageal reflux in patients with primary ciliary dyskinesia.

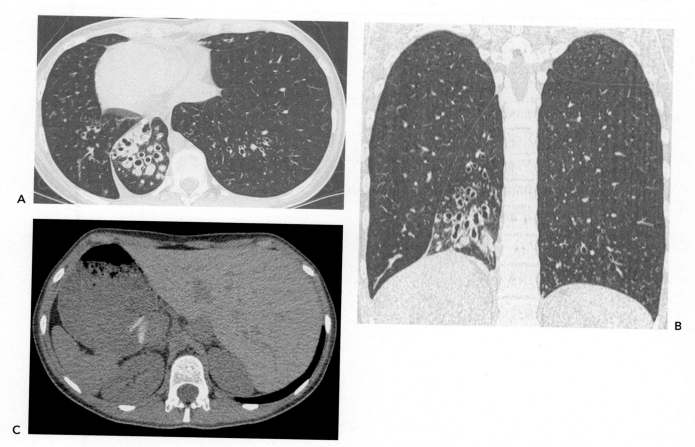

FIGURE 4-38 A, B: Transverse and coronal HRCT images show right lower lobe bronchiectasis with bronchial wall thickening, bronchial mucoid impaction, and volume loss. The cardiac apex is on the right. **C:** Unenhanced CT image through the upper abdomen (mediastinal window settings) demonstrates abdominal situs inversus. Chronic sinusitis, bronchiectasis, and situs inversus totalis comprise Kartagener's syndrome, which is part of the spectrum of ciliary motility disorders.

5

Small Airways Diseases

Constrictive bronchiolitis
Postinfectious constrictive bronchiolitis: Swyer-James syndrome
Asthma
Bronchocentric granulomatosis
Hypersensitivity pneumonitis
Hypersensitivity pneumonitis—subacute
"Tree-in-bud"
Juvenile laryngotracheal papillomatosis
Yellow nail syndrome

Constrictive bronchiolitis

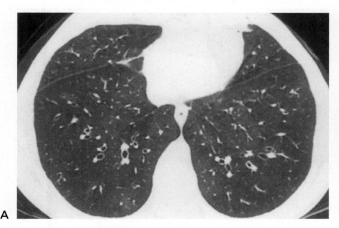
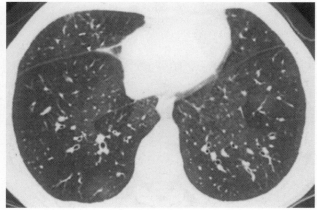

A   B

FIGURE 5-1 A: HRCT scan obtained at full-suspended inspiration. There is a slight heterogeneity to the attenuation of the lung parenchyma. This represents air trapping, which, when severe, can be visible on inspiratory CT scans.

Air trapping that occurs as a result of disease of the small airways may be classified as *fixed* or *reactive*. In fixed obstruction, there is narrowing or occlusion of the small airways; this is a common feature in diffuse panbronchiolitis and constrictive bronchiolitis. Reactive disease is an intermittent process in which the small airways narrow, producing a temporary increase in resistance to air flow: Asthma and other forms of bronchospasm, including that which occurs in conjunction with chronic obstructive pulmonary disease, are classified as *reactive airways disease*. **B:** HRCT scan obtained at suspended full expiration at the same anatomic level as above shows multiple focal lucencies. These lucencies correspond to multiple secondary lobules and represent extensive air trapping in them. This indicates severe obstructive disease of the small airways in this patient with constrictive bronchiolitis.

Constrictive bronchiolitis is a disease that can lead to progressive chronic respiratory failure. The underlying causes and predisposing factors for the development of constrictive bronchiolitis are protean and include penicillamine therapy; previous infection, especially by measles or adenoviruses; toxic fume inhalation (e.g., anhydrous ammonia); graft-versus-host disease; collagen vascular disease, such as rheumatoid arthritis and polymyositis; and chronic lung allograft rejection.

In constrictive bronchiolitis, noncartilaginous bronchioles are occluded by granulation tissue and destroyed. The characteristic combination of clinical and physiologic features, as well as evidence of air trapping at suspended full expiration HRCT, will often suggest the diagnosis of constrictive bronchiolitis.

Constrictive bronchiolitis *(continued)*

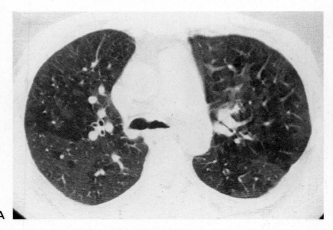
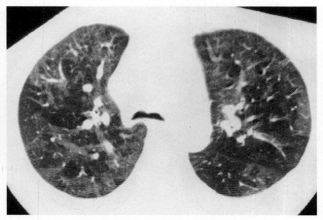

A **B**

FIGURE 5-2 Inspiratory **(A)** HRCT scans from a dyspneic patient with constrictive bronchiolitis shows a mosaic pattern of lung attenuation. Note the small caliber and paucity of vessels within the low-density regions, reflecting vasoconstriction consequent to bronchiolitis and impaired ventilation. Expiratory HRCT scan **(B)** at the same level as **A** shows increased density and decreased volume in the normal regions, whereas hypoattenuation and volume are maintained in the affected areas. This confirms regional air trapping.

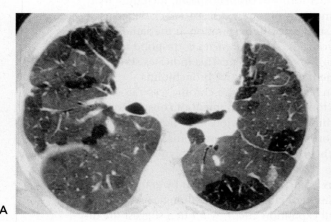
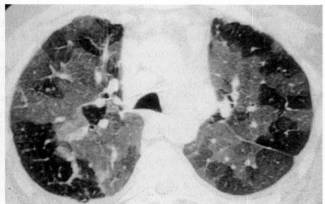

A **B**

FIGURE 5-3 Paired inspiratory-expiratory HRCT scans from a patient with constrictive bronchiolitis after toxic fume inhalation show a heterogeneous pattern of attenuation on the inspiratory CT scans **(A)**. HRCT performed at end expiration shows areas of air trapping in both lungs, resulting in a mosaic pattern of lung attenuation **(B)**. Air trapping is best shown and confirmed on the expiratory CT scan series.

Constrictive bronchiolitis *(continued)*

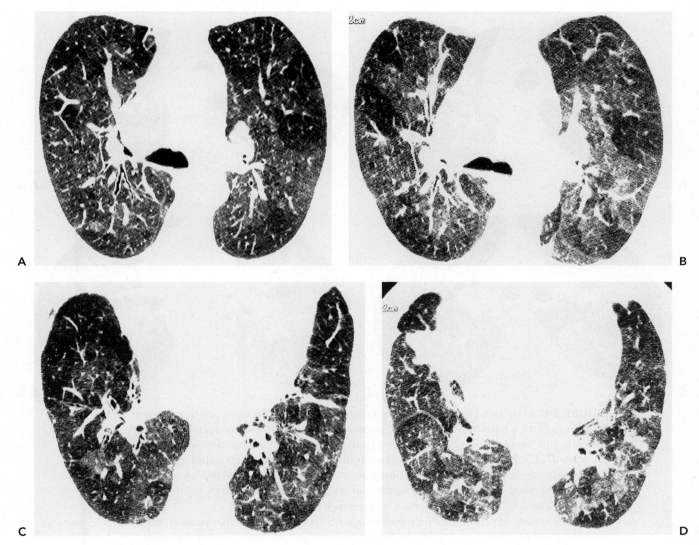

FIGURE 5-4 **A–D:** Two paired inspiratory-expiratory HRCT scans obtained at the mid and lower lungs from a patient with constrictive bronchiolitis suffered after severe smoke inhalation again show a heterogeneous (mosaic) pattern of attenuation on the inspiratory CT scans **(A,C)**. HRCT performed at end expiration shows areas of air trapping in both lungs, resulting in a mosaic pattern of lung attenuation **(B,D)**. Air trapping is, again, best shown and confirmed on the expiratory CT scan series.

Constrictive bronchiolitis *(continued)*

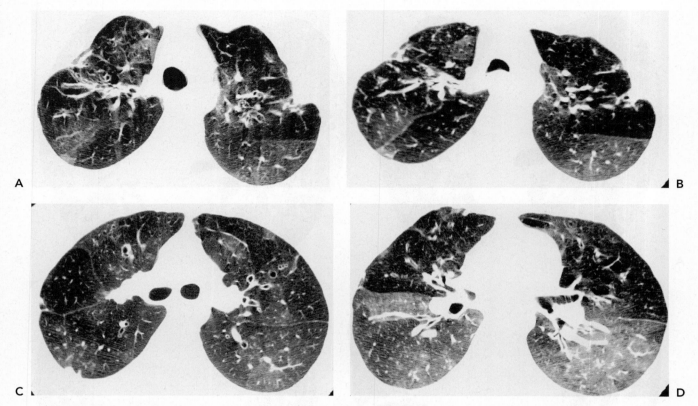

FIGURE 5-5 A–D: Two paired inspiratory-expiratory HRCT scans obtained at the upper and mid lungs from a patient with juvenile rheumatoid arthritis and subsequent constrictive bronchiolitis again show a heterogeneous (mosaic) pattern of attenuation on the inspiratory CT scans **(A,C)**. HRCT performed at end expiration shows areas of air trapping in both lungs, resulting in a mosaic pattern of lung attenuation **(B)**. Also note the bronchiectasis of the medium-sized airways that often accompanies small airways diseases. Bronchiectatic airways will "collapse" on end exhalation, as seen in **B** and **D**.

A wide variety of pulmonary histopathologic features are seen in rheumatoid arthritis, including constrictive bronchiolitis, pulmonary rheumatoid nodules, usual interstitial pneumonia, organizing pneumonia, lymphoid hyperplasia, follicular bronchiolitis, and nonspecific interstitial pneumonia.

Constrictive bronchiolitis *(continued)*

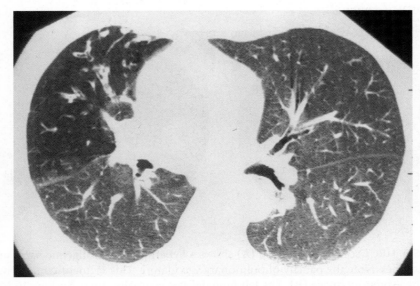

FIGURE 5-6 HRCT scan shows thick-walled dilatated bronchi, with and without mucus impaction, in the right middle lobe. The low-attenuation parenchyma of the right middle lobe has sparse vascular markings, even in areas without frank bronchiectasis. This suggests lobar hypoxia, with consequent vasoconstriction and shunting from this region. The pattern suggests underlying small airways disease, likely constrictive bronchiolitis, associated with the larger airways disease, namely, bronchiectasis.

Postinfectious constrictive bronchiolitis: Swyer-James syndrome

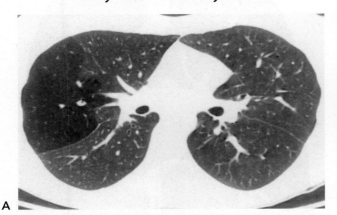

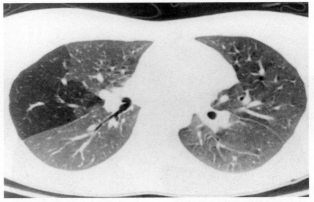

A   B

FIGURE 5-7 **A,B:** HRCT scans at inspiration **(A)** and expiration **(B)** show a markedly hyperlucent oligemic and expanded lateral segment of the middle lobe. This segment remains hyperlucent on the expiratory image **(B)**. The rest of the right lung and left lung deflate normally. These findings indicate obstruction of the lateral segmental bronchus of the middle lobe. Although asymmetric, they are compatible with the clinical diagnosis of Swyer-James syndrome consequent to constrictive bronchiolitis. Swyer-James syndrome is usually caused by a childhood adenovirus infection that results in bronchiectasis and constrictive bronchiolitis. On the chest radiograph, patients with Swyer-James classically have unilateral hyperlucent lung. On CT, the findings are often bilateral but asymmetric (case courtesy of J. Takasugi, University of Washington, Seattle, WA).

Postinfectious constrictive bronchiolitis: Swyer-James syndrome *(continued)*

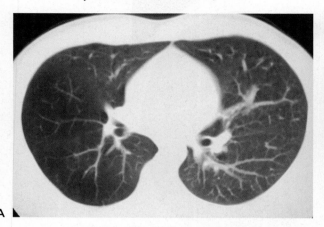
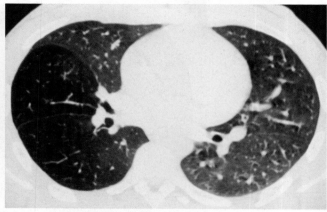

A   B

FIGURE 5-8 HRCT scan at inspiration **(A)** shows a hyperlucent and oligemic right, middle, and lower lobes. Note the paucity of pulmonary vasculature. This segment remains hyperlucent on the expiratory image **(B)**. The left lung deflates normally. These findings indicate obstruction of the right bronchus intermedius or a small airways disease. In this case, bronchoscopy showed normal airways, and the clinical diagnosis of Swyer-James syndrome consequent to constrictive bronchiolitis was made (case courtesy of C. Clagget, Madigan Army Medical Center, Tacoma, WA).

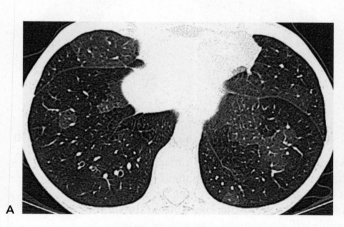
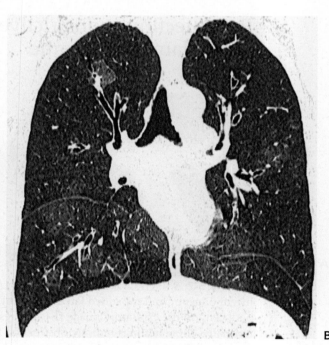

A   B

FIGURE 5-9 Constrictive bronchiolitis (Crohn disease) **A,B:** Transverse and coronal HRCT images from a patient with Crohn disease and progressive airflow obstruction show pulmonary hyperinflation and a mosaic pattern of attenuation. Hypoattenuating regions reflect extensive air trapping, whereas foci of ground-glass opacity represent hyperperfused normal lung. Constrictive bronchiolitis is an uncommon complication of inflammatory bowel diseases and can occur with both ulcerative colitis and Crohn disease. Pulmonary manifestations of inflammatory bowel disease most commonly occur later in the course of disease.

Asthma

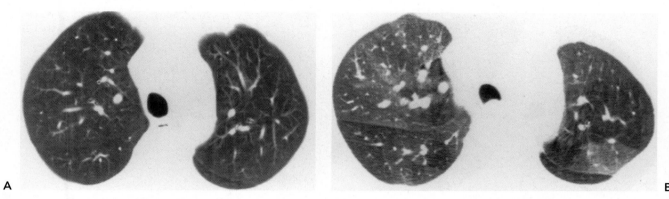

A   B

FIGURE 5-10 HRCT scan from a patient with asthma obtained at suspended full inspiration (**A**) produced images without detectable disease. However, repeat HRCT examination at suspended full expiration (**B**) shows patchy, heterogeneous lung attenuation consistent with air trapping, a nonspecific but key finding that reflects obstruction to airflow in small bronchi and bronchioli.

In patients with small airways diseases, HRCT scans obtained at suspended full inspiration may be entirely normal, as in this patient. Expiratory CT scanning can play an important role in the diagnostic workup of patients with small airways diseases. It is very sensitive in detecting subtle air trapping, in many cases more sensitive than spirometry; the detection of air trapping can provide clues to an otherwise unsuspected or underappreciated small airways disease. Expiratory CT scanning provides anatomic and physiologic information that is complementary to conventional suspended full-inspiration CT and pulmonary function testing. Depending on the clinical scenario, the extent and distribution of air trapping are useful in indicating or directing further diagnostic workup, such as transbronchial, thoracoscopic, or open lung biopsy.

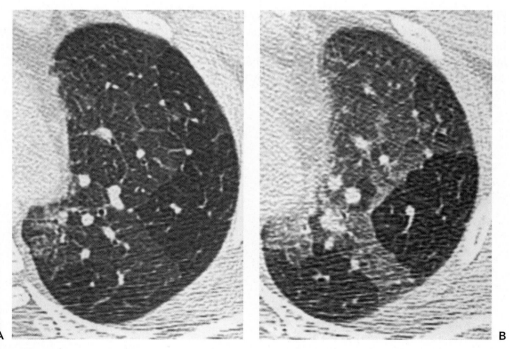

A   B

FIGURE 5-11 Inspiratory HRCT scan through the left upper lobe (**A**) from a patient with asthma shows a subtle mosaic pattern of lung attenuation. Expiratory HRCT scan (**B**) at approximately the same level shows air trapping in a multilobular distribution characteristic of small airways disease. These findings can be seen in diseases that obstruct the small airways, including asthma, constrictive bronchiolitis, and other forms of chronic bronchiolitis.

Asthma *(continued)*

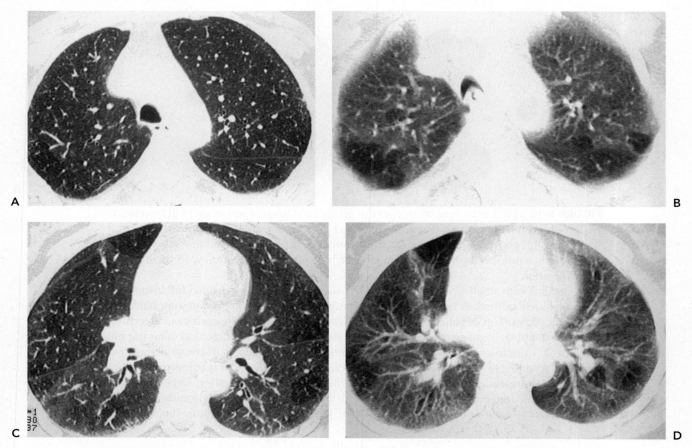

A   B   C   D

FIGURE 5-12 Inspiratory **(A,C)** and expiratory **(B,D)** HRCT scans through the upper and lower lungs from a patient with asthma show a very subtle heterogeneous mosaic pattern on inspiratory images that is markedly accentuated on expiratory images where there are lobular and multilobular regions of air trapping characteristic of small airways obstruction and consistent with asthma or reactive airways disease. Differential diagnosis includes constrictive bronchiolitis.

Bronchocentric granulomatosis

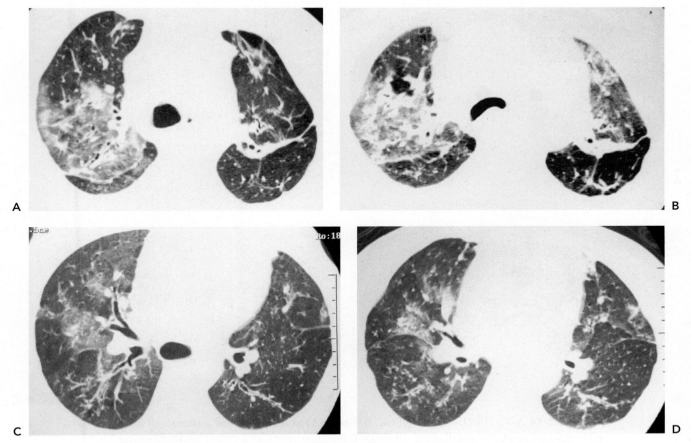

FIGURE 5-13 Inspiratory **(A,C)** and expiratory **(B,D)** HRCT scans through the mid and lower lungs from a patient with bronchocentric granulomatosis (BCG). The HRCT manifestations of BCG include multifocal areas of bronchiectasis and lung scarring from the intense inflammatory insult within the bronchial lumen. Note the extensive air trapping on the end-exhalation images.

BCG can be categorized as one of five distinct clinical syndromes of pulmonary angiitis and granulomatosis: *Wegener's granulomatosis, lymphomatoid granulomatosis, necrotizing sarcoid granulomatosis, BCG,* and *allergic angiitis and granulozmatosis* (Churg-Strauss syndrome). Some authors have classified BCG as part of the spectrum of allergic bronchopulmonary aspergillosis. There are two different clinical subgroups of BCG: those patients with asthma and those without.

Hypersensitivity pneumonitis

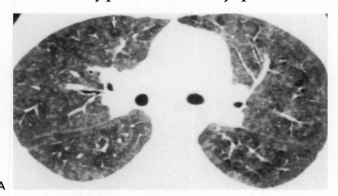

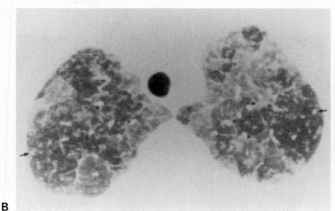

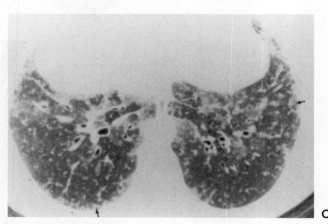

FIGURE 5-14 A–C: HRCT scans from two patients **(A)** and **(B,C)** show a mosaic of ground-glass opacification and small, hazy, ill-defined nodular opacities (*arrows*) centered around peripheral bronchovascular bundles—small airways—consistent with hypersensitivity pneumonitis. Depending on chronicity, the ground-glass opacity can be caused by noncaseating granulomas, filling of the air spaces with macrophages, interstitial pneumonitis, and bronchiolitis.

Hypersensitivity pneumonitis (also called *extrinsic allergic alveolitis*) occurs in response to the inhalation of organic particles in the home or workplace. It may be acute, subacute, or chronic. This immunologically mediated disease is often difficult to distinguish clinically and physiologically from other idiopathic diffuse lung diseases. The diagnosis is usually based on a constellation of findings that include antigen exposure, characteristic signs and symptoms, abnormal physical examination, and physiologic and radiographic evaluation.

In patients with hypersensitivity pneumonitis, the chest radiograph commonly appears normal. HRCT is more sensitive than chest radiograph for the detection of this disease.

Two widely recognized types of hypersensitivity pneumonitis are farmer's lung and bird-breeder's lung. Numerous other antigenic substances have also been recognized.

Hypersensitivity pneumonitis—subacute

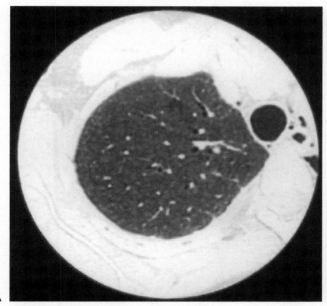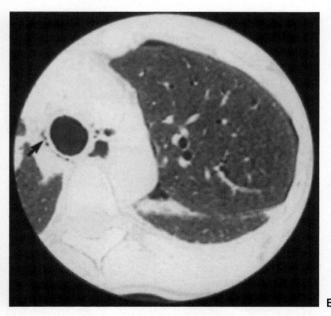

A   B

FIGURE 5-15

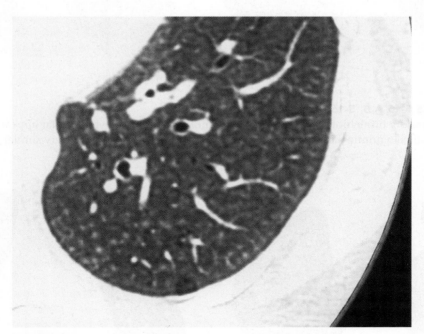

FIGURE 5-16

FIGURES 5-15 A,B, 5-16, and 5-17 A–C HRCT scans from three patients with subacute bird fancier's lung show common characteristic findings: diffuse, poorly circumscribed, small, nodular opacities that involve peribronchiolar tissues (centrilobular). Also noted are regions of poorly circumscribed ground-glass opacity that correlate histologically with interstitial pneumonitis, cellular bronchiolitis, and small, noncaseating granulomas. Air trapping may be also present in some patients. Note the air trapping in a single lobule in Figure 5-16 and multiple acinar-sized areas in Figure 5-17 **C**. Also note the pneumothorax and pneumomediastinum (*arrow*) in Figure 5-15 **B**. These were presumed to have been caused by paroxysmal coughing.

Hypersensitivity pneumonitis—subacute *(continued)*

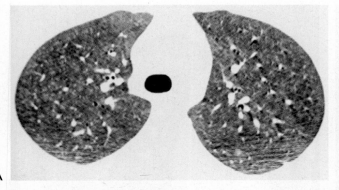

A

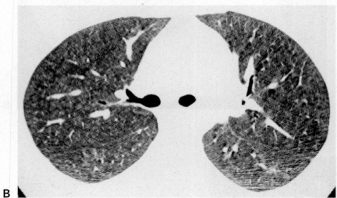

B

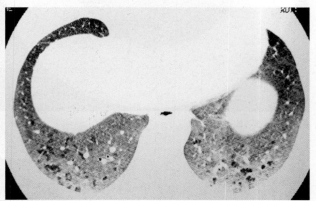

C

FIGURES 5-17

FIGURES 5-15 A,B, 5-16, and 5-17 A–C *(continued)*
Respiratory bronchiolitis, seen in cigarette smokers, can have a very similar appearance because the anatomic distribution of the inciting inflammatory agents is very similar.

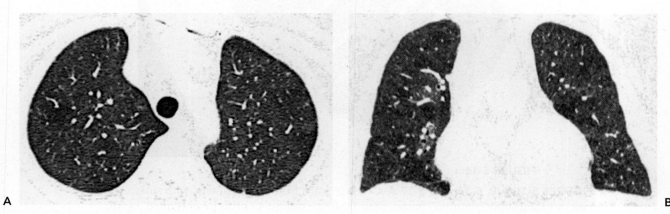

A   B

FIGURE 5-18 Transverse and coronal HRCT images from a patient with hypersensitivity pneumonitis from a pet bird show patchy ground-glass opacity and hypoattenuation lobules, the latter of which represents air trapping. Bronchiolitis is a component of hypersensitivity pneumonitis.

Hypersensitivity pneumonitis—subacute *(continued)*

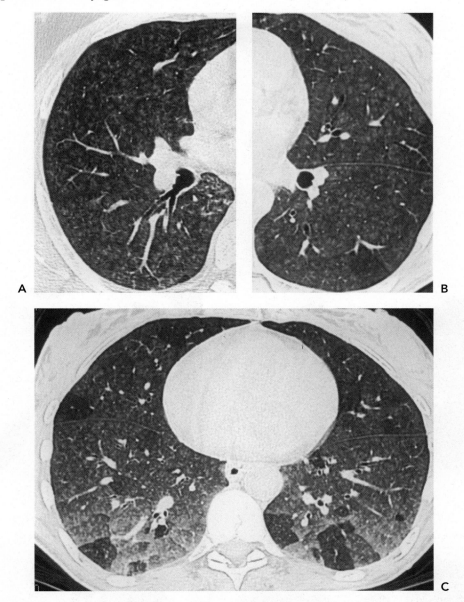

FIGURE 5-19 Inspiratory **(A,B)** and expiratory **(C)** HRCT scans from a patient with parakeet breeder's hypersensitivity pneumonitis. Note fuzzy, poorly circumscribed centrilobular nodular opacities characteristic of hypersensitivity pneumonitis (extrinsic allergic alveolitis). In **C**, expiratory HRCT image shows mosaic pattern of lung attenuation with lobular regions of air trapping consistent with small airways obstruction. A pathologic component of hypersensitivity pneumonitis is bronchiolitis. Mosaic pattern of lung attenuation with air trapping is characteristic of bronchiolitis. This case exemplifies the spectrum of airways diseases that can have air trapping as a component.

Hypersensitivity pneumonitis—subacute *(continued)*

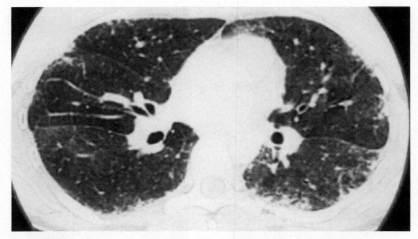

FIGURE 5-20

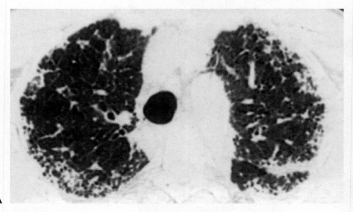
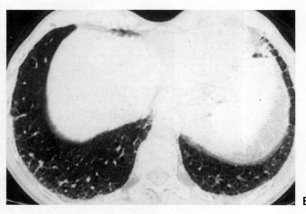

A   B

FIGURE 5-21

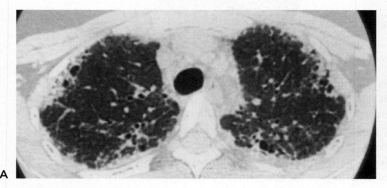
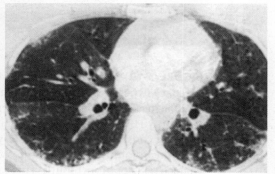

A   B

FIGURE 5-22

FIGURES 5-20, 5-21 A,B, and 5-22 A,B: HRCT scans from three patients whose symptoms have persisted for at least 12 months and shown to have bird fancier's disease causing chronic hypersensitivity pneumonitis show a peripheral fibrotic process affecting the mid and upper lungs predominantly, with relative sparing of the apices and bases. However, other patients with chronic hypersensitivity pneumonitis can show diffuse disease without zonal predominance. It is this nonbasal distribution of fibrosis that allows distinction of chronic hypersensitivity pneumonitis from other causes of fibrosis, such as idiopathic pulmonary fibrosis.

Hypersensitivity pneumonitis—subacute *(continued)*

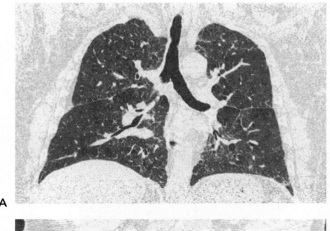

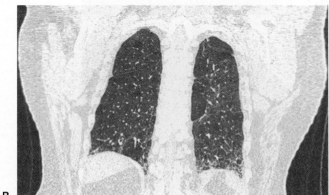

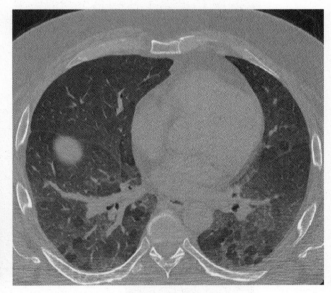

FIGURE 5-23 A–C: Coronal HRCT scans through the posterior **(A)** and mid **(B)** chest, and transverse HRCT through the lower chest **(C)** from a patient with chronic hypersensitivity pneumonitis for at least 5 years show mild diffuse residual interstitial lung fibrosis with mild distortion of the lung anatomy, diffusely, but predominantly in the lower lungs. Note the very mild scattered lobular air trapping seen in **A** and **C**.

"Tree-in-bud"

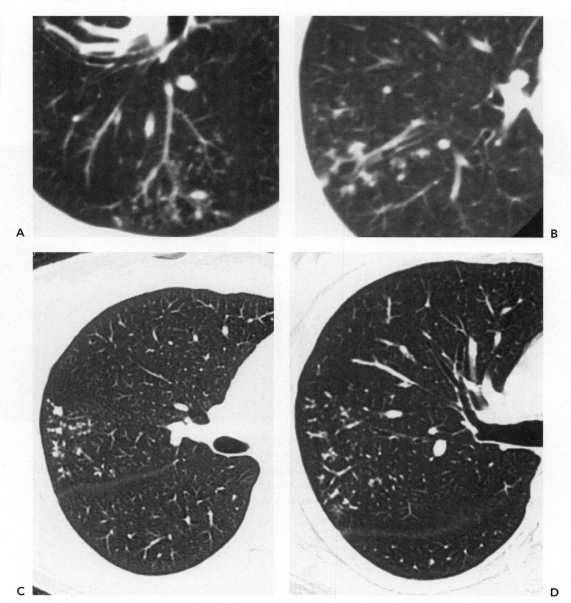

FIGURE 5-24 A–D: HRCT scans from a patient with the clinical diagnosis of *Histoplasmosis* bronchiolitis show the tree-in-bud (TIB) pattern of a small airways disease. Note branched Y- and V-shaped centrilobular opacities characteristic of bronchiolar filling.

Bronchiolitis and bronchiolectasis are nonspecific inflammatory processes of the small airways caused by many different insults. The TIB pattern is a direct CT scan finding of bronchiolar disease for the CT scan finding of endobronchial spread of *Mycobacterium tuberculosis*. This pattern is analogous to the larger airway "finger-in-glove" appearance of bronchial impaction but on a much smaller scale. The *TIB pattern* has become a popular descriptive term for many bronchiolar disease processes, all with similar appearances, although it is still often used inappropriately to imply a pathognomonic finding for tuberculosis.

The list of diseases associated with the bronchioles potentially producing a TIB pattern at CT scanning is extensive. The more common disease processes can be grouped as follows: (a) infection, (b) immunologic disorders, (c) congenital disorders, (d) aspiration, and (e) idiopathic condition.

Indirect CT scan signs of bronchiolar disease include air trapping, especially with expiratory CT scanning, and subsegmental atelectasis.

"Tree-in-bud" *(continued)*

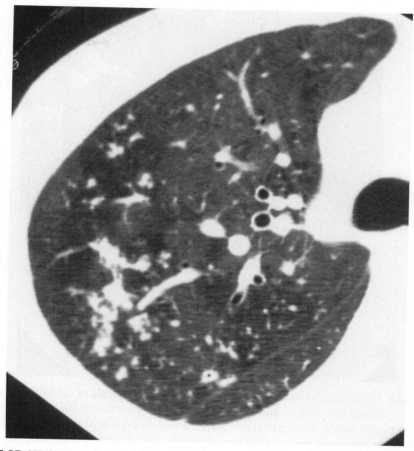

FIGURE 5-25 HRCT scan through the right upper lobe from a patient with active endobronchial tuberculosis shows impacted peripheral bronchioles in a typical TIB pattern. This appearance can be seen with inflammatory or infectious small airway disease of any etiology but is typical of tuberculous bronchitis. Note the relatively decreased attenuation in the parenchyma surrounding these areas, likely caused by air trapping.

"Tree-in-bud" *(continued)*

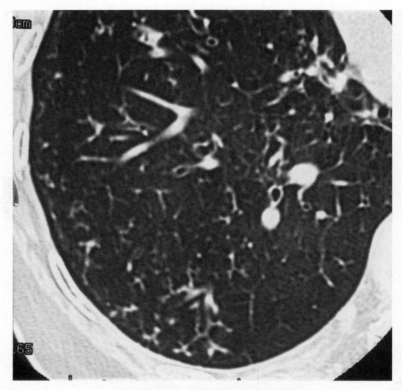

FIGURE 5-26 HRCT scan from a patient with the clinical diagnosis of viral bronchiolitis shows a TIB pattern. Note the V- and Y-shaped opacities in the centrilobular location, characteristic of bronchiolitis. There are also regions of bronchiectasis. The TIB pattern can be seen with many infectious etiologies of bronchiolitis, including viral, bacterial, parasitic, mycobacterial, and fungal agents.

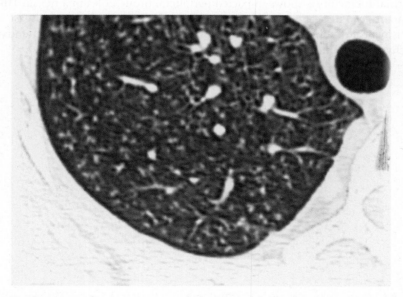

FIGURE 5-27 HRCT scan from a patient with bronchiolitis from Silo Filler's disease. Note the centrilobular nodular opacities that are well circumscribed. Many of them are Y or V shaped. They are relatively well circumscribed compared with the poorly circumscribed nodular opacities seen in the centrilobular regions in patients with hypersensitivity pneumonitis. Silo Filler's disease involves bronchiolitis secondary to toxic fume inhalation. The fumes are from decaying silage and are composed of nitrogen dioxide.

"Tree-in-bud" *(continued)*

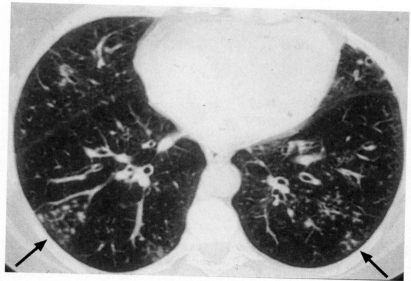

FIGURE 5-28 HRCT scan obtained at the level of the lower lobes from a 48-year-old asymptomatic woman with primary Sjögren's syndrome (SS) shows two foci of peripheral branching structures caused by impaction of inflammatory material in distal bronchioles with the characteristic TIB appearance (*arrows*).

Patients with primary SS are more susceptible to bronchiolar damage and recurrent respiratory tract infections. The appearance of SS on thin-section CT scans includes septal and nonseptal lines, parenchymal nodules, patchy areas of ground-glass and honeycombing, signs of small airways, and cysts (see Fig. 6-25). Bronchial abnormalities in SS were not selective but part of a more generalized interstitial lung disease, as is well known for other connective tissue disorders.

The coexistence of interstitial and bronchiolar disease may explain the sometimes complex abnormalities found with pulmonary function tests in such patients. A study of 50 patients with primary SS showed that abnormal findings were present on HRCT scans in 17 patients (34%) compared with only 7 patients (14%) on conventional chest radiograph. Also, CT scan depicted abnormalities in 7 (19%) of the 37 patients free of respiratory symptoms. These results suggest that parenchymal abnormalities detected on CT scans may not interfere with the functional status of such patients and that early detection of subtle pulmonary changes may precede the appearance of symptoms by a number of years.

In the lungs, two pathologic processes, such as multinodular amyloid and lymphoid interstitial pneumonia have been described in association with SS. Lymphoid infiltration of extranodal sites is a prominent feature of SS, and the risk of occurrence of lymphoma is much greater in such patients than in the general population. Radiologically, pulmonary lymphoma associated with SS can present as a diffuse interstitial process or as multiple nodular infiltrates.

Juvenile laryngotracheal papillomatosis

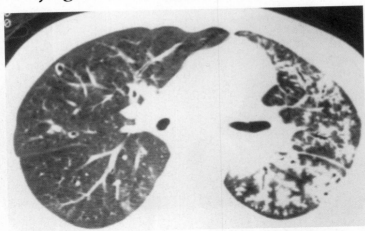

FIGURE 5-29 HRCT scan from a patient with juvenile laryngotracheobronchial papillomatosis shows multiple, small, solid, and cavitary/cystic nodules throughout the lower lungs. The nodules are worse in the left lung. The lesions tend to be centered within the bronchovascular bundles.

Juvenile laryngotracheobronchial papillomatosis is a recurrent, prolonged disease usually confined to the upper airway. Although pulmonary involvement is present in only 1% of patients with this infection, the presence of lung disease carries a poor prognosis. The lung lesions appear cystic or solid and represent benign squamous cell proliferations or papillomas with or without central cavities containing debris or air. Papillomas may spread from the larynx to the bronchi and bronchioles. This occurs by direct extension—lesions develop in the lungs many years after the onset of laryngeal papillomatosis. Although the laryngeal lesions may regress spontaneously, it is uncommon for the lung lesions to do so. Lung cancer has been reported to occur with increased frequency in these patients.

Yellow nail syndrome

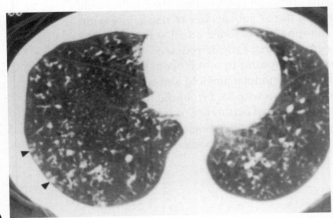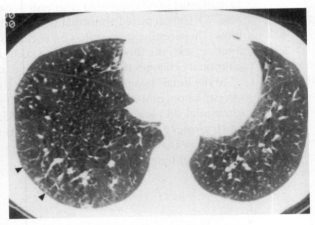

A   B

FIGURE 5-30 A: HRCT scan shows multiple, peripheral, irregular nodules in both lower lobes. In this patient with the diagnosis of yellow nail syndrome, these nodules represent mildly dilatated, mucus-filled bronchioles.

Yellow nail syndrome is an unusual lymphangitic disorder that may be caused by congenital hypoplasia of the lymphatics. It is characterized by the classic triad of physical findings: yellow nail discoloration, lymphedema, and pleural effusion that may be chylous or exudative. Bronchiectasis with bronchial wall thickening, bronchial dilatation, and mucus plugging is an associated pulmonary feature. **B:** After medical treatment of this patient, mucus plugging resolved and HRCT could demonstrate the dilatated patent bronchi.

6

Cystic Lung Diseases

Lymphangioleiomyomatosis
Tuberous sclerosis
Pulmonary Langerhans cell histiocytosis
Sjögren's syndrome
Neurofibromatosis
Hydrocarbon aspiration
Pulmonary Placental Transmogrification

Lymphangioleiomyomatosis

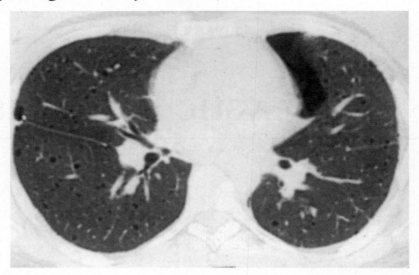

FIGURE 6-1 HRCT scan shows multiple, evenly distributed, small cystic spaces, with well-defined walls, throughout the lungs, typical for mild lymphangioleiomyomatosis (LAM). Also note the left anteromedial pneumothorax, a common complication of LAM.

LAM is a rare disease of unknown etiology affecting women of reproductive age. Pathologically, LAM is characterized by progressive proliferation of smooth muscle in the airways, arterioles, venules, and lymphatics of the lung, leading to progressive shortness of breath, lung cysts, pneumothorax, hemoptysis, and chylous effusion.

The HRCT and pathologic appearances of LAM are indistinguishable from the cystic lung disease of tuberous sclerosis. Pleural effusions are common with LAM.

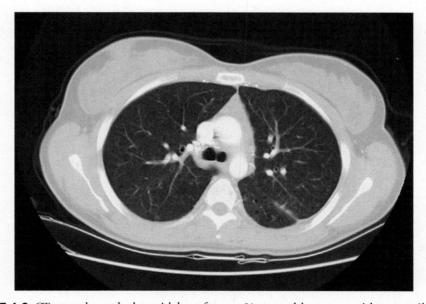

FIGURE 6-2 CT scan through the midchest from a 21-year-old woman with very mild LAM, obtained after a thoracentesis. Note a small left pleural effusion and subtle diffuse small lung cysts. The patient initially presented with a massive left chylothorax.

Lymphangioleiomyomatosis *(continued)*

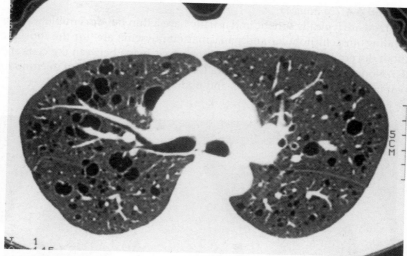

FIGURE 6-3

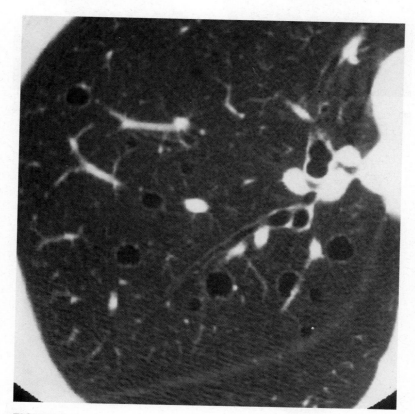

FIGURE 6-4

FIGURES 6-3 and 6-4 HRCT scans from two different patients with LAM of moderate severity show cystic spaces that are larger, but still relatively spheric, with well-defined walls. They are distributed diffusely throughout all regions of the parenchyma. Note that the lesions have no vessels within them. The findings are characteristic of LAM.

Although Langerhans cell histiocytosis (LCH) can also have a predominantly cystic appearance, it is distinguished from LAM by the upper-zone predominance of cysts, with relative sparing of the lung bases. In LAM, the distribution is diffuse and uniform. The "cysts" of LCH often become bizarrely shaped and are actually regions of paracicatricial emphysema.

(continued)

Lymphangioleiomyomatosis *(continued)*

FIGURES 6-3 and 6-4 *(continued)*
The "cysts" in LAM are typically spheric and usually have a thin but discernible wall. In contrast, the HRCT findings in centrilobular and panacinar emphysema are, for the most part, lucent regions without discernible walls. In LAM, the lung parenchyma between the cysts appears normal on HRCT. Nodules are common in LCH. In LAM, they are very rare, but micronodular pneumocyte hyperplasia is associated with LAM, and nodules can be seen with CT.

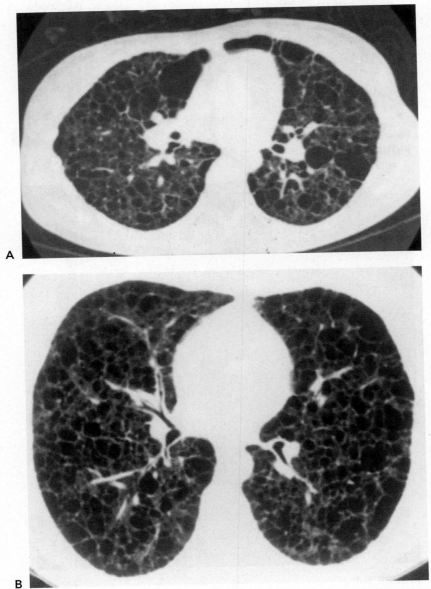

FIGURE 6-5 A,B: HRCT scans from two different patients with severe cystic lung disease of LAM show innumerable cysts ranging from a few millimeters to 5 cm in diameter.

Lymphangioleiomyomatosis *(continued)*

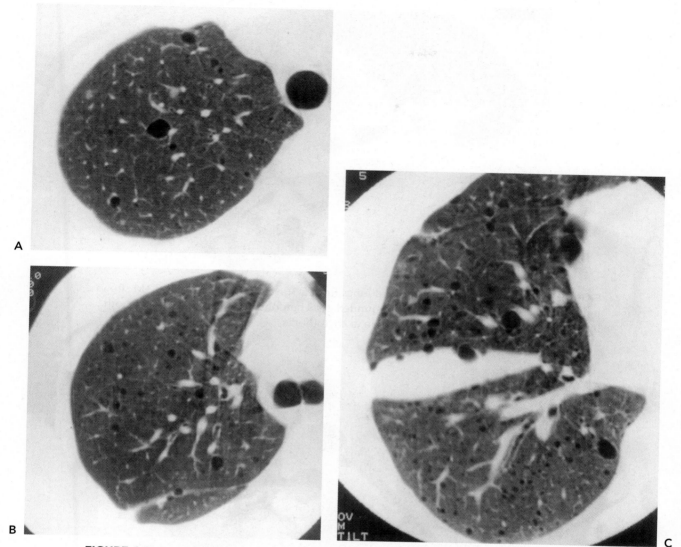

FIGURE 6-6 A–C: HRCT scans from a patient with mild LAM show the diffuse, random distribution of cysts of various sizes. These are distributed throughout all zones of the lungs, but, in this case, predominate in the bases. The cysts have thin discrete walls, unlike emphysema. Also, there is never a centrilobular core structure present in the center of the cyst, unlike that seen with centrilobular emphysema. Note the effusion in the major fissure—likely chylous.

Lymphangioleiomyomatosis *(continued)*

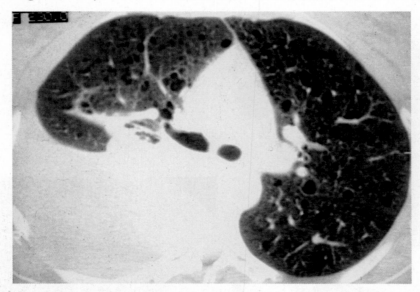

FIGURE 6-7 HRCT scan through the mid lungs from a 36-year-old woman with LAM shows multiple, well-defined, and thin-walled rounded cysts randomly scattered throughout both lungs. Also note large right pleural effusion, a chylothorax.

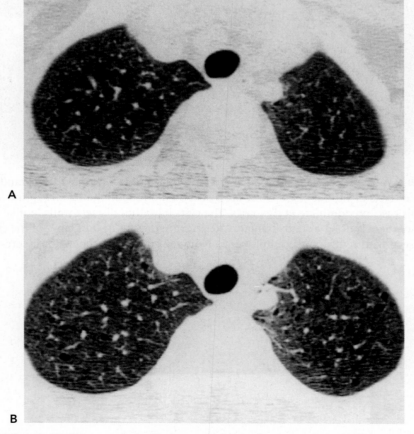

FIGURE 6-8 A,B: HRCT scans through the upper lobes from a patient with LAM performed at an interval of 4 months show more and larger cysts, indicating progression of the disease. Note the increase in the size and number of typical thin-walled cysts.

Lymphangioleiomyomatosis *(continued)*

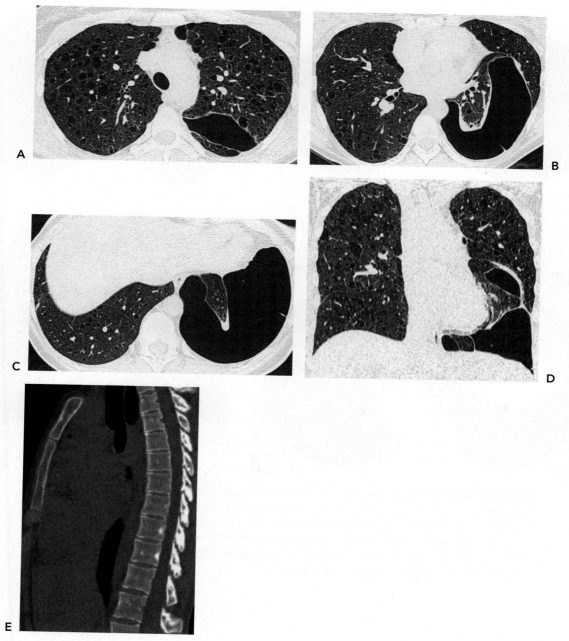

FIGURE 6-9 A–D: Transverse and coronal HRCT images show diffuse thin wall cysts in both lungs. A loculated pneumothorax is present on the left. Recurrent pneumothoraxes can lead to pleural adhesions, and over time the affected lung may fail to re-expand, leading to chronic pneumothorax. Sagittal reconstruction shows numerous sclerotic lesions in the spine that represent bone islands. Osteopoikilosis can develop in patients with tuberous sclerosis and LAM.

Lymphangioleiomyomatosis *(continued)*

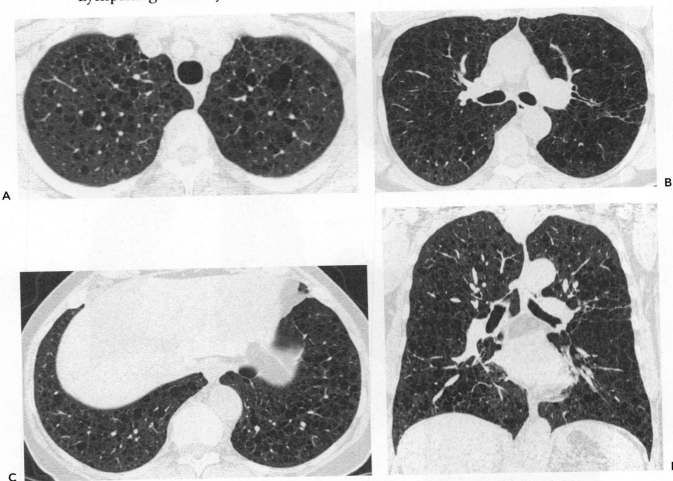

FIGURE 6-10 A–D: Transverse and coronal HRCT images show pulmonary hyperinflation with diffuse thin wall cysts. The cysts in LAM range from 2 to 20 mm and lack a zonal predilection. The intervening lung is usually normal. Over time, the number and size of cysts increase. Patients may develop spontaneous pneumothorax or chylothorax. Extrathoracic findings that may help make the diagnosis of LAM include retroperitoneal and mediastinal lymphangiomas and renal angiomyolipomas.

Lymphangioleiomyomatosis *(continued)*

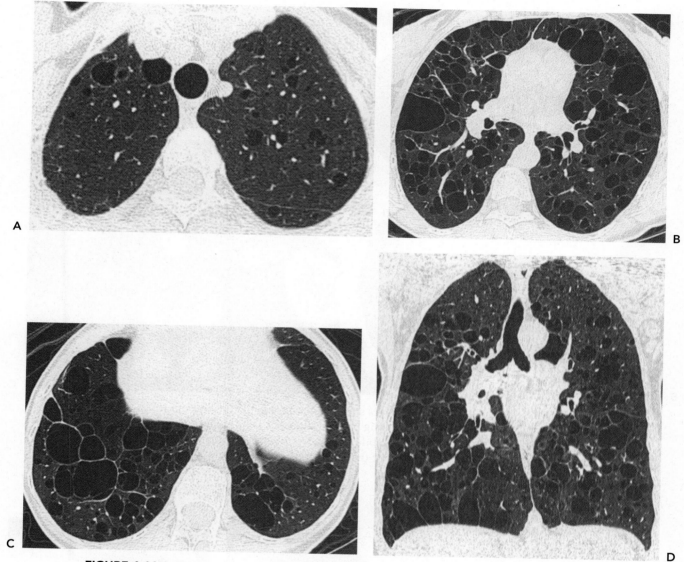

FIGURE 6-11 A–D: Transverse and coronal HRCT images demonstrate hyperinflated lungs with diffuse thin wall cysts in a patient with LAM.

Lymphangioleiomyomatosis *(continued)*

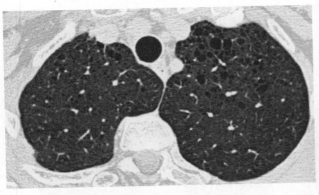

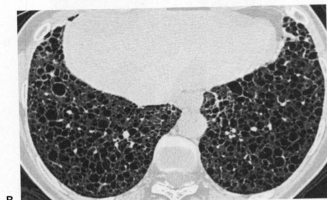

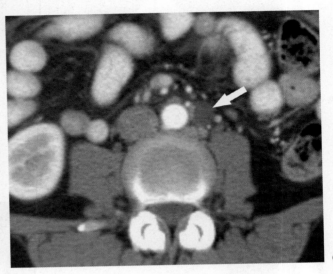

FIGURE 6-12 LAM 4—**A,B:** HRCT images show numerous small cysts in both lungs with partial sparing of the lung apices. The lung between the cysts is normal. **C:** Contrast-enhanced CT image through the upper abdomen shows a water-attenuation cystic nodule in the retroperitoneum (*arrow*) to the left of the aorta, representing a lymphangioma.

Tuberous sclerosis

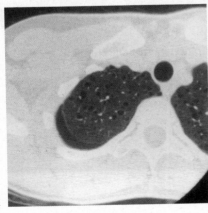

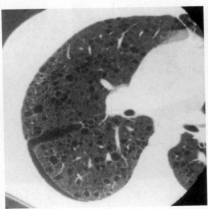

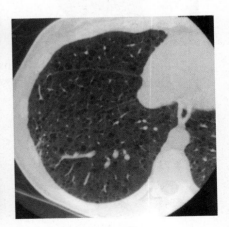

FIGURE 6-13 A–C: HRCT scans from a woman with tuberous sclerosis show moderate cystic lung disease. Cysts are distributed diffusely from apex to base in a random pattern. Note the pneumothorax **(B)**, one of the complications of this disease as with LAM. Also note that the pneumothorax extends into an incomplete major fissure.

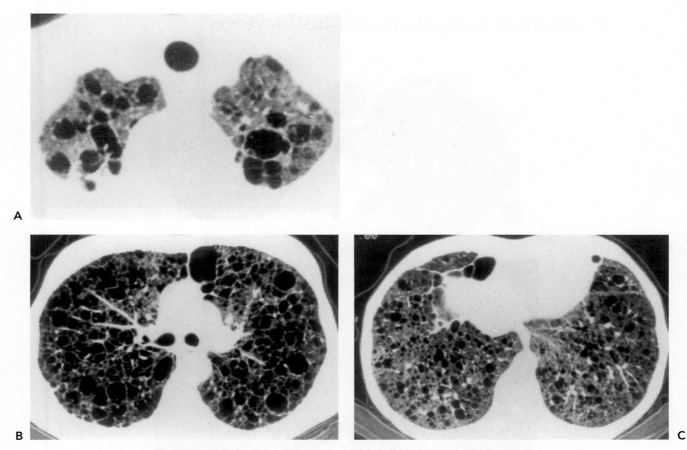

FIGURE 6-14 A–C: HRCT scans from a woman with tuberous sclerosis show extensive, end-stage cystic lung disease. HRCT findings are indistinguishable from LAM.

Pulmonary Langerhans cell histiocytosis

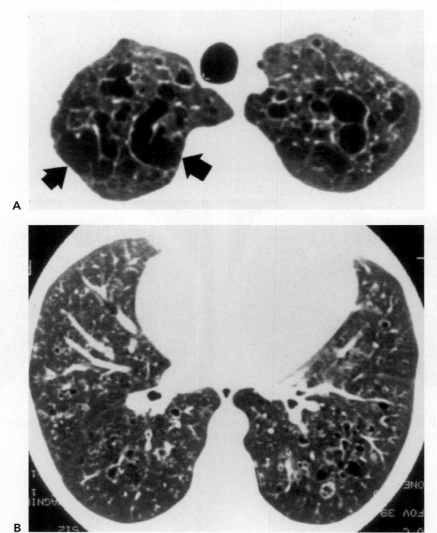

FIGURE 6-15 A,B: HRCT scans from a patient with Pulmonary Langerhans cell histiocytosis (PLCH) show lung cysts that are larger and more extensive in the apex, much less severe in the mid lung, and absent in the lung bases (not shown). The cysts can attain unusual shapes, perhaps from coalescence of regions of paracicatricial emphysema (*arrows*). Small peripheral lung nodules are also present in **B**. PLCH is a disease of unknown etiology that usually affects multiple organs. When the disease process is isolated to the lung, usually in adults, it is often referred to as *PLCH*. PLCH is more common in whites, and most of those affected are cigarette smokers. Indeed, a close temporal relationship between smoking cessation and radiologic improvement has been demonstrated.

HRCT scans can show a variety of patterns of disease in PLCH. Cysts, nodules, or cysts and nodules can be identified. Cysts are usually less than 10 mm in diameter. Nodules are usually less than 5 mm in diameter. Cysts may attain bizarre or unusual shapes (*large arrows*); the cysts are caused by paracicatricial emphysema. Like LAM, the interstitial patterns that appear on chest radiographs are actually innumerable overlapping lung cysts. Lung cysts have no central or peripheral distribution, but nodules may be seen in association with the central bronchovascular bundles of secondary lobules.

Pulmonary Langerhans cell histiocytosis *(continued)*

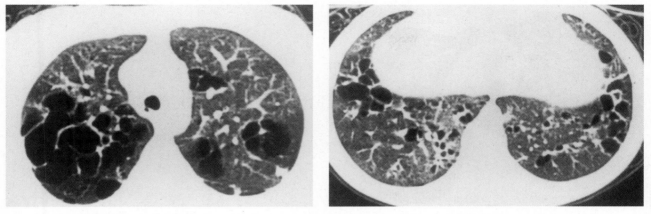

FIGURE 6-16 A,B: HRCT scans in a 10-year-old boy with PLCH show typical features, with apical coalescence of cystic lung disease. In addition, the patient had multiple organ system involvement with diabetes insipidus and a lytic sphenoid bone lesion.

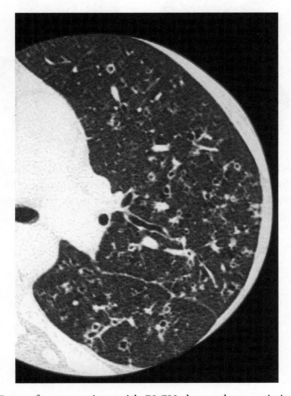

FIGURE 6-17 HRCT scan from a patient with PLCH shows characteristic findings that include a cystic infiltrative process with an upper lung predilection. The lung bases are characteristically spared. The cysts have a tendency to be less spheric and smooth walled than those seen in LAM.

In PLCH, HRCT scans can show a variety of patterns of disease, including lung cysts only, the combination of cysts and nodules, or predominately nodules.

Pulmonary Langerhans cell histiocytosis *(continued)*

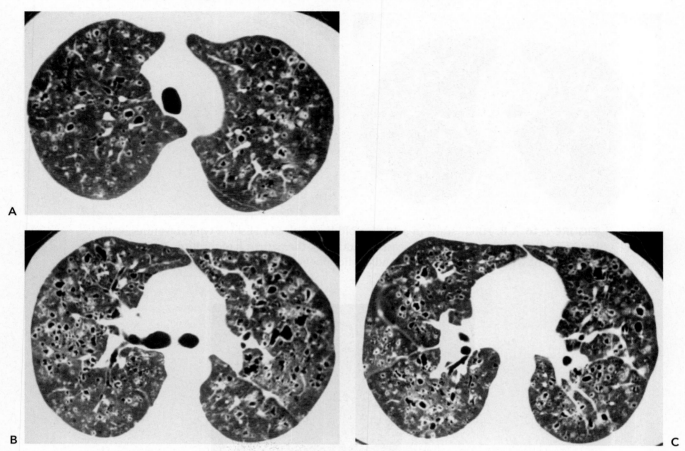

FIGURE 6-18 A–C: HRCT scans through the upper, mid, and lower lungs from this patient with PLCH show diffuse, mixed, small cysts and nodules throughout the lungs, typically without a central, peripheral, or bronchovascular distribution. In this somewhat atypical case, the abnormalities are more diffusely disseminated.

Pulmonary Langerhans cell histiocytosis *(continued)*

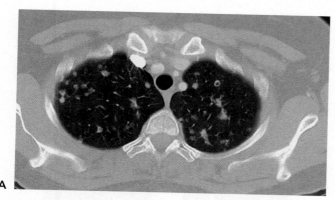

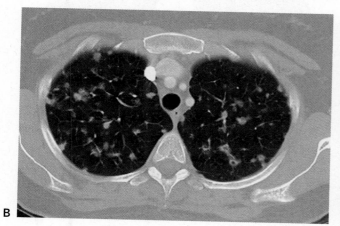

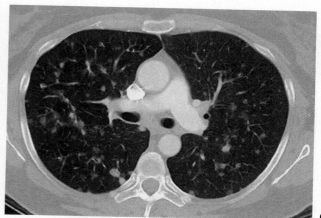

FIGURE 6-19 Characteristic findings of middle and upper lobe cysts often with nonspherical bizarre shapes and/or nodules with interstitial thickening are characteristic of this disease. High-resolution CT findings from this patient show a spectrum of well circumscribed and irregular solid nodules to cystic changes with a mid and upper-lung distribution. The cystic lesions are thought to be the result of paracicatricial emphysema and not cavitated nodules. Pulmonary LCH is a disorder in which histiocytes proliferate and accumulate within the lung, often resulting in scarring. The cause is unknown but occurs most commonly in patients who smoke cigarettes.

Pulmonary Langerhans cell histiocytosis *(continued)*

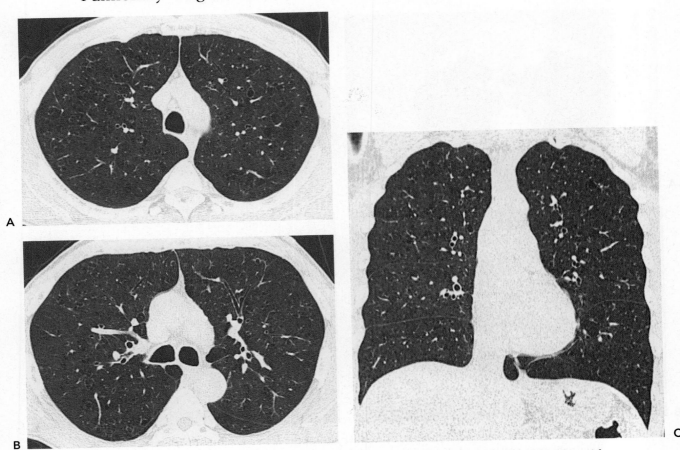

A

B

C

FIGURE 6-20 Transverse and coronal HRCT images show scattered thin wall cysts in the mid and upper lung zones. Several poorly defined nodules are also present. With disease progression, the cysts enlarge and can coalesce. The nodules can also enlarge and undergo central cavitation, developing into cysts. The hyperlucent foci without perceptible walls represent centrilobular emphysema.

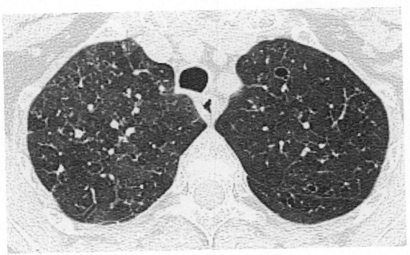

FIGURE 6-21 HRCT image through the upper lobes shows thin wall cysts in the left upper lobe and small nodules in both lungs. Patchy ground-glass opacity is also present in the right upper lobe. As PLCH occurs almost exclusively in smokers, findings of respiratory bronchiolitis such as poorly defined centrilobular nodules and patchy ground-glass opacity may also be present on HRCT.

Pulmonary Langerhans cell histiocytosis *(continued)*

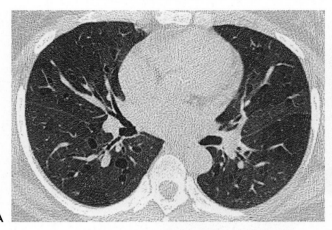 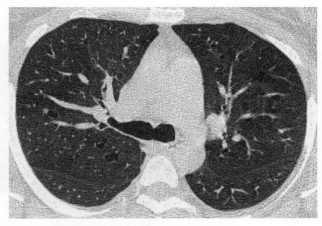

A   B

FIGURE 6-22 A–B: HRCT images through the mid lung zones show scattered thin wall cysts, some of which have irregular shapes. At the level of the carina are a few scattered small nodules. Larger hyperlucent regions in the lungs represent areas of air trapping, reflecting chronic small airways disease, presumably related to smoking.

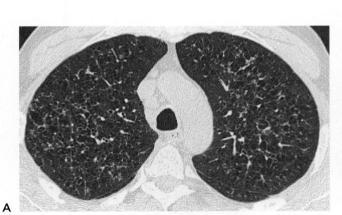 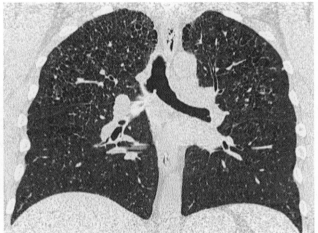

A   B

FIGURE 6-23 A–B: Transverse and coronal HRCT images show diffuse cysts predominantly in the upper lobes with sparing of the lung bases. Scattered small nodules are also present. Patients with PLCH can present with spontaneous pneumothorax when subpleural cysts rupture into the pleural space.

Pulmonary Langerhans cell histiocytosis *(continued)*

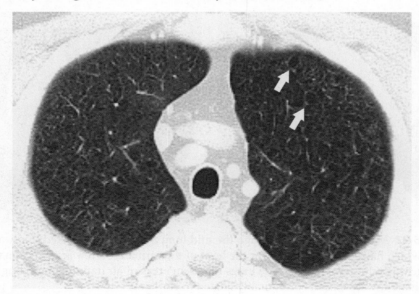

FIGURE 6-24 LCH 6—Transverse HRCT image shows innumerable cysts throughout both lungs (*arrows*). End-stage PLCH can be difficult to distinguish from severe emphysema. The cysts in PLCH usually have thin walls, whereas small emphysematous bullae usually lack perceptible walls.

Sjögren's syndrome

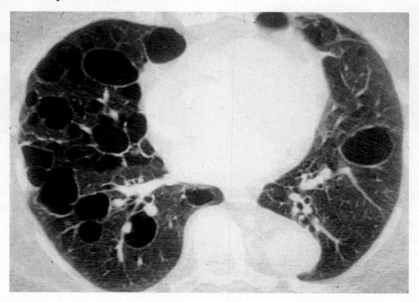

FIGURE 6-25 HRCT scan through the mid lungs from a patient with primary Sjögren's syndrome shows multiple, thin-walled cysts of varying sizes. The lung parenchyma between the cystic spaces is normal. This appearance is similar to that of lymphangiomyomatosis. Although the mechanism of cyst formation is unclear, a "ball-valve" mechanism is advocated because of the existence of a lymphocytic and plasma cell infiltration around bronchiolar walls.

Sjögren's syndrome *(continued)*

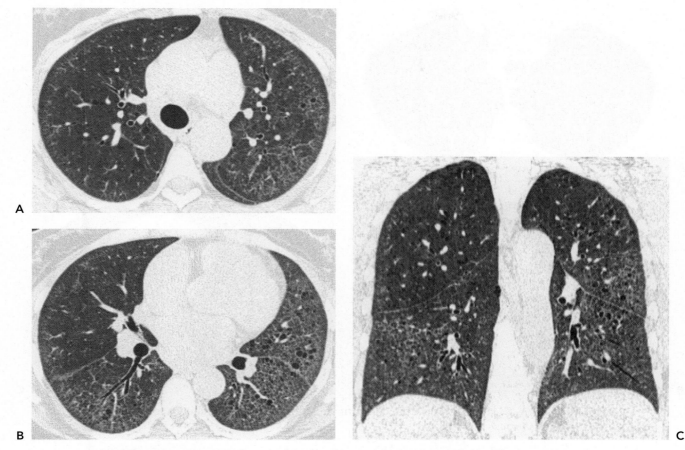

FIGURE 6-26 A–C: HRCT images from a patient with Sjögren syndrome show numerous small cysts with thin walls on a background of ground-glass opacity. The cysts have a slight basal predominance. Small nodules may also develop in lymphoid interstitial pneumonia (LIP)

Sjögren's syndrome *(continued)*

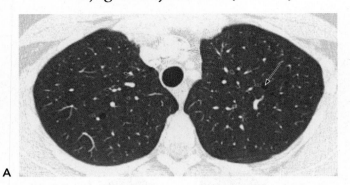

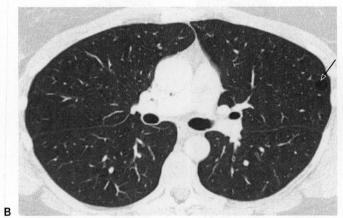

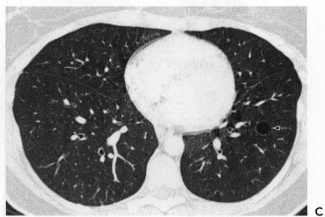

FIGURE 6-27 A–C: HRCT images from a patient with Sjögren syndrome show a few small thin wall cysts (*arrows*).

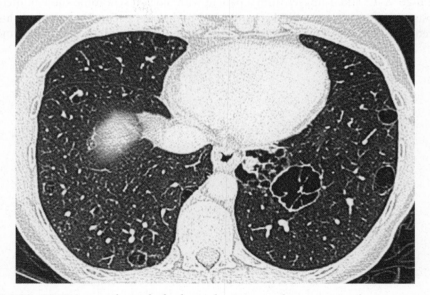

FIGURE 6-28 HRCT image through the lower lung zones shows scattered cysts, some of which have septations and vessels. The cysts in LIP usually have a basal predominance and are usually fewer in number and larger than those occurring in LAM and PLCH.

Sjögren's syndrome *(continued)*

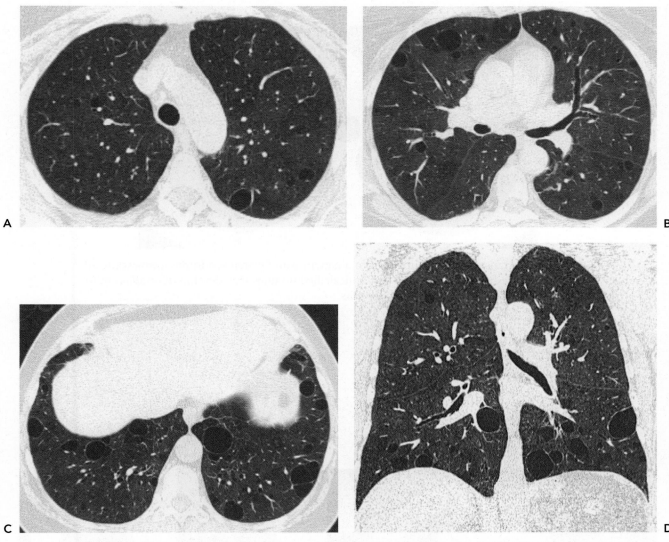

FIGURE 6-29 A–D: Transverse and coronal HRCT images from a patient with Sjögren syndrome demonstrate scattered cysts of varying sizes predominating in the lower lobes. Many cysts have vessels coursing along their walls, a feature not typical of the cysts of PLCH and LAM. The subpleural cysts can rupture and lead to spontaneous pneumothorax.

Sjögren's syndrome *(continued)*

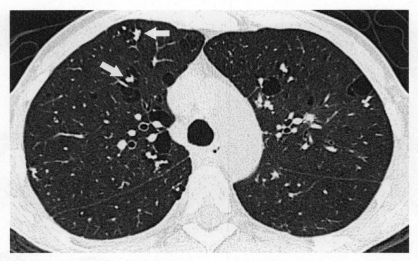

FIGURE 6-30 Transverse HRCT image from a patient with Sjögren syndrome shows scattered cysts and nodules (*arrows*). Calcified and noncalcified nodules may develop in or adjacent to the cysts in LIP, representing amyloid deposits.

Neurofibromatosis

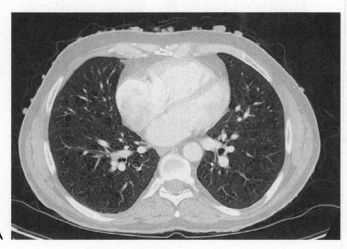

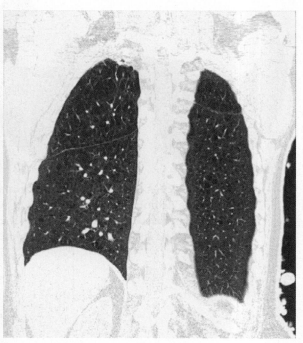

A   B

FIGURE 6-31 A,B: Transverse (**A**) and coronal (**B**) reformat CT scans from the chest from a nonsmoking patient with neurofibromatosis 1 and diffuse lung disease show innumerable lung cysts with an upper lobe predominance. Note the presence of innumerable neurofibromas on the chest wall. The presence of upper lobe predominant cysts and bulla distinct from typical centrilobular pulmonary emphysema is a reported clinical manifestation of neurofibromatosis.

Hydrocarbon Aspiration

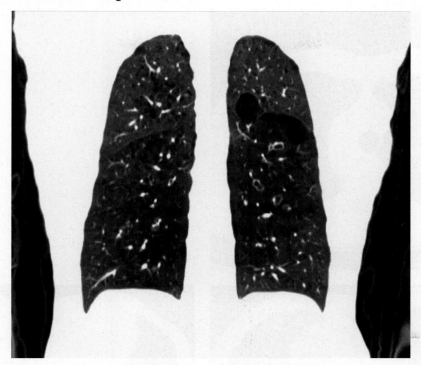

FIGURE 6-32 Coronal reformat CT scan through the posterior chest from an older patient who suffered hydrocarbon aspiration (petroleum distillate) 40 years earlier shows cystic changes in the superior segment of the left lower lobe and mild diffuse perihilar air trapping. Acute hydrocarbon aspiration, often an occupational hazard seen with fire-eaters, can result in necrotizing pneumonia and pneumatocele formation.

Pulmonary Placental Transmogrification

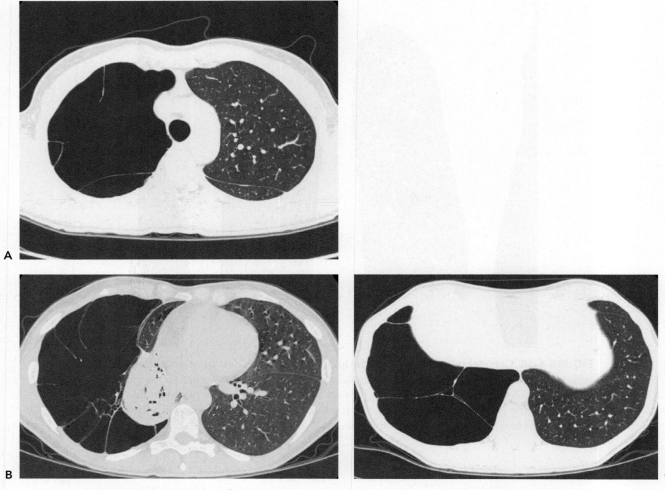

FIGURE 6-33 HRCT scan from an aysmptomatic, nonsmoking, 43-year-old woman with presumed pulmonary placental transmogrification shows near complete emphysematous/cystic destruction of the right lung. There is a right perihilar mass (in **B**) that is also described with this disorder. The left lung was entirely normal. Placental transmogrification of the lung is a very rare disorder that describes a peculiar histologic pattern characterized by formation of placental villous-like structures within the lung parenchyma that results in several appearances ranging from a solitary pulmonary nodule, small pulmonary cystic lesions, to striking bullous emphysema, as in this case. This disorder has been reported to be associated with fibrochondromatous hamartomas and pulmonary lipomatosis.

7

Obstructive Lung Diseases

Panlobular emphysema
Centrilobular emphysema
Centrilobular emphysema and the trachea
Distribution of centrilobular emphysema
Effects of patient position on appearance of centrilobular
  emphysema
Asymmetric emphysema
Fibrosis associated with emphysema
Paraseptal or distal lobular emphysema
Paraseptal emphysema—spectrum of severity
Giant bullous emphysema (vanishing lung syndrome)
Atypical bullous emphysema
Paracicatricial emphysema
Congenital lobar emphysema
Intralobar pulmonary sequestration

Panlobular emphysema

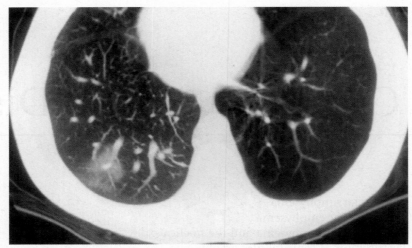

FIGURE 7-1

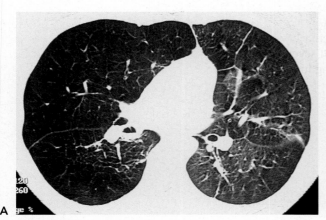

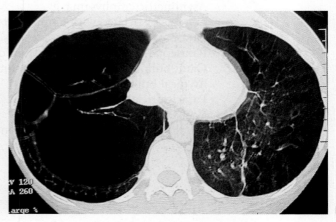

A

B

FIGURE 7-2

FIGURES 7-1 and 7-2 A,B: HRCT scans from two patients with alpha$_1$-antitrypsin (antitrypsin) deficiency. The patient in Figure 7-1, having undergone a right lung transplant, shows diffuse low attenuation lung parenchyma with a diminution of the vascular structures, typical of panlobular emphysema. Also note the large bulla formation in Figure 7-2**B** in the right lung that can occur with alpha$_1$-antitrypsin deficiency.

Panlobular emphysema characteristically has a lower lobe distribution, although it can occur anywhere in the lung. Panlobular emphysema is seen with alpha$_1$-antitrypsin (antitrypsin) deficiency and in obliterative bronchiolitis. In smokers, panlobular emphysema can be seen in conjunction with centrilobular emphysema, but it is not the dominant morphologic abnormality and is probably just advanced centrilobular emphysema. Panlobular emphysema may also be a normal senescent finding in nonsmokers.

Four different morphologic subtypes of emphysema have been described: (i) panlobular, (ii) centrilobular, (iii) paraseptal (also called *distal lobular*), and (iv) paracicatricial (irregular or scar). As the terms imply, emphysema within the secondary pulmonary lobule can be a diffuse lobular process, as in panlobular emphysema, and may be locally selective with proximal (centrilobular) or peripheral (distal lobular) lobular involvement.

Panlobular emphysema *(continued)*

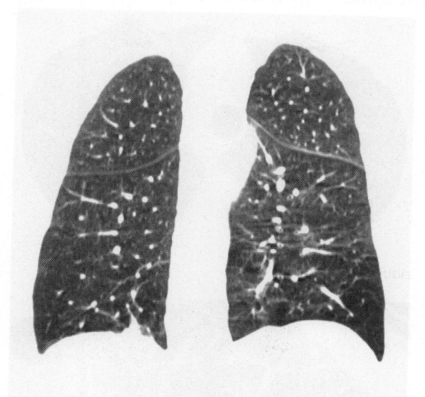

FIGURE 7-3 Coronal reformat CT scan through the posterior chest from a patient who abused intravenous methylphenidate (Ritalin) shows diffusely decreased lung attenuation throughout the parenchyma of the lower lungs, representing panlobular pulmonary emphysema. Intravenous injection of the crushed methylphenidate hydrochloride tablets can lead to this basilar predominant panlobular emphysema, identical to that seen in alpha-1-antitrypsin deficiency. It is believed that the nonsoluble particulate filter (often talc) becomes trapped within the pulmonary arterioles and capillaries when the drugs are crushed and injected. The particles then migrate through the vessel wall into the interstial tissue and lead to aggregations of multi-nucleated giant cells. The pathophysiology of the basilar predominant emphysema is unknown.

Centrilobular emphysema

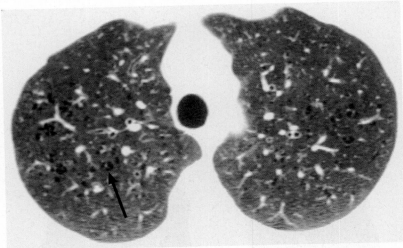

FIGURE 7-4

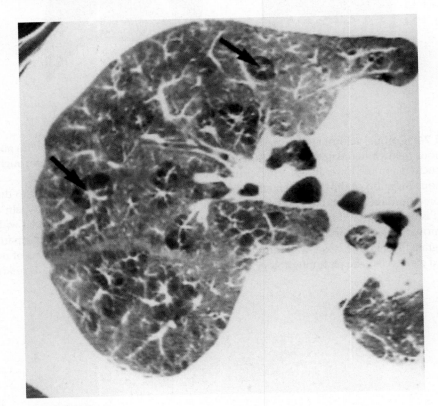

FIGURE 7-5

FIGURES 7-4, 7-5, 7-6, and 7-7 HRCT scans from four patients with centrilobular emphysema show multiple, focal, rounded lucencies of various size (generally ranging from 5 to 10 mm) surrounded by normal parenchyma, without discrete walls. Note that small, white dots in the center of these lucencies are the preserved centrilobular core structures (*arrows*). The appearance of a partial "wall" may be seen when an emphysematous space abuts a vessel, usually a vein. In these examples, note the milder extent and severity of disease in Figure 7-3 and the more diffuse disease in Figure 7-6, with extensive involvement of the right lower lobe.

The most common form of pulmonary emphysema is centrilobular emphysema. Strongly associated with cigarette smoking, centrilobular emphysema results from destruction of alveoli surrounding the proximal respiratory bronchiole. This disease has a predilection for the

(continued)

Centrilobular emphysema *(continued)*

FIGURES 7-4, 7-5, 7-6, and 7-7 *(continued)*
upper-lung zones, including the apical and posterior segments of the upper lobes and the superior segments of the lower lobes, although, when severe, can be quite diffuse.

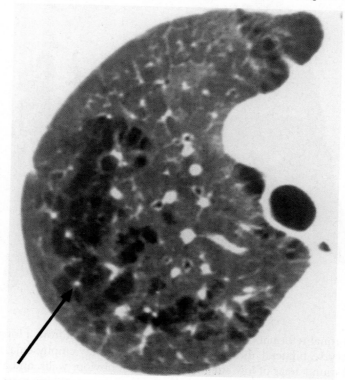

FIGURE 7-6

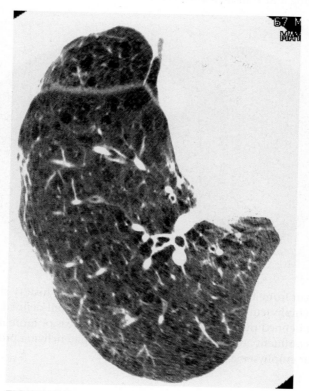

FIGURE 7-7

Centrilobular emphysema *(continued)*

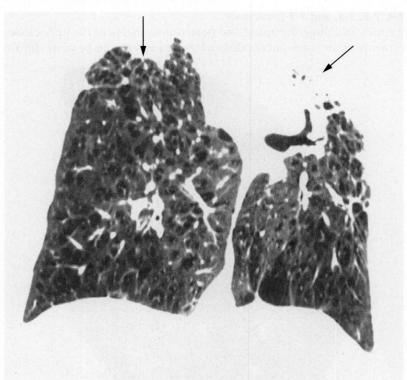

FIGURE 7-8 Coronal reformat CT scan through the anterior chest from a long-term cigarette smoker shows severe, bilateral, diffuse centrilobular pulmonary emphysema. Note the innumerable typical round areas of low attenuation, without obvious walls, and a white centrilobular core structure in the center. Also note the right apical lung mass and left upper lobe extensive scarring and volume loss *(arrows)*.

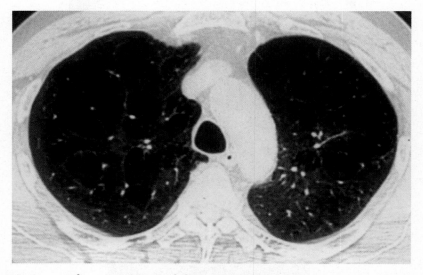

FIGURE 7-9 CT scan from a patient with long cigarette smoking history shows severe bilateral centrilobular emphysema in upper lobes. Note multiple, well-defined, confluent lucencies, most without defined margins, surrounded by patchy areas of more normal-appearing parenchyma. The confluent areas of low-attenuation lung parenchyma probably represent areas of panlobular emphysema, as well as centrilobular

(continued)

Centrilobular emphysema *(continued)*

FIGURE 7-9 *(continued)*

emphysema. When severe, centrilobular emphysema can involve the entire lobule and appear like panlobular emphysema; there is much more extensive lung destruction. However, pathologically, the dominant form of emphysema is centrilobular. When any emphysematous space is larger than 1 cm, it can be defined as a *bulla*.

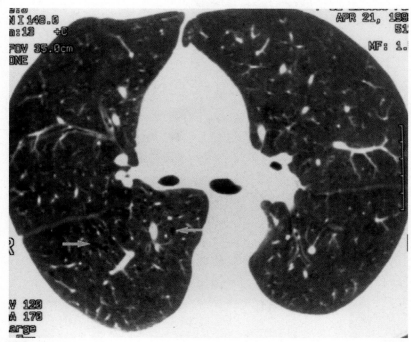

FIGURE 7-10

FIGURES 7-10, 7-11, and 7-12 HRCT scans through the mid lungs from three patients show centrilobular emphysema in the superior segments of the lower lobes (*arrows*). Centrilobular emphysema has a predilection for the upper portion of the individual lobes—that is, the apical and posterior segments of the upper lobes and the superior segments of the lower lobes.

(continued)

Centrilobular emphysema *(continued)*

FIGURES 7-10, 7-11, and 7-12 *(continued)*

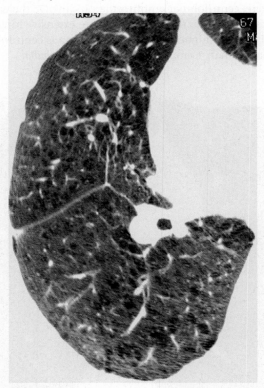

FIGURE 7-11

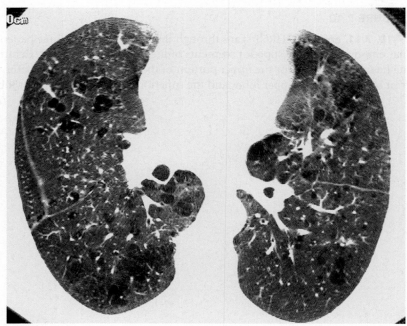

FIGURE 7-12

Centrilobular emphysema and the trachea

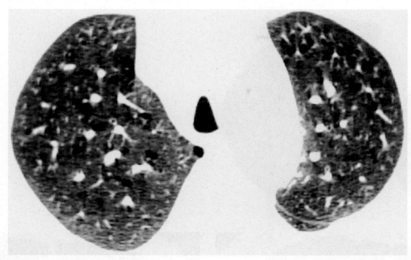

FIGURE 7-13

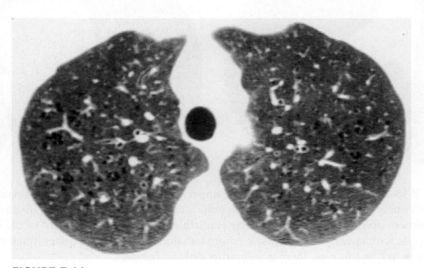

FIGURE 7-14

FIGURES 7-13 and 7-14 HRCT scans through the upper lungs from two patients with centrilobular emphysema show a saber-sheath tracheal deformity in Figure 7-13 but not in Figure 7-14.

The saber-sheath tracheal deformity is a radiologic finding for the diagnosis of chronic obstructive pulmonary disease, with a specificity of approximately 95% but with a low sensitivity (40% to 50%). This finding supports the hypothesis that the increase in volume of both lungs pressing on the mediastinum in patients with chronic obstructive pulmonary disease will exert a lateral pressure on the trachea, resulting in an increase in the antero-posterior and decrease in the transverse tracheal diameters.

Distribution of centrilobular emphysema

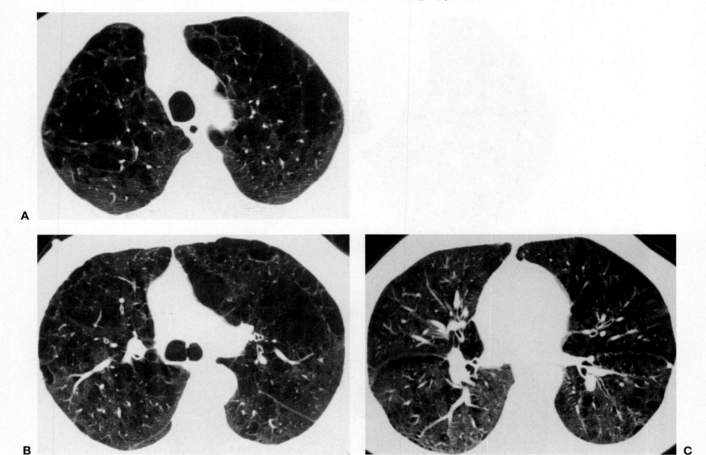

FIGURE 7-15 A–C: HRCT scans through the upper, mid, and lower lungs from a patient with moderately severe centrilobular emphysema show the typical upper-lung distribution of the emphysematous spaces. Note that there is much more severe involvement of the lung parenchyma, with larger, more extensive emphysematous spaces in the upper lungs than lower lungs. Yet, in this case, there is still rather diffuse disease.

Effects of patient position on appearance of centrilobular emphysema

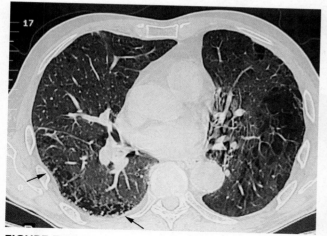
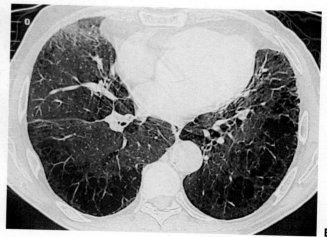

FIGURE 7-16

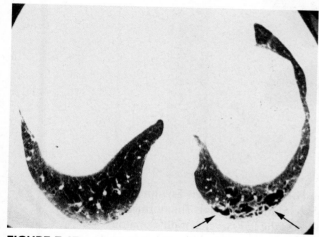
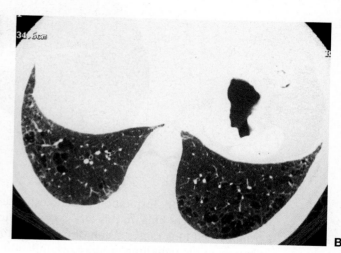

FIGURE 7-17

FIGURES 7-16 A,B and 7-17 A,B: Paired supine and prone HRCT scans through the lower lungs from two patients show the effects of patient position on the CT scan appearance of centrilobular emphysema. In both cases, the supine scans show thick-walled, distorted lucencies in the posterobasal peripheral lung that have an appearance suggestive of honeycomb lung fibrosis (*arrows*). On prone positioning, these areas of "fibrosis" are shown to be nothing more than emphysematous spaces that were distorted and collapsed in gravity-dependent areas of the lung.

Asymmetric emphysema

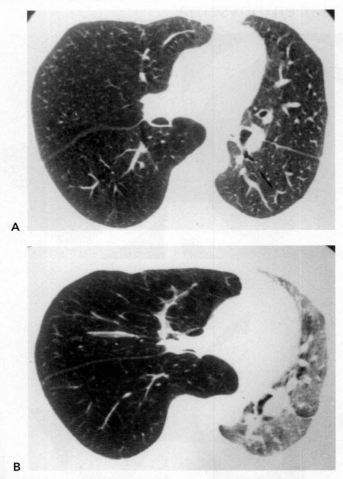

FIGURE 7-18 **A,B:** Inspiration **(A)** and expiration HRCT scans **(B)** show asymmetric emphysema of the right lung, in this case, secondary to a left lung transplant. The normal exit of air from the left lung causes a shift of the mediastinum to the left. Severe emphysematous changes in the right lung produce overinflation. The expiratory image reveals air trapping in the right lung. Note the mobility of the mediastinum as it swings to the left on expiration.

Fibrosis associated with emphysema

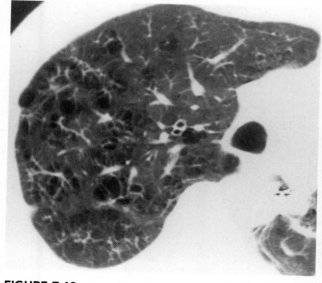
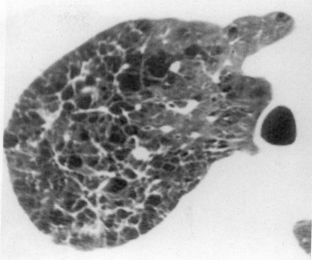

A

FIGURE 7-19

B

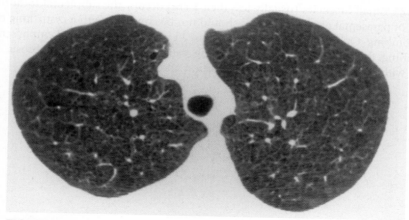

FIGURE 7-20

FIGURES 7-19 A,B and 7-20 HRCT scans from two patients who smoke cigarettes. The caudal regions of the right upper lobe (Fig. 7-19**A**) show areas of typical centrilobular pulmonary emphysema whose walls are characteristically undefinable. By contrast, in the more apical regions of the same lobe (Fig. 7-19**B**), the emphysematous spaces have discrete walls that are thicker than normal interlobular septa or other linear pulmonary structures. Similar but more subtle findings of fibrosis associated with centrilobular emphysema are noted in Figure 7-20. Because cigarette smoking causes inflammation at the terminal bronchiole and alveolar level, fibrosis can coexist with emphysema, although it may be difficult to detect on radiographic or even CT images. This appearance rarely could be confused with pulmonary Langerhans cell histiocytosis.

Paraseptal or distal lobular emphysema

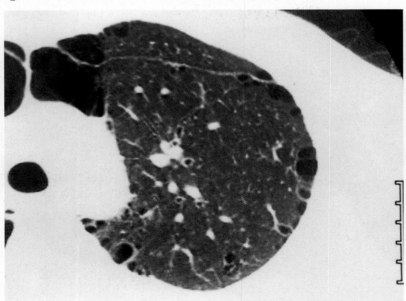

FIGURE 7-21 Small lucencies (usually less then 1 cm) occupy the subpleural location. These are typical of paraseptal emphysema and should not be confused with a cystic lung disease or honeycombing. On occasion, patients can be seen with both paraseptal emphysema and honeycombing. In such cases, the honeycombing, caused by end-stage lung fibrosis, is associated with much more architectural distortion and wall thickening.

Paraseptal emphysema—spectrum of severity

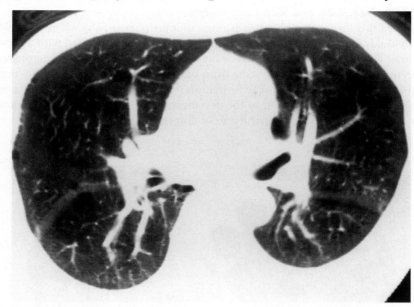

FIGURE 7-22

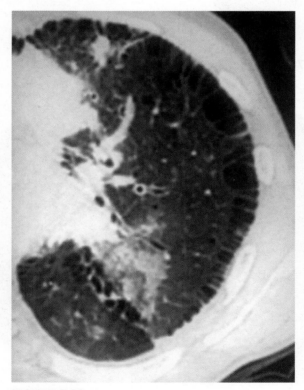

FIGURE 7-23

FIGURES 7-22, 7-23, 7-24, and 7-25 HRCT scans from four patients show the spectrum pulmonary involvement that may result from paraseptal emphysema, typically less than 1-cm peripheral lucencies, often with well-circumscribed borders. This form of emphysema may be focal or multifocal and has a predilection for the fissures and sharp pleural reflections, as along the azygous fissure in Figure 7-25 (*arrow*).

(continued)

Paraseptal emphysema—spectrum of severity *(continued)*

FIGURES 7-22, 7-23, 7-24, and 7-25 *(continued)*

The cause of this form of emphysema is often unknown, especially when it develops in young individuals who appear otherwise normal. It may be unassociated with airflow obstruction or chronic clinical symptoms or may coexist with centrilobular emphysema.

Coalescence of this type of emphysema from unknown influences is generally regarded as a mechanism of bullae and giant bullae formation (vanishing lung syndrome). Paraseptal emphysema appears to be important in the development of spontaneous pneumothoraces but is not associated with airflow obstruction or chronic clinical symptoms.

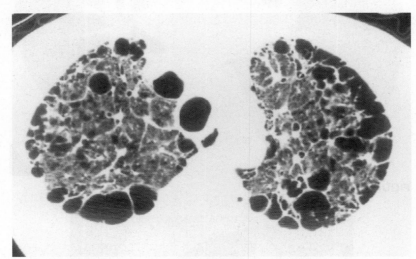

FIGURE 7-24

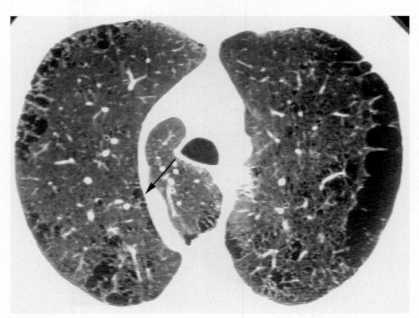

FIGURE 7-25

Paraseptal emphysema—spectrum of severity *(continued)*

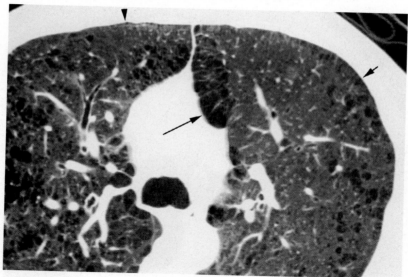

FIGURE 7-26

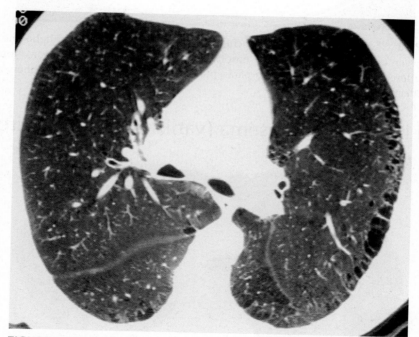

FIGURE 7-27

FIGURES 7-26 and 7-27 HRCT scans through the mid lung from two different patients show the spectrum of paraseptal emphysema that can be seen even within the same patient. In Figure 7-26, note the very small paraseptal spaces (*arrowhead*), the somewhat larger paraseptal spaces (*small arrow*), and the largest paraseptal spaces (*large arrow*). There is centrilobular pulmonary emphysema as well. In Figure 7-27, note the asymmetric involvement of the left lung.

Paraseptal emphysema—spectrum of severity *(continued)*

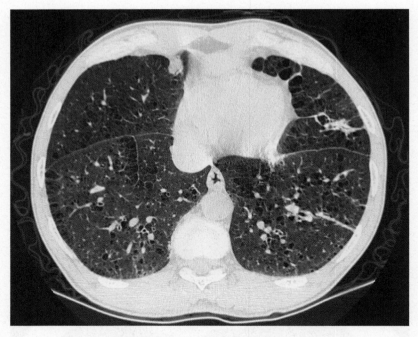

FIGURE 7-28 CT scan through the lower chest from a cigarette smoker highlights the differ-ences between centrilobular pulmonary emphysema and paraseptal emphysema. Note the distinct differences in distribution with paraseptal emphysema in the lung periphery and pleural reflections.

Giant bullous emphysema (vanishing lung syndrome)

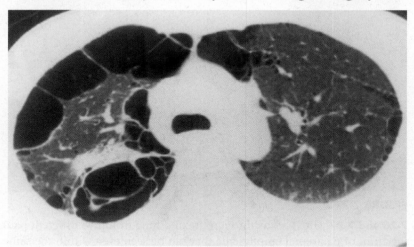

FIGURE 7-29

FIGURES 7-29 and 7-30 A,B: HRCT scans from two patients show extensive lung destruction with multiple, large, peripheral bullae occupying the hemithoraces. Note the marked asymmetry. In Figure 7-29, the more normal-appearing lung shows paraseptal emphysema in the left lung, whereas in Figure 7-30, there is associated mild intraparenchymal centrilobular emphysema, an-teromedially in right lung. These findings are typical of idiopathic giant bullous emphysema,

(continued)

Giant bullous emphysema (vanishing lung syndrome) *(continued)*

FIGURES 7-29 and 7-30 A,B *(continued)*

also called *vanishing lung syndrome*. This is a severe, precocious, giant bullous emphysema in the upper lungs, often asymmetric, in cigarette-smoking, young, dyspneic men. The syndrome can be seen, however, in nonsmokers. The dominant and consistent HRCT feature in both smokers and nonsmokers is that of extensive paraseptal emphysema coalescing into the giant bullae.

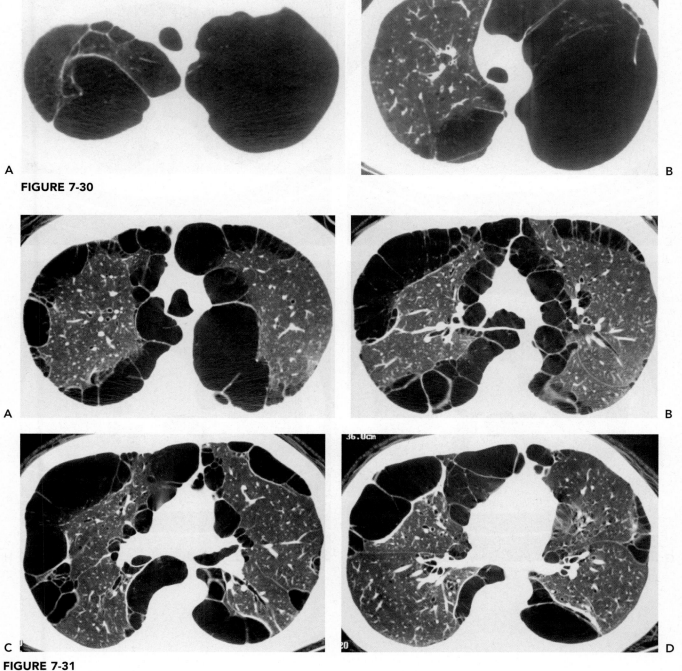

FIGURE 7-30

FIGURE 7-31

FIGURE 7-31 A–H: HRCT scans in Figure 7-31, obtained at four levels (A–D) through the upper and lower lungs in this patient with vanishing lung syndrome, shows the asymmetric distribution of the giant bulla throughout the periphery of the lungs, again with no underlying

(continued)

Giant bullous emphysema (vanishing lung syndrome) *(continued)*

FIGURE 7-31 A–H *(continued)*
centrilobular emphysema. Repeat HRCT 5 years later (**E–H**), shown here at the same
anatomic levels as **A–D**, shows progression of disease, with increased size of the giant bulla.

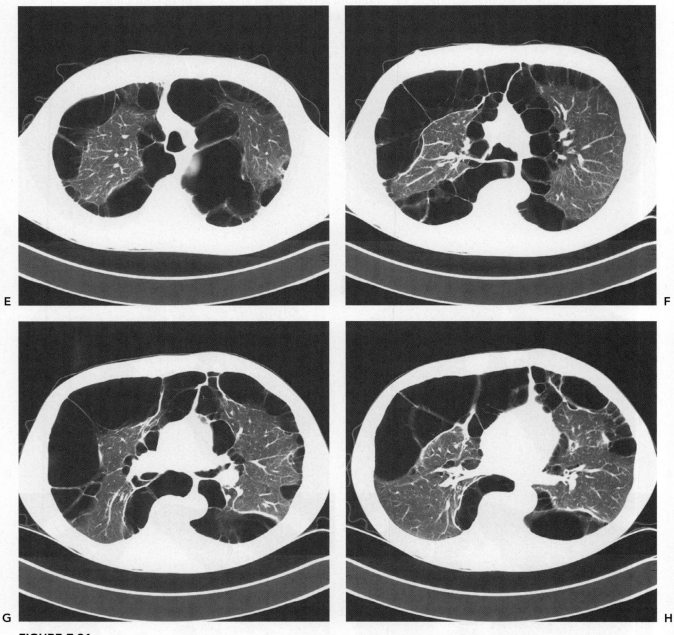

FIGURE 7-31

Giant bullous emphysema (vanishing lung syndrome) *(continued)*

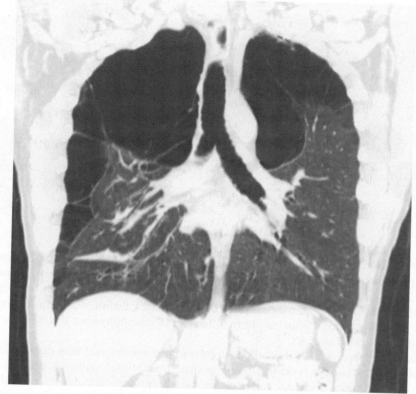

FIGURE 7-32 Coronal reformat CT scanned through the midchest from a patient with vanishing lung syndrome shows bilateral giant bulla in the upper lobes.

Atypical bullous emphysema

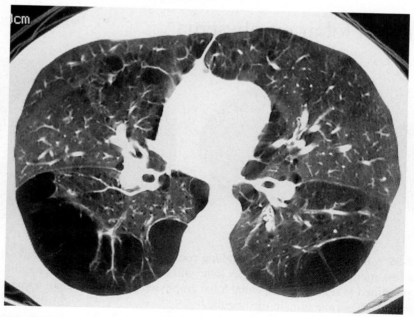

FIGURE 7-33 HRCT scan from a patient with bullous emphysema show a distinctly unusual posterior distribution. These are likely enlarged paraseptal emphysematous spaces, similar to that seen in patients with giant bullous emphysema. The cause for this peculiar distribution of bullae is unknown.

Paracicatricial emphysema *(continued)*

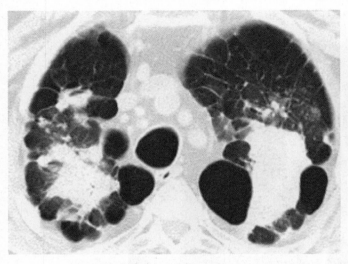
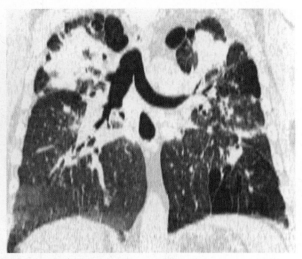

A   B

FIGURE 7-34 Transverse **(A)** and coronal **(B)** HRCT images from a patient with complicated silicosis (progressive massive fibrosis) show multiple large subpleural bullae adjacent to the masslike foci of fibrotic tissue. As the small silicotic nodules coalesce to form large opacities, paracicatricial emphysema often develops in the periphery, a feature that helps distinguish progressive massive fibrosis from carcinoma. Paracicatricial emphysema can be quite severe in cases of complicated silicosis.

Paracicatricial emphysema (also called *irregular* or *scar emphysema*) may develop in any part of the lung and usually is quite variable in size. In addition to silicosis, other causes of paracicatricial emphysema include tuberculosis, radiation injury, sarcoidosis, and other postinflammatory conditions. It is always associated with adjacent fibrosis that may be focal (e.g., apical scarring of old granulomatous disease) or diffuse (progressive massive fibrosis due to silicosis). However, the emphysematous changes usually are of no functional or clinical significance; the "cystic" changes seen in pulmonary Langerhans cell histiocytosis (PLCH) are also caused by paracicatricial emphysema.

Congenital lobar emphysema

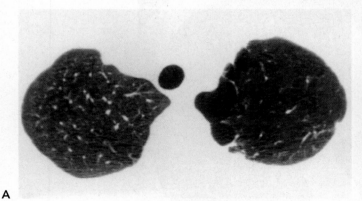
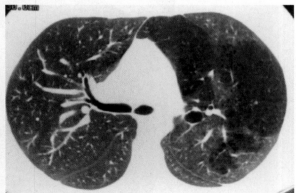

A   B

FIGURE 7-35 **A,B:** HRCT scan of a nonsmoking young adult shows multiple, well-demarcated regions of low attenuation in the left upper lobe with minimal bullous change at the apex. This was presumed to represent congenital lobar emphysema. Note the sharp transition from emphysematous to normal lung in the lingula.

Intralobar pulmonary sequestration

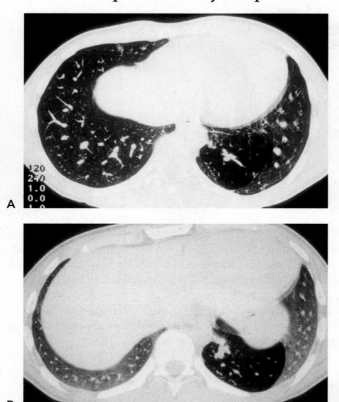

FIGURE 7-36 A: CT scan obtained at suspended full inspiration from a 28-year-old man complaining of left lower chest pain, mild dyspnea, and low fever shows a hyperlucent focal area in the left lower lobe, outlined by normal lung. **B:** HRCT obtained at suspended end expiration at the same level as in **A** shows air trapping within the abnormal lung. Adjacent to the descending thoracic aorta, a subtle tubular structure representing an anomalous aortic vessel was demonstrated (not shown). These findings are typical for an intralobar sequestration.

Pulmonary sequestration is defined as a segment of lung tissue that is separate from the tracheobronchial tree and receives its blood supply from a systemic artery. The vascular supply is from the thoracic aorta in 80% to 90% of cases, coursing within the inferior pulmonary ligament. Origin of the vascular supply from beneath the diaphragm is not rare.

Intralobar sequestrations account for 75% of cases of sequestration and affect the posterior basal segment of the left lung in 60% of cases. The radiographic appearance depends on the degree of aeration and the presence of infection. The lack of communication of the sequestered lung with the normal tracheobronchial tree is associated with a continued accumulation of secretions accompanied by acute inflammation and infection.

CT and magnetic resonance image scanning are useful in noninvasive evaluation of pulmonary sequestration. Systemic arterial supply is an essential feature of pulmonary sequestration and differentiates it from other focal lesions with similar characteristics. The vascular supply is usually well demonstrated by CT or magnetic resonance imaging. Venous drainage is via the inferior pulmonary vein to the left atrium.

Intralobar pulmonary sequestration *(continued)*

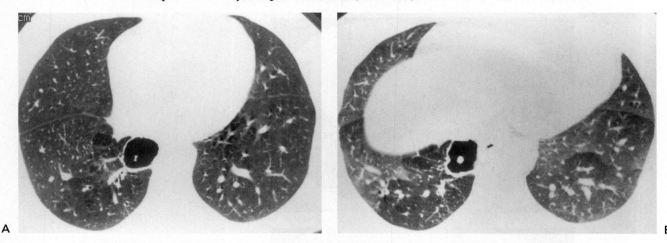

A   B

FIGURE 7-37 A,B: Inspiration and expiration HRCT scans show a nonsegmental area in the right lower lobe containing multiple cysts and low-attenuation parenchyma typical for an intralobar sequestration. The lucency of the surrounding lung is a particular characteristic of intralobar sequestrations.

Intralobar bronchopulmonary sequestration lacks normal communications with the tracheobronchial tree; however, they can be ventilated by collateral air drift or through fistulous bronchial communications, as suggested by the air trapping at expiration HRCT.

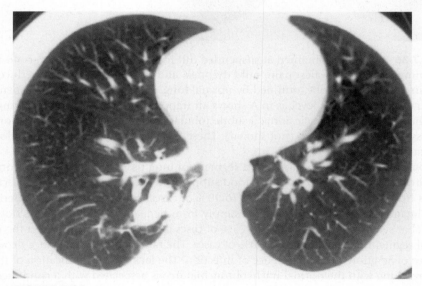

FIGURE 7-38

FIGURES 7-38, 7-39, and 7-40 HRCT scans from three different patients each show a multicystic mass centered in the posterior basal segment of the right lower lobe. The location and appearance are typical of intralobar sequestration, a congenital malformation consisting of nonfunctioning, abnormal lung tissue contained within otherwise normal lung tissue.

A bronchopulmonary sequestration is a congenital anomaly in which a portion of lung develops abnormally and without normal or direct continuity to the tracheobronchial tree. Such sequestered regions of lung always receive systemic arterial supply, often from

(continued)

Intralobar pulmonary sequestration *(continued)*

FIGURES 7-38, 7-39, and 7-40 *(continued)*

anomalous vessels that arise below the diaphragm. Sequestrations are further classified as *intralobar* or *extralobar* types: Intralobar sequestrations drain to the pulmonary venous system, do not have a separate pleural investment, are usually aerated, and present in childhood or adulthood. Extralobar sequestrations drain systemically, have a separate pleural investment, are not aerated and, therefore, are more masslike, and often present during infancy. Sequestrations are most often identified in the left lower lobe adjacent to the diaphragm.

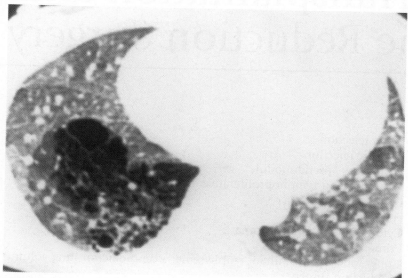

FIGURE 7-39

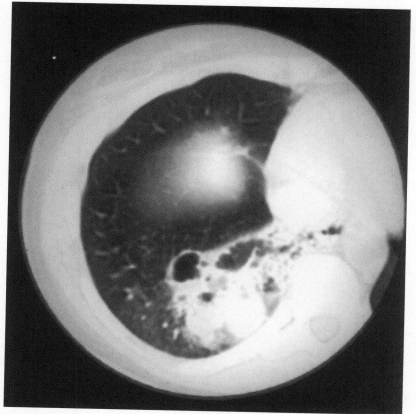

FIGURE 7-40

8

Lung Transplantation and Lung Volume Reduction Surgery

Acute rejection

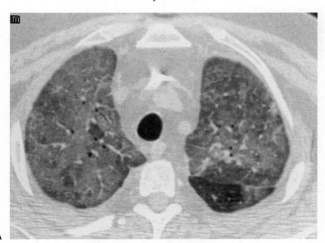 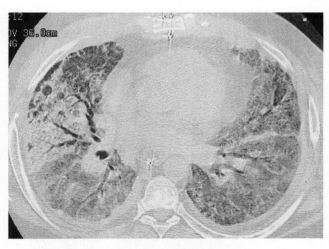

A   B

FIGURE 8-1 A: HRCT scan, 3 weeks after bilateral lung transplantation and now with severe acute rejection, shows diffuse ground-glass opacification. The extensive nature of the ground-glass opacification on CT scanning correlates histologically with a higher grade of acute rejection. HRCT is 65% sensitive and 85% specific in making the diagnosis of acute rejection in the lung transplant population. The only significant HRCT finding in acute rejection is ground-glass opacification, which is patchy and localized in mild rejection and widespread in severe rejection. **B:** HRCT scan 1 month later, when the patient developed cryptogenic organizing pneumonia and diffuse alveolar damage, shows bilateral areas of consolidation and ground-glass opacification and dilatated airways. Patients with severe acute rejection can recover completely or develop severe graft dysfunction, cryptogenic organizing pneumonia, or adult respiratory distress syndrome.

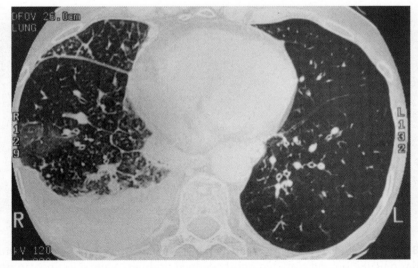

FIGURE 8-2 HRCT scan from a patient with a right lung transplant and acute rejection shows right pleural effusion, scattered areas of ground-glass opacification, and interlobular septal thickening. These findings, without a concomitant increase in cardiac size or vascular pedicle width or evidence of vascular redistribution, have been shown to correlate with acute rejection when seen on chest radiographs.

Acute rejection *(continued)*

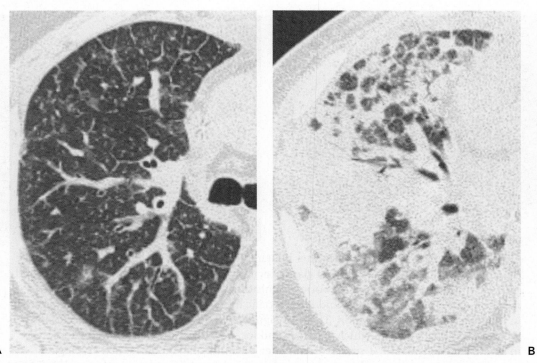

A   B

FIGURE 8-3 A: HRCT image of the right lung at the level of the carina shows diffuse interlobular septal thickening, patchy ground-glass opacity, and a few scattered poorly defined nodules. **B:** HRCT image through the right lung base demonstrates extensive consolidation with sparing of some secondary pulmonary lobules.

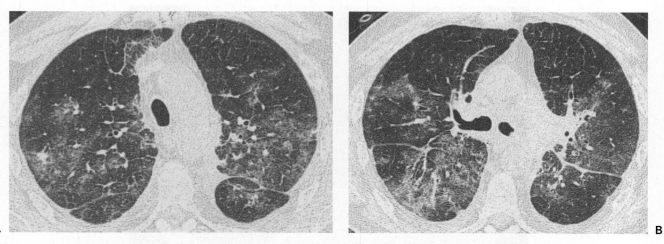

A   B

FIGURE 8-4 A–D: HRCT image shows patchy peribronchial ground-glass opacity with intralobular reticulation and scattered poorly defined nodules. Acute rejection can mimic infection such as viral pneumonia.

(continued)

Acute rejection *(continued)*

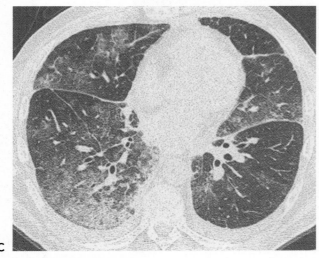
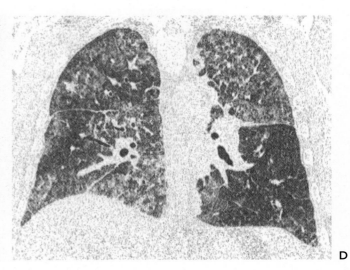

FIGURE 8-4 *(continued)*

Chronic rejection

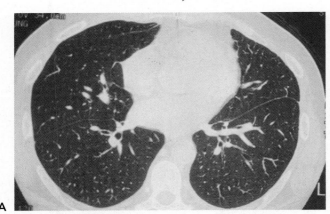
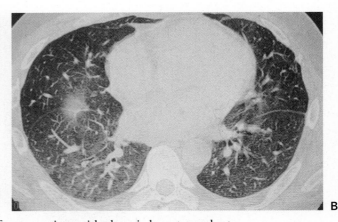

FIGURE 8-5 A: HRCT scan during inspiration from a patient with chronic lung transplant rejection shows normal-appearing bilateral lung transplants. **B:** HRCT scan during expiration shows bilateral areas of abnormal lucency, representing air trapping from obliterative bronchiolitis (OB). OB is the major long-term complication after lung transplantation, occurring in more than 50% of transplant recipients. The pathologic lesions of OB are widely presumed to be a manifestation of chronic rejection. Air trapping, as detected on expiratory HRCT, is the most sensitive and accurate radiologic indicator of OB in the lung transplant patient.

Chronic rejection *(continued)*

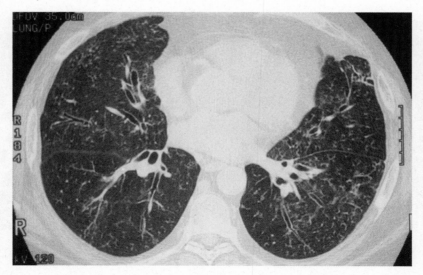

FIGURE 8-6 HRCT scan from a patient with bilateral lung transplants and severe chronic rejection shows dilatated bronchi and bronchioles and small, linear, nodular branching opacities in a bronchiolar distribution. On HRCT, bronchiectasis is a frequent, although often late, finding in lung transplant recipients with OB.

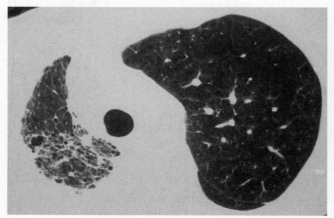
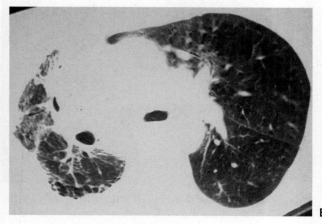

A   B

FIGURE 8-7 A-B: HRCT scans from a patient with a single right lung transplant for pulmonary emphysema show a sequelae of severe chronic rejection with extensive lung fibrosis and bronchiectasis. Note the marked shift of the mediastinum to the right secondary to the right lung volume loss and the hyperinflation of the native emphysematous lung.

Chronic rejection *(continued)*

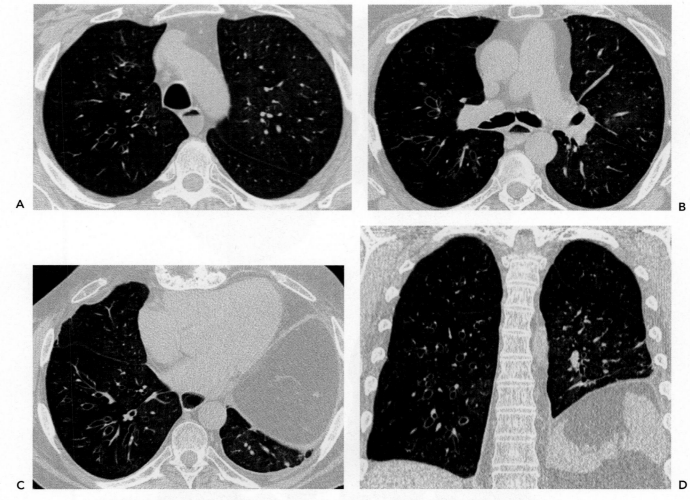

FIGURE 8-8 A–D: Transverse and coronal CT images show diffuse central cylindrical bronchiectasis with a mosaic pattern of attenuation. Hypolucent areas of lung reflect underlying air trapping. Chronic rejection in lung transplant manifests as OB, which results in progressive airflow obstruction. Bronchiectasis is usually a late finding. Infection and chronic rejection are the leading causes of graft failure, and the mean graft survival is approximately 5 years.

Chronic rejection *(continued)*

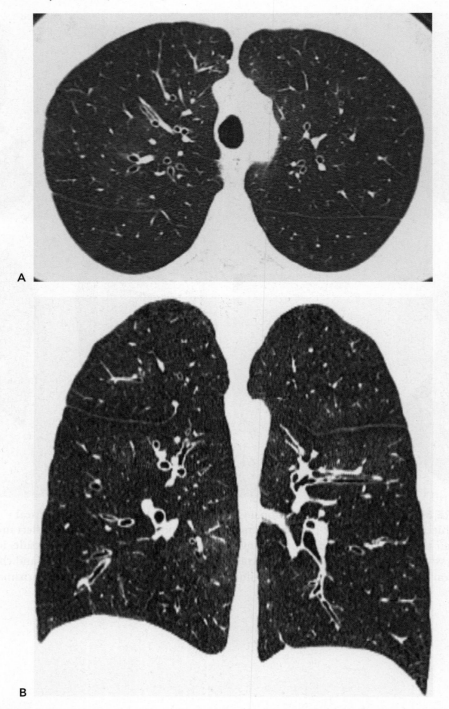

FIGURE 8-9 A-B: Transverse and coronal CT images show pulmonary hyperinflation with marked decreased attenuation of the lung parenchyma. Foci of apparent ground-glass opacity represent regions of normal ventilation and perfusion.

Chronic rejection *(continued)*

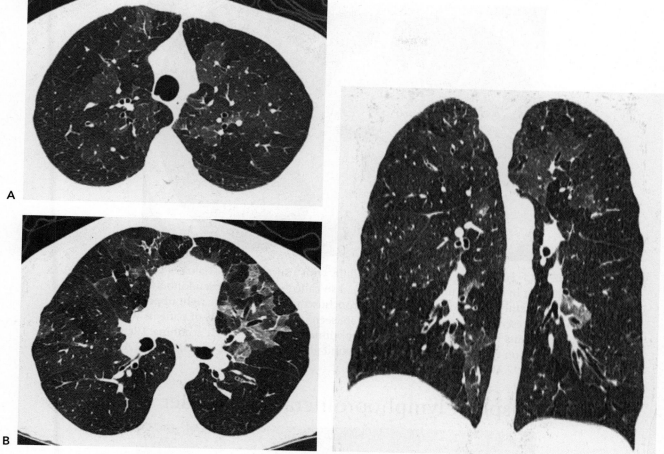

FIGURE 8-10 A–C: Transverse and coronal CT images show a striking mosaic pattern of attenuation. Hyperlucent areas represent localized air trapping as a manifestation of chronic rejection. Ground-glass areas represent localized hyperperfusion as the lungs shunt blood to areas of adequate ventilation.

Postbiopsy "pseudonodule"

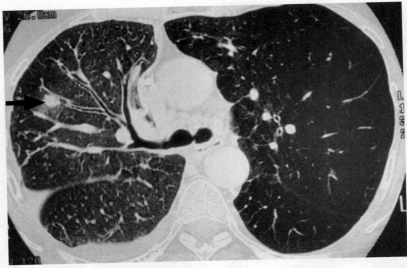

FIGURE 8-11 HRCT scan shows a small nodule, with a surrounding "halo" of ground-glass opacification in the right upper lobe (*arrow*), a so-called postbiopsy pseudonodule. The patient had recently undergone surveillance bronchoscopic biopsy of the right upper lobe. Nodules representing biopsy-related injury are seen in as many as 30% of patients with lung transplants who have undergone biopsy within a few weeks of CT scanning. (Reprinted with permission from Collins J, Stern EJ. Ground-glass opacity at CT: the ABCs. *AJR Am J Roentgenol* 1997;169:355–367.)

Posttransplant lymphoproliferative disorder

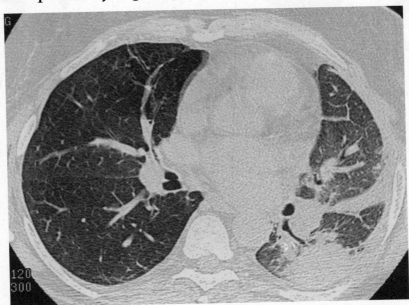

FIGURE 8-12 HRCT scan from a patient with a left lung transplant shows a mass in the left lower lobe and left pleural effusion. Left lung volume is small relative to the right native emphysematous lung. Most cases of posttransplant lymphoproliferative disorder (PTLD), including this case, are associated with Epstein-Barr virus (EBV) infection. EBV-associated lymphoproliferative disease can range from benign lymphoid hyperplasia to high-grade lymphoma. The most common CT scan findings are multiple nodules, frequently in a predominantly peribronchovascular or subpleural distribution.

Posttransplant lymphoproliferative disorder *(continued)*

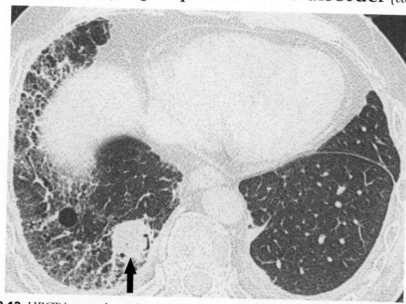

FIGURE 8-13 HRCT image shows large nodule (*arrow*) in the lower lobe of the fibrotic native lung. Transthoracic needle biopsy revealed PTLD. PTLD can range from polyclonal lymphocyte proliferation to high-grade lymphoma. It occurs in 5% to 20% of lung transplant recipients and is the result of EBV infection or reactivation, usually in patients treated with cyclosporin. Lung transplant recipients who are EBV-antibody seronegative at the time of transplant are at much greater risk of developing PTLD than those infected before transplant. PTLD most commonly develops in the second month after transplant and rarely after 1 year.

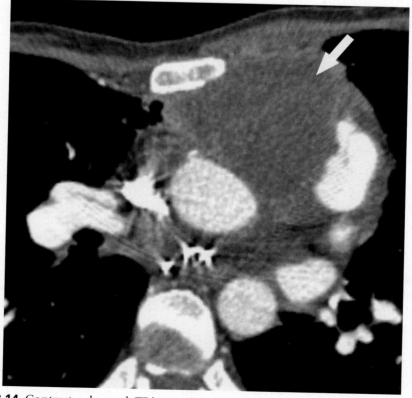

FIGURE 8-14 Contrast-enhanced CT image (mediastinal window settings) shows large infiltrating mediastinal mass (*arrow*) in a double lung transplant recipient. Transthoracic core needle biopsy showed high-grade B-cell lymphoma, which was attributed to PTLD.

Bacterial pneumonia

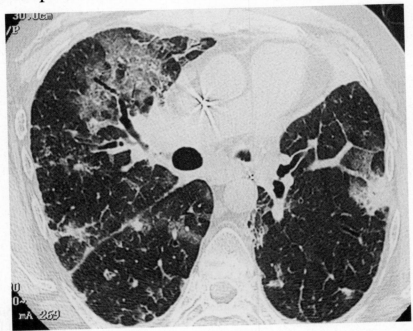

FIGURE 8-15 HRCT scan from a patient with bilateral lung transplants and *Staphylococcus aureus* pneumonia shows scattered areas of consolidation, ground-glass opacification, and bronchial dilatation.

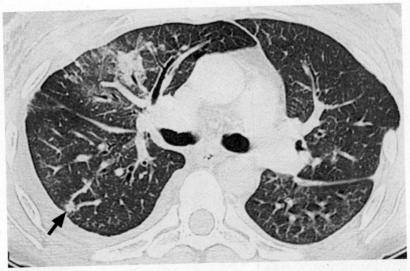

FIGURE 8-16 HRCT scan from a patient with bilateral lung transplants and *Pseudomonas* pneumonia shows an irregular nodule in the right lower lobe (*arrow*), patchy consolidation in the right upper lobe with surrounding ground-glass opacification, and interlobular septal thickening.

Bacterial pneumonia *(continued)*

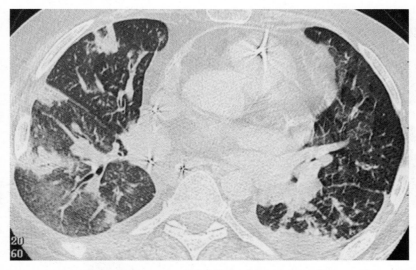

FIGURE 8-17 HRCT scan from a patient with bilateral lung transplants and *Pseudomonas* pneumonia shows bilateral areas of consolidation in a subpleural and bronchovascular distribution and ground-glass opacification. Although the incidence of bacterial pneumonia is highest in the first month after transplantation, bacterial pneumonia continues to be a major infectious complication throughout the transplant recipient's life. Bacterial pneumonia is usually caused by *S. aureus*, Enterobacteriaceae, *Pseudomonas aeruginosa*, or other gram-negative organisms. Although bacterial infections are more common, they are less fatal than viral and fungal infections. Nodules, consolidation, ground-glass opacification, and septal thickening are all common manifestations of bacterial infection on CT scanning of lung transplant recipients, occurring in 52%, 74%, 83%, and 61% of patients, respectively.

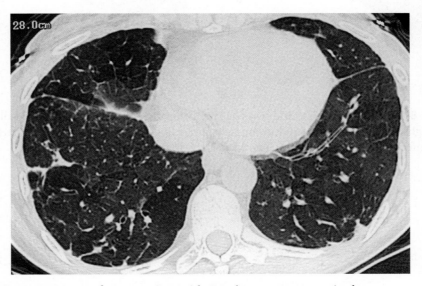

FIGURE 8-18 HRCT scan from a patient with *Pseudomonas* pneumonia shows peribronchovascular thickening, subtle ground-glass opacification, septal thickening, dilatated bronchioles, and small subpleural opacities. These findings were new compared with prior CT scan and resolved on follow-up CT scan after antibiotic treatment. This case illustrates the importance of not attributing new bronchiolar dilatation to OB when the patient has other new, potentially reversible, parenchymal abnormalities.

Bacterial pneumonia *(continued)*

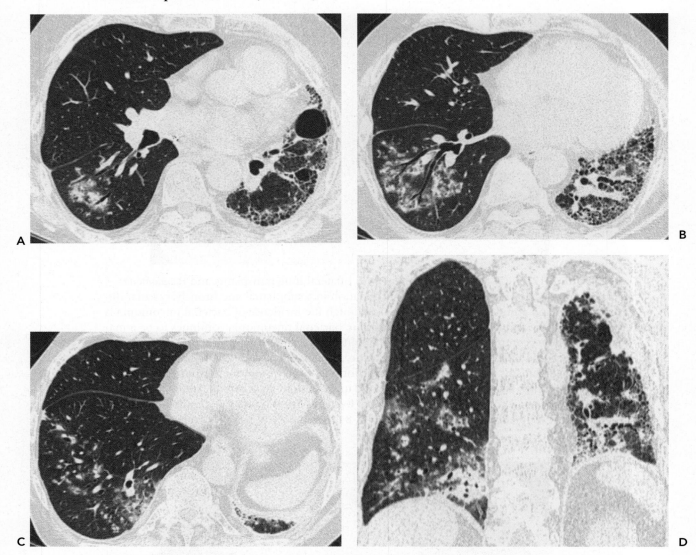

FIGURE 8-19 A–D: Transverse and coronal HRCT images show peribronchial consolidation, ground-glass opacity, and nodules in the right lung allograft secondary to mycobacterium avium infection. The native left lung is extensively fibrotic.

Fungal pneumonia

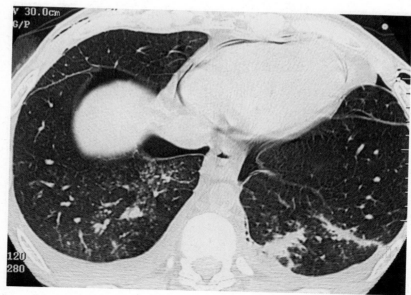

FIGURE 8-20 HRCT scan from a patient with *Aspergillus* pneumonia shows patchy areas of consolidation and the "tree-in-bud" pattern of bronchiolar impaction. The pneumothoraces were related to the bilateral transplant surgery. The nonspecific tree-in-bud pattern can be seen in viral, bacterial, and fungal infections.

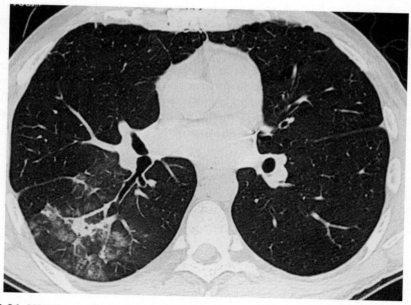

FIGURE 8-21 HRCT scan from a patient with *Aspergillus* pneumonia shows areas of consolidation and ground-glass opacification in the right lower lobe in this patient with bilateral lung transplants.

Fungal pneumonia *(continued)*

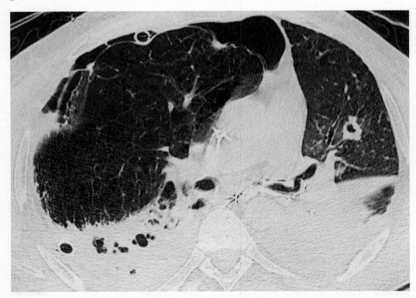

FIGURE 8-22 HRCT scan from a patient with *Aspergillus* pneumonia shows bilateral pleural effusions, consolidation at the lung bases, and a small cavitary nodule in the left upper lobe. The patient has a left lung transplant and severe emphysema of the native right lung. There is a chest tube on the right for a persistent pneumothorax. The rounded lucencies at the right lung base are thought to be caused by underlying emphysema and not lung necrosis.

Fungal pneumonias, usually caused by *Aspergillus*, are less common than cytomegalovirus or bacterial pneumonia after transplantation but are associated with a higher mortality. Infection with *Aspergillus* occurs most commonly 2 to 6 months after transplantation. Locally invasive or disseminated *Aspergillus* infection accounts for 2% to 33% of post–lung transplant infections and 4% to 7% of all lung transplant deaths. The total number of *Aspergillus* infections does not differ between patients with and without cystic fibrosis, and the isolation of *Aspergillus* from the respiratory tract occurs in 30% to 50% of patients in both groups. Nodules, consolidation, and ground-glass opacification are common findings on CT scanning of lung transplant recipients, occurring in 90%, 60%, and 90%, respectively, of lung transplant recipients with fungal pneumonia.

Fungal pneumonia *(continued)*

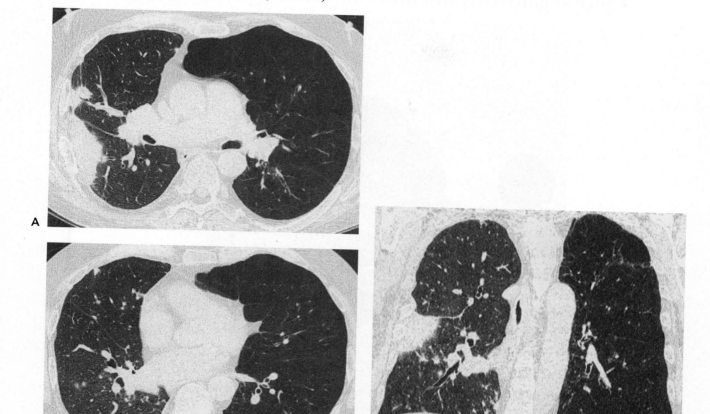

FIGURE 8-23 A–C: Transverse and coronal HRCT images show subpleural consolidation and scattered small nodules in the right lung allograft, due to histoplasmosis infection.

Cytomegalovirus pneumonia

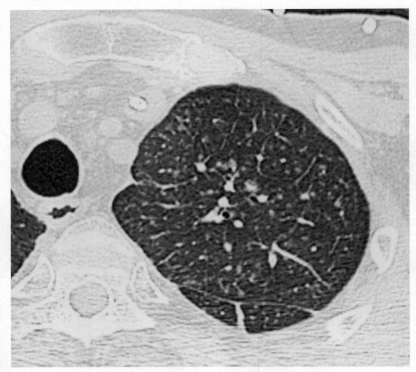

FIGURE 8-24 HRCT scan from a patient with cytomegalovirus pneumonia shows multiple 1- to 2-mm nodules randomly scattered throughout the left lung transplant and interlobular septal thickening.

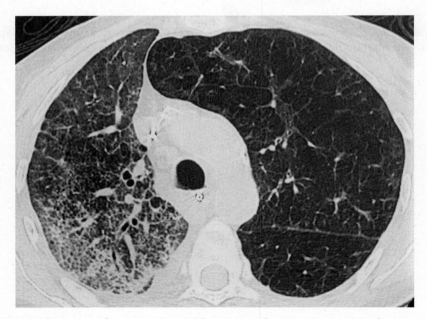

FIGURE 8-25 HRCT scan from a patient with cytomegalovirus pneumonia shows extensive interlobular septal thickening, ground-glass opacification, and bronchiolar dilatation of the right transplant lung. The left native lung is emphysematous.

Cytomegalovirus pneumonia *(continued)*

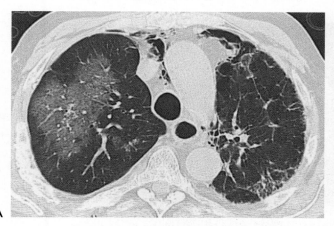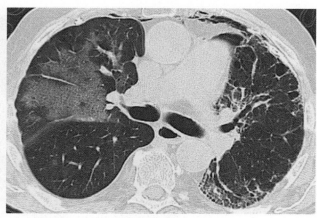

A   B

FIGURE 8-26 A-B: HRCT images through the right lung allograft show relatively confluent ground-glass opacity with superimposed tiny discrete nodules. There is considerable overlap of HRCT findings in immunocompromised patients with various viral pneumonias and include ground-glass opacity, consolidation, tiny nodules, and septal thickening.

Cytomegalovirus (CMV) is the most commonly diagnosed viral infection in patients with lung transplants. Acute and chronic allograft rejection is managed with increasing the dose of immunosuppressive drugs, which increases susceptibility to cytomegalovirus infection. The viral infection creates a state of immune activation, increasing the risk of rejection. The cycle generates significant diagnostic and management dilemmas. Cytomegalovirus infection most commonly develops between 1 and 4 months after transplantation, and it varies from asymptomatic infection to fulminant pneumonia. Nodules, consolidation, and ground-glass opacification are common findings on CT scanning of lung transplant recipients with cytomegalovirus infection, occurring in 53%, 63%, and 74% of cases, respectively.

Pneumonia is the most common thoracic infection in lung transplant recipients, and *Pseudomonas*, cytomegalovirus, and *Aspergillus* are the most common single responsible agents. Nodules, consolidation, ground-glass opacification, septal thickening, and pleural effusion are common CT scan findings of bacterial, viral, and fungal infections. However, when these findings are seen on CT scanning of a patient after lung transplant surgery, they are not helpful in making a specific infectious diagnosis.

CT scan abnormalities in patients with a single lung transplant and pneumonia involve predominantly the transplanted lung. This does not help distinguish infection from rejection or lymphoproliferative disease, both of which also tend to involve predominantly the transplant lung.

Primary lung carcinoma

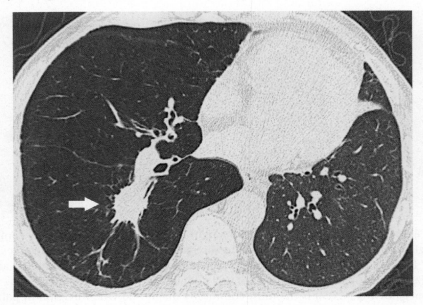

FIGURE 8-27 HRCT image shows a large spiculated nodule (*arrow*) in the lower lobe of the emphysematous native right lung. Lung transplant recipients, particularly those with smoking-related or fibrotic lung disease, are at increased risk of developing primary lung carcinoma because of underlying predisposition in addition to chronic immunosuppression.

Upper lobe—predominant emphysema: a candidate for lung volume reduction surgery

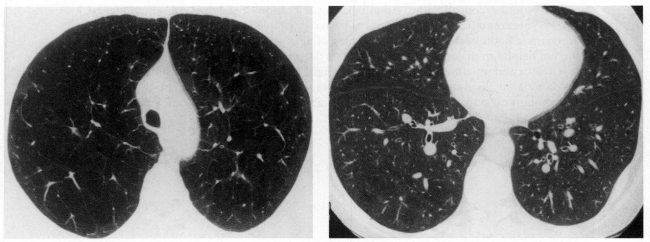

FIGURE 8-28 HRCT scans through the upper (**A**) and lower (**B**) portions of the lungs from a candidate for lung volume reduction surgery show low-attenuation lung parenchyma with thinning of pulmonary blood vessels that is more severe in the upper lungs than the lower lungs.

(continued)

Upper lobe—predominant emphysema: a candidate for lung volume reduction surgery *(continued)*

FIGURE 8-28 *(continued)*
The target areas with the most severe lung destruction are at the lung apices. This patient may undergo lung volume reduction surgery through the preferred approach of a median sternotomy for access to the target areas for resection. Patients with areas of preserved lung parenchyma and targets of relatively focal upper lobe–predominant emphysema or lower lobe–predominant emphysema have better clinical outcomes after lung volume reduction surgery.

Lower lobe—predominant emphysema: a candidate for lung volume reduction surgery with severe panlobular emphysema

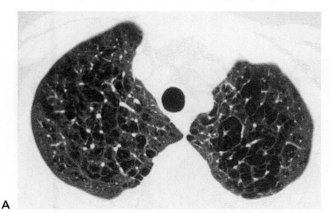

A

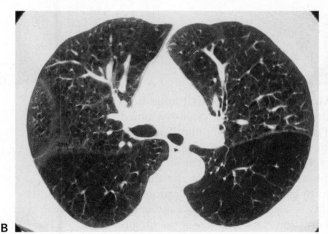

B

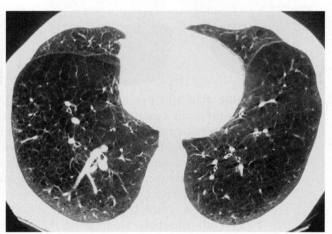

C

FIGURE 8-29 HRCT scans through the upper **(A)**, mid **(B)**, and lower **(C)** lungs from a patient who is a candidate for lung volume reduction surgery show extensive lung destruction with low-attenuation lung parenchyma and marked thinning of pulmonary vessels that is more severe at the lung bases than the lung apices. This patient with severe lower lobe–predominant panlobular emphysema secondary to alpha$_1$-antitrypsin deficiency has areas of relatively preserved lung parenchyma at the lung apices.

The target areas with the most severe lung destruction are at the lung bases. This patient may undergo lung volume reduction surgery through the preferred approach of bilateral thoracotomies or bilateral video-assisted thoracoscopy, rather than median sternotomy, to have better access to the target areas for resection. Patients without any preserved lung parenchyma or no targets of relatively focal upper lobe–predominant emphysema or lower lobe–predominant emphysema have poorer clinical outcomes after lung volume reduction surgery. With extensive emphysema, there is also a greater risk of operative or perioperative mortality.

Diffuse severe centrilobular emphysema

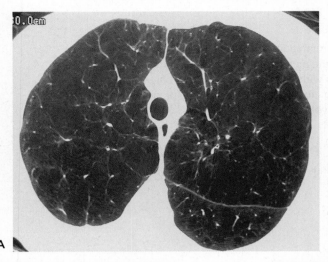

A

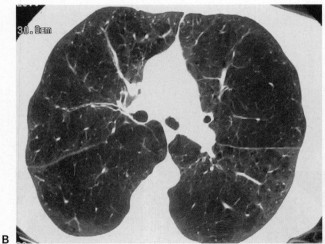

B

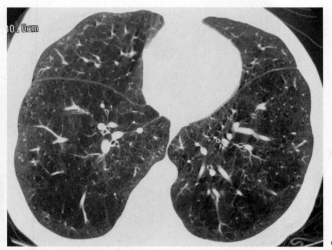

C

FIGURE 8-30 HRCT scans through the upper **(A)**, mid **(B)**, and lower **(C)** lungs from a patient who is not a candidate for lung volume reduction surgery show extensive lung destruction with low-attenuation lung parenchyma and marked thinning of pulmonary vessels extending almost uniformly from the lung apices to the lung bases. Although diffuse and uniform low attenuation is more characteristic of alpha$_1$-antiprotease deficiency–related panlobular emphysema, when centrilobular emphysema becomes severe, the abnormality may involve the lung in a more diffuse and uniform pattern. The only indication that the emphysema is centrilobular is that the abnormality is slightly less extensive at the lung bases. With panlobular emphysema, the lung destruction is more severe at the lung bases. Using CT attenuation–based densitometry, 60% of this patient's lung parenchyma fell below an attenuation value of –950 Hounsfield units on HRCT. This attenuation threshold has been demonstrated to be the optimum threshold to use on thin-section CT for quantification of emphysema severity.

Patients without any preserved lung parenchyma, without targets of relatively focal upper lobe–predominant emphysema, or with lower lobe–predominant emphysema have poorer clinical outcomes after lung volume reduction surgery. With extensive emphysema, there is also a greater risk of operative or perioperative mortality.

Noncandidate for lung volume reduction surgery with severe fixed airflow obstruction

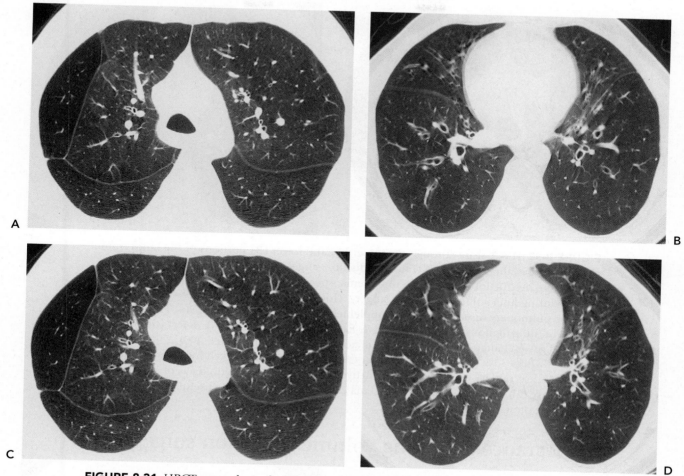

FIGURE 8-31 HRCT scans through the upper and lower portions of the lungs obtained during inspiration **(A,B)** and expiration **(C,D)** from a patient who is not a candidate for lung volume reduction surgery show extensive and diffuse low-attenuation lung parenchyma. In addition, there is moderate cylindrical bronchiectasis. On expiration, there is very little, if any, change in lung attenuation caused by severe fixed airflow obstruction. Unlike patients with emphysema, the blood vessels are not thinned or distorted in their branching pattern.

Chronic obstructive pulmonary disease includes asthma, chronic bronchitis, and emphysema. Asthma is classically characterized by airway obstruction and wheezing that are reversible with bronchodilators. Chronic bronchitis is characterized by excessive sputum production, whereas emphysema is characterized by fixed airflow obstruction. All are characterized by shortness of breath. In many patients, these clinical features overlap. For example, patients with emphysema may have a lesser component of reactive airway disease. However, when asthma is long-standing, the initially reversible airflow obstruction may become fixed. This may make it difficult to distinguish emphysema using pulmonary function testing. This non–cigarette-smoking patient had a nearly 50-year history of asthma since childhood, which gradually became fixed. Pulmonary function testing demonstrated a very severe obstructive ventilatory defect with air trapping and impaired gas exchange [1-second forced expiratory volume (FEV_1), 22% predicted; forced vital capacity (FVC), 49% predicted; FEV_1/FVC, 44% predicted; diffusing capacity of the lung (Dlco), 56% predicted]. There was no reversibility of the obstruction after the administration of a bronchodilator. In this patient, the lack of change in lung attenuation on expiratory HRCT supports the fixed nature of the airflow obstruction, and the lack of architectural distortion of the pulmonary vasculature confirms that this is not emphysema. The lack of emphysema makes this patient ineligible for lung volume reduction surgery.

Noncandidate for lung volume reduction surgery with severe fixed airflow obstruction *(continued)*

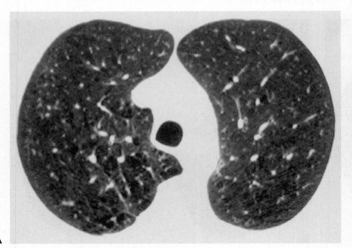
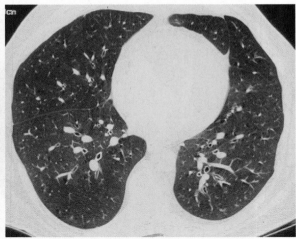

A

B

FIGURE 8-32 HRCT scans through the upper **(A)** and lower **(B)** portions of the lungs from a patient being evaluated for lung volume reduction surgery show no focal areas of low-attenuation lung destruction to indicate emphysema; specifically, there are no target areas for resection during lung volume reduction surgery. This patient had a long history of chronic obstructive pulmonary disease requiring supplemental oxygen for the past years. Pulmonary function testing demonstrated a very severe, fixed obstructive ventilatory defect with impaired gas exchange (FEV$_1$, 13% of predicted; FVC, 26% of predicted; FEV$_1$/FVC, 36% of predicted; Dlco, 35% of predicted). Further evaluation revealed marked hypercarbia (Pco$_2$ = 67 mm Hg) secondary to untreated obstructive sleep apnea. Other etiologies of obstructive lung disease can be confused for emphysema clinically. HRCT may be useful to confirm or exclude the presence of emphysema.

Appearance after lung volume reduction surgery

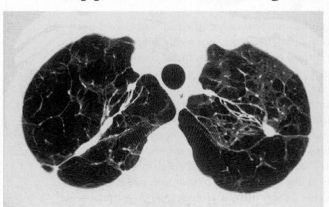
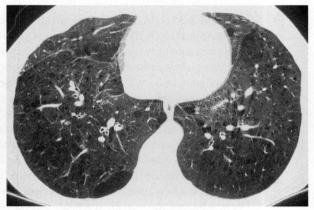

A

B

FIGURE 8-33 HRCT scans through the upper **(A)** and lower **(B)** portions of the lungs from a patient who had undergone bilateral upper lobe lung volume reduction surgery through a median sternotomy 1 year earlier show staple lines at the lung apex. Note that moderately severe upper lobe–predominant emphysema remains, with relative sparing of the lung bases. Lung volume reduction surgery is not a cure for emphysema but improves shortness of breath, exercise tolerance, and pulmonary function in patients with severe emphysema that is refractory to medical management.

Appearance after lung volume reduction surgery *(continued)*

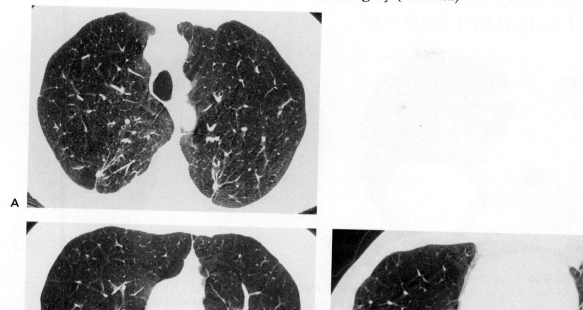

FIGURE 8-34 HRCT scans through the upper **(A)**, middle **(B)**, and lower **(C)** portions of the lungs from a patient who had undergone bilateral lung volume reduction surgery show staple lines, in cross section, in a subpleural location at the lung apices **(A)**, whereas in the superior segments of the lower lobes, particularly on the left side, the staple line is seen within the axial plane of the HRCT image. When seen in cross section on a single image, the appearance mimics a spiculated nodule *(arrow)*. Note that small bronchi and pulmonary vessels are pulled toward the staple line. In this patient, staple lines are also noted in the basilar segments of the lower lobes **(C)**. On the right side, the staple line is along the major fissure. Severe diffuse emphysema remains.

Appearance after lung volume reduction surgery and lung transplantation

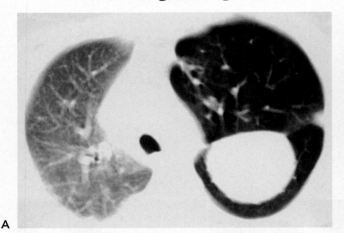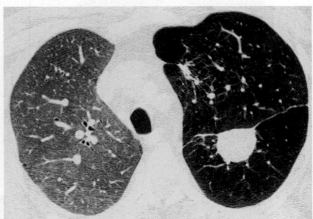

A   B

FIGURE 8-35 CT scans through the upper thorax 3 days after right lung transplantation **(A)** and left lung volume reduction surgery and HRCT image 4 months later **(B)** show a large, loculated fluid collection in the left major fissure representing a postoperative hemothorax. Complications after lung volume reduction surgery are largely related to air leaks across the pleural surface with persistent pneumothoraces that may be loculated. Hemothorax is less commonly encountered. Note the normal attenuation of the transplanted right lung 4 months after surgery compared with the diffuse low attenuation of the native left lung after lung volume reduction surgery. In this patient, hyperinflation of the left lung at the time of transplantation was believed to compromise the function of the lung allograft, and the decision was made to reduce the size of the left lung to reduce the volume of the left lung and thereby decrease the severity of mediastinal shift toward the right side.

9

Diffuse Lung Diseases

Usual interstitial pneumonia
Lower lung zones
Advanced pulmonary fibrosis
Nonspecific interstitial pneumonia
Rheumatoid interstitial lung disease/Nonspecific interstitial pneumonia
Mixed connective tissue disease/Nonspecific interstitial pneumonia
Dermatomyositis/Nonspecific interstitial pneumonia
Scleroderma/Nonspecific interstitial pneumonia
Spontaneous pneumomediastinum in IPF
Unusual manifestation of pulmonary fibrosis
Desquamative interstitial pneumonia
Respiratory bronchiolitis–associated interstitial lung disease
Acute interstitial pneumonia
Acute respiratory distress syndrome—acute/subacute phase
Acute respiratory distress syndrome—pulmonary fibrosis
Bone marrow transplant recipient with graft-versus-host disease
Cryptogenic organizing pneumonia
Bronchioloalveolar cell carcinoma in scleroderma
Hard metal pneumoconiosis
Primary systemic amyloidosis
Cyclophosphamide (Cytoxan) drug toxicity
Amiodarone toxicity
Pulmonary drug toxicity
Acute eosinophilic pneumonia
Chronic eosinophilic pneumonia
Plumonary lymphangiomatosis
Sarcoidosis
Lofgren's syndrome
End-stage sarcoidosis
Sarcoidosis and air trapping
Berylliosis
Silicosis
Alveolar microlithiasis
Metastatic calcification
Lymphangitic carcinomatosis
Erdheim-Chester disease
Idiopathic pulmonary hemosiderosis

Usual interstitial pneumonia

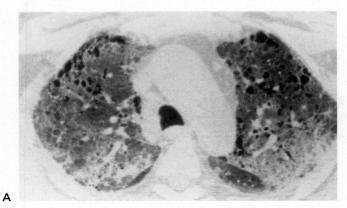

A

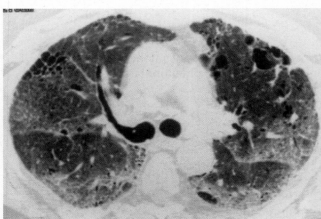

B

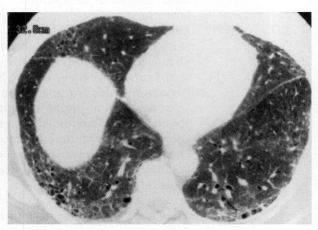

C

FIGURE 9-1

FIGURES 9-1 A–C and 9-2 HRCT scans from two patients with typical usual interstitial pneumonia (UIP) show the characteristic findings of a reticular infiltrative process, architectural distortion, and honeycombing in a peripheral distribution. It is important to evaluate for architectural distortion as a sign of chronicity and fibrosis. UIP usually is more profuse in the bases. In later stages of UIP, there are cicatricial changes that may result in traction bronchiectasis and bronchiolectasis. By HRCT, this pattern should be called UIP; idiopathic pulmonary fibrosis (IPF) is a clinical diagnosis. The HRCT pattern of UIP is nonspecific and is seen in patients with IPF, asbestosis, and many connective tissue diseases involving the lung especially rheumatoid arthritis.

(continued)

Usual interstitial pneumonia *(continued)*

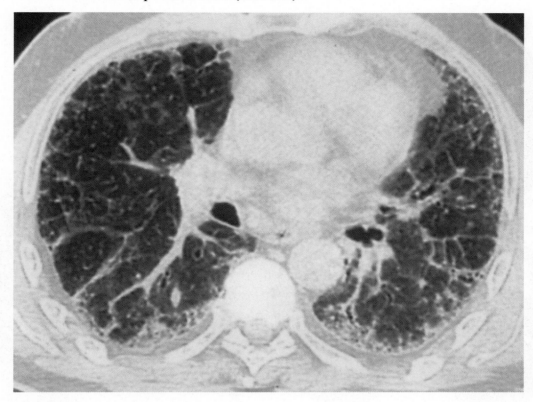

FIGURE 9-2

FIGURES 9-1 A–C and 9-2 *(continued)*

Usual interstitial pneumonia *(continued)*

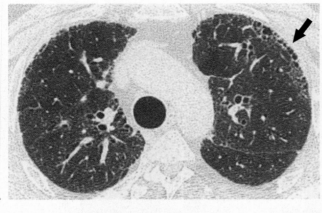

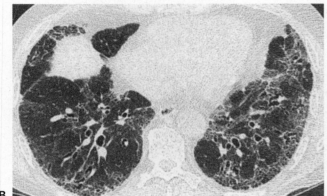

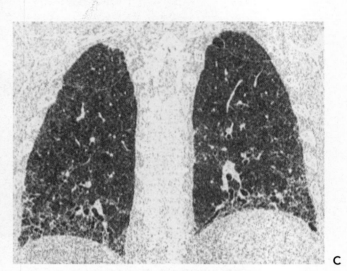

FIGURE 9-3 A–C: Transverse and coronal HRCT images from a patient with IPF show peripheral and basal predominant reticulation with traction bronchiectasis. Mild honeycombing is present in the left upper lobe (*arrow*). Note the relatively normal lung elsewhere. It is important to note these changes in nondependent regions of lung, as atelectasis in dependent lung can mimic these mild changes of fibrosis. Obtain prone scans as needed to evaluate the posterior portions of the lungs to distinguish the two conditions.

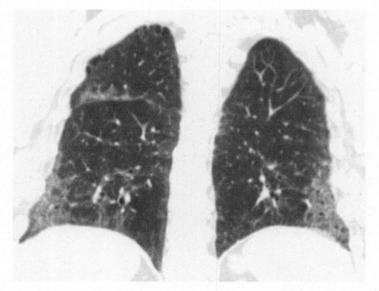

FIGURE 9-4 Coronal HRCT scan from a patient with IPF shows peripheral, basilar predominant ground-glass opacity with some reticulation in and architectural distortion as a milder form of UIP without overt honeycomb formation.

Lower lung zones

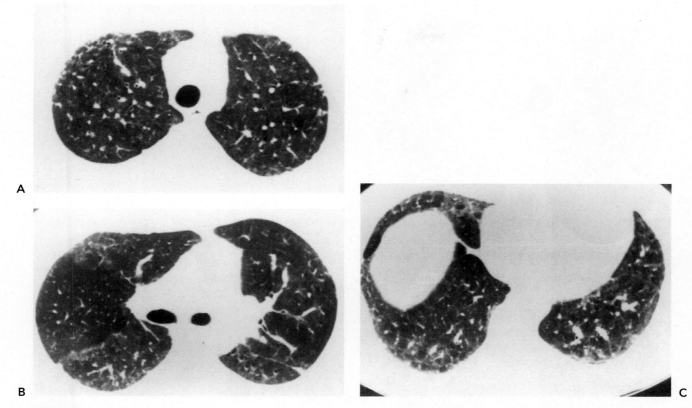

FIGURES 9-5

FIGURES 9-5 A–C: HRCT scan from a patient with UIP shows ill-defined centrilobular nodular opacities, interlobular septal thickening, hazy ground-glass opacities and basilar distribution of this infiltrative process. If the ground-glass opacity is associated with signs of architectural distortion, it is probably irreversible, representing fibrosis beyond the resolution of the CT scan. Clinically, this patient had IPF.

Advanced pulmonary fibrosis

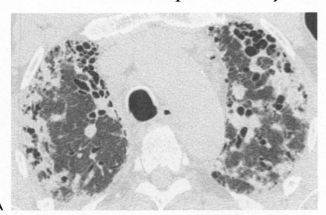

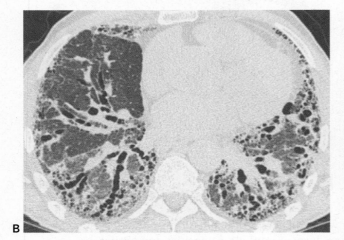

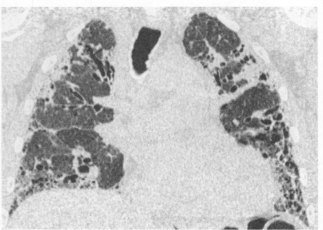

FIGURE 9-6 A–C: Transverse and coronal HRCT images show extensive lung fibrosis. There is extensive traction bronchiectasis. As typical of UIP, the fibrosis is basal and peripheral predominant. This case shows characteristic findings of advanced idiopathic UIP. Specific features of advanced disease include a peripheral and basilar predilection of marked lung architectural distortion with honeycombing and traction bronchiectasis. When the disease is this advanced, the HRCT signs of milder fibrosis, namely thickened interlobular septa, thickened intralobular core structures (ill-defined centrilobular nodular opacities), nondependent subpleural lung opacity, and ground-glass lung opacities, may not be evident.

Advanced pulmonary fibrosis *(continued)*

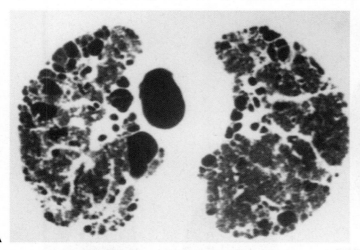
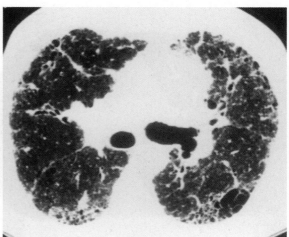

A   B

FIGURE 9-7 **A,B:** HRCT scans from a patient with advanced IPF show severe honeycombing and traction dilatation of the trachea and main bronchi. Peripheral honeycombing can have a "cystic" appearance, but in this case, there is extensive architectural distortion not usually associated with cystic lung diseases.

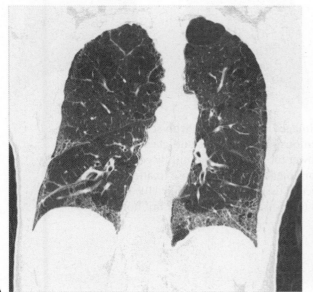
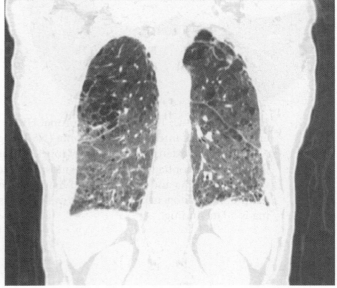

A   B

FIGURE 9-8 **A,B:** Coronal HRCT scans from two patients, both longtime cigarette smokers with increasingly progressive dyspnea, IPF, and superimposed centrilobular pulmonary emphysema show both peripheral basilar reticulation, architectural distortion, and mild honeycomb formation as well as superimposed upper lobe predominant moderately severe centrilobular emphysema. Note the distinct difference in appearance between the emphysema and the honeycombing.

Nonspecific interstitial pneumonia

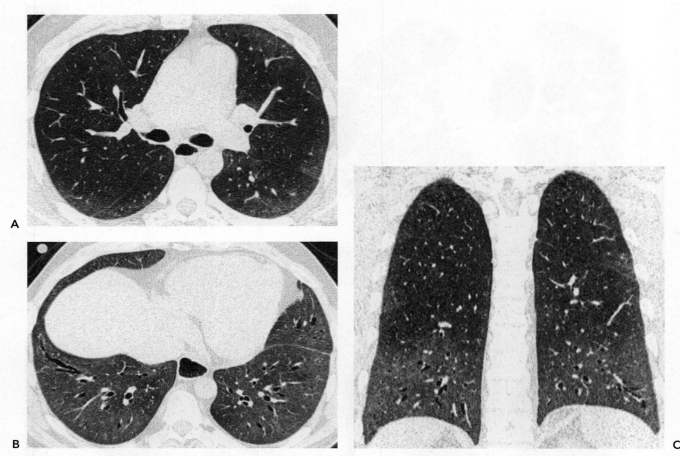

FIGURE 9-9 A–C: Transverse and coronal HRCT images from a patient with scleroderma and nonspecific interstitial pneumonia (NSIP) demonstrate patchy ground-glass opacity, which is more extensive in the lower lobes. The lower lobe bronchi are mildly ectatic. Note the patulous esophagus. NSIP is the most common interstitial lung disease to affect patients with scleroderma and is common in many connective tissue diseases. Unlike UIP, NSIP is a temporally homogeneous process. It can progress to end-stage lung fibrosis, but honeycombing is a late finding.

Nonspecific interstitial pneumonia *(continued)*

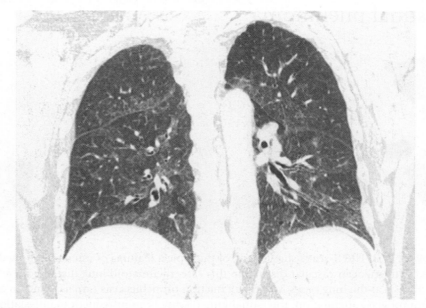

FIGURE 9-10 Coronal HRCT scan through the posterior chest from a patient with NSIP shows diffuse ground-glass opacities and mild reticulations somewhat nonspecific findings. Note the lack of honeycombing or peripheral distribution typical for UIP.

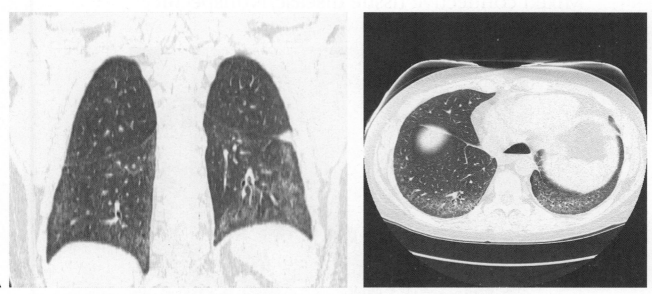

FIGURE 9-11 A,B: Transverse and coronal HRCT images from a patient with scleroderma and NSIP demonstrate patchy ground-glass opacity with mild reticulation, more extensive in the lower lobes, but with some very peripheral sparing.

Rheumatoid interstitial lung disease/Nonspecific interstitial pneumonia

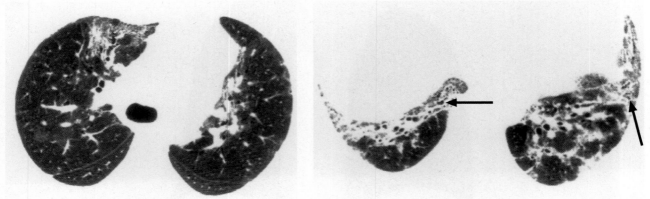

A

B

FIGURE 9-12 A,B: HRCT scans show many of the typical features of interstitial lung disease associated with collagen vascular disease; in this case, rheumatoid lung disease. There is pulmonary fibrosis at the lung bases, secondary traction bronchiectasis (*arrows*), and an area of patchy ground-glass attenuation. Interstitial lung disease is an infrequent manifestation of rheumatoid arthritis.

Mixed connective tissue disease/Nonspecific interstitial pneumonia

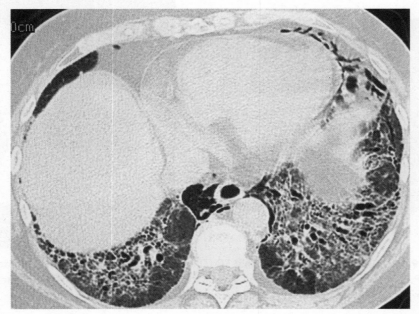

FIGURE 9-13 HRCT scan through the lower lungs from this patient with mixed connective tissue disease and calcinosis cutis, Raynaud's phenomenon, esophageal motility disorder, sclerodactyly, and telangiectasis syndrome (CREST) shows fibrotic changes in the lung bases, with honeycombing. There is architectural distortion and traction bronchiectasis. Note the mild dilatation of the lower esophagus. There is also a small amount of pneumomediastinum. These findings are consistent with mixed connective tissue disease involving the lung and esophagus.

Dermatomyositis/Nonspecific interstitial pneumonia

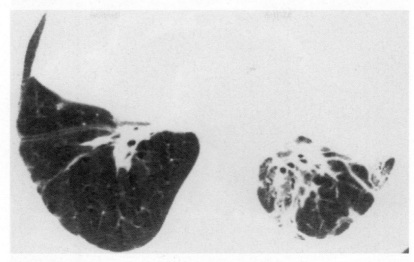

FIGURE 9-14

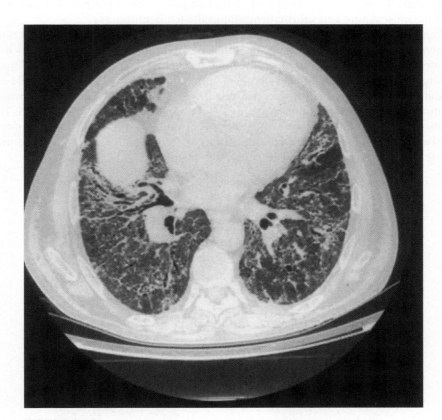

FIGURE 9-15

FIGURES 9-14 and 9-15 HRCT scans from two patients with dermatomyositis show a reticular infiltrative process in the lung bases with architectural distortion, including traction bronchiectasis. The upper lungs were spared. The findings are compatible with the pathologic diagnosis of NSIP associated with dermatomyositis.

Dermatomyositis/Nonspecific interstitial pneumonia *(continued)*

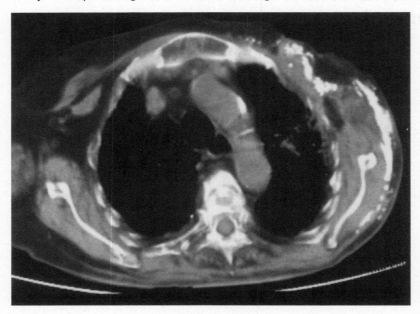

FIGURE 9-16 CT scan from a patient with dermatomyositis shows platelike calcification of some of the musculature and subcutaneous fat in the left hemithorax.

Dermatomyositis is characterized by proximal muscle weakness and a violaceous skin rash. Polymyositis is similar but spares the skin. Coexistent malignant disease occurs in approximately 15% of patients. Tumors of the lung, ovary, breast, and gastrointestinal track predominate. Interstitial lung fibrosis occurs in approximately 5% of patients and like other interstitial fibroses, most often involves the lung bases. Subcutaneous calcification, which can be quite striking, can affect the extremities, abdominal wall, pelvis, or chest wall. These calcifications are often fine, reticular, or streaky early in the disease and become coarser as the disease progresses. Soft tissue calcifications can be seen in patients with dermatomyositis, chronic renal failure, myositis ossificans, and other conditions.

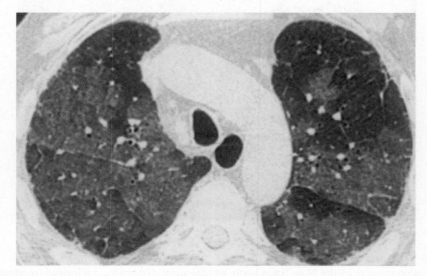

FIGURE 9-17 HRCT scan from a patient with dermatomyositis shows bilateral confluent regions of ground-glass opacity. Ground-glass opacity on HRCT is a nonspecific finding and can be seen in desquamative interstitial pneumonia (DIP), NSIP, hypersensitivity pneumonitis, cardiogenic and noncardiogenic edema, and so forth.

Scleroderma/Nonspecific interstitial pneumonia

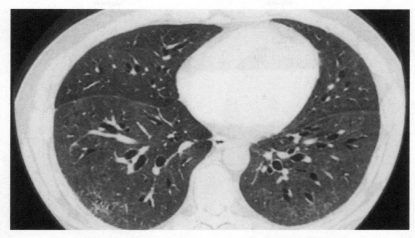

FIGURE 9-18 HRCT scan from a patient with scleroderma shows diffuse ground-glass opacity throughout the lungs. Note the marked dilatation of the basilar bronchi due to traction. In this case, the ground-glass opacity should be caused by fibrosis because there is architectural distortion. The patient's mid and upper lungs were uninvolved. HRCT findings are typical for NSIP

Specific sites of disease associated with multisystemic scleroderma (progressive systemic sclerosis) include skin changes, Raynaud's phenomenon, esophageal dysmotility, and lung fibrosis. The female-to-male distribution is approximately 3 to 1.

Spontaneous pneumomediastinum in IPF

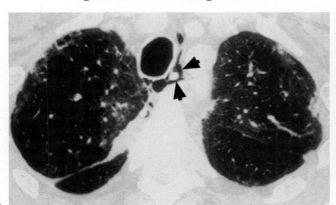
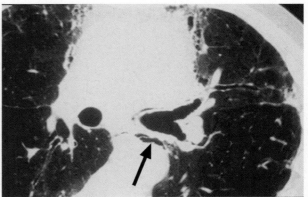

A   B

FIGURE 9-19 **A,B:** HRCT scan from a 70-year-old woman with IPF and acute onset of dyspnea and chest pain shows, in **A**, gas in the mediastinum, around the esophagus (*arrowheads*). In **B**, HRCT scan through the upper lobes shows gas into the peribronchovascular bundle (interstitial emphysema), outlining left main bronchus and descending aorta (*arrow*).

IPF has a poor prognosis, with 50% of patients dying 5 years after the onset of symptoms. Several specific complications have been described in patients with IPF, including respiratory failure, heart failure, spontaneous pneumothorax and pneumomediastinum, and bronchogenic carcinoma. The clinical manifestations of spontaneous extra-alveolar air in IPF are varied and range from radiographic findings alone in asymptomatic patients to severe respiratory insufficiency. Symptoms are variable and include dyspnea, cough, and chest pain.

Unusual manifestation of pulmonary fibrosis

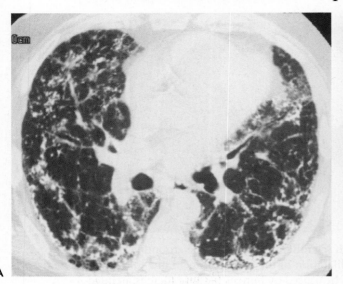
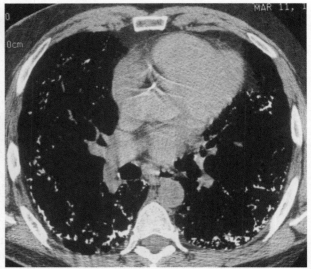

A

B

FIGURE 9-20 A,B: HRCT scans through the lower lungs, with lung **(A)** and soft tissue **(B)** windows, from a patient with idiopathic UIP show a typical distribution of peripheral and basilar lung fibrosis, with extensive reticulation and honeycombing. The unusual feature in this case is that the infiltrative lung disease has regions of ossification. This is rarely seen in idiopathic UIP and is probably an osseous metaplasia.

Desquamative interstitial pneumonia

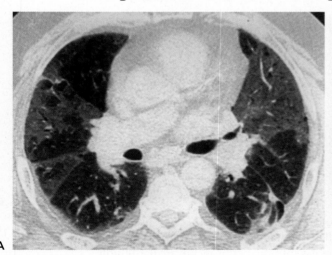
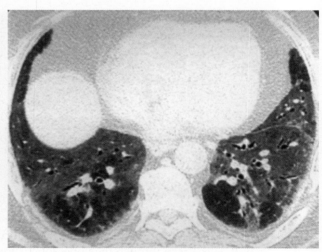

A

B

FIGURE 9-21

FIGURES 9-21 A,B and 9-22 HRCT scans from two patients with DIP show patchy ground-glass opacities associated with some architectural distortion (e.g., mild traction bronchiectasis, lobular distortion) probably indicative of fibrosis. DIP is a distinct form of interstitial pneumonia characterized by a more benign clinical course and specific morphologic and cellular cytologic features. Without treatment, median survival in DIP is more than 10 years, whereas in UIP it is between 3 and 5 years. DIP is generally considered a cigarette smoking-related interstitial lung disease.

(continued)

Desquamative interstitial pneumonia *(continued)*

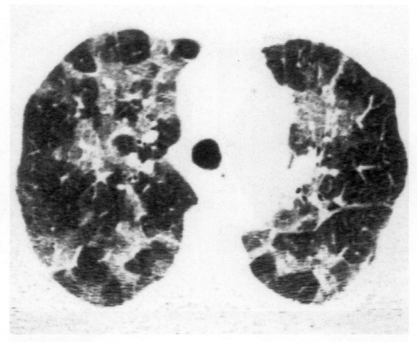

FIGURE 9-22

FIGURES 9-21 A,B and 9-22 *(continued)*

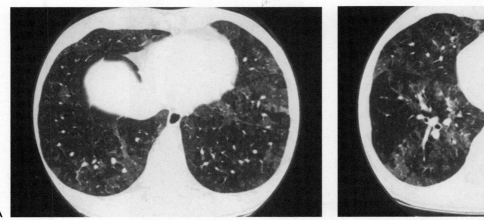

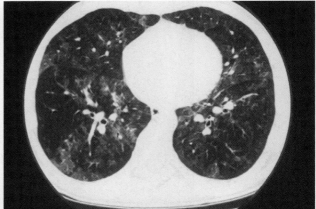

A   B

FIGURE 9-23

FIGURES 9-23 A,B, 9-24 A,B, and 9-25 HRCT scans from three patients with DIP. In Figures 9-23 and 9-24, note multiple patchy regions of ground-glass attenuation, with a lobular or mosaic pattern of distribution. In Figure 9-25, again note patchy bilateral regions of ground-glass attenuation but with superimposed patchy regions of denser reticulation (fibrosis). DIP is now usually considered on the spectrum of lung injury with respiratory bronchiolitis (RB) and RB–associated interstitial lung disease, as a smoking-related interstitial lung disease, reflecting varying responses to alveolar macrophage pneumonia.

(continued)

Desquamative interstitial pneumonia *(continued)*

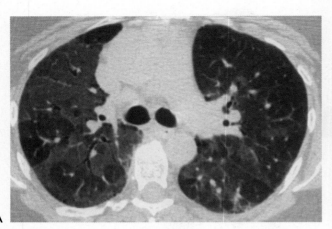

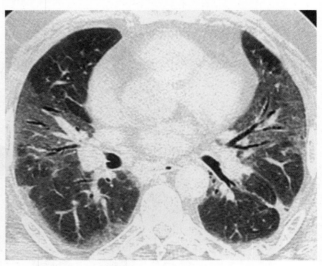

A

B

FIGURE 9-24

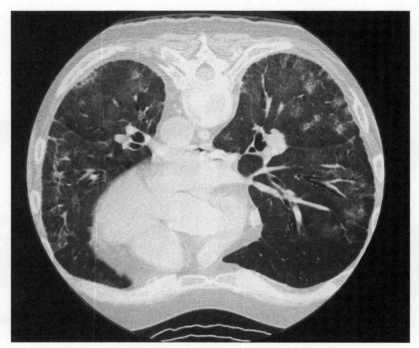

FIGURE 9-25

FIGURES 9-23 A,B, 9-24 A,B, and 9-25 *(continued)*

Desquamative interstitial pneumonia *(continued)*

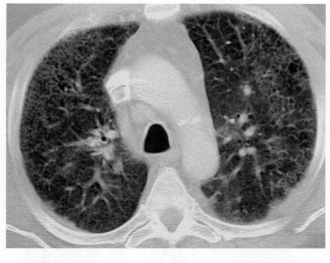

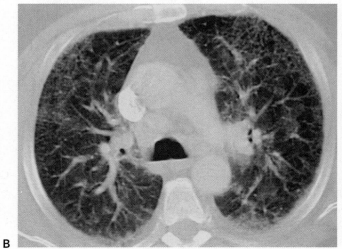

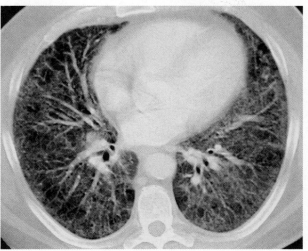

FIGURE 9-26 A–C: Three HRCT scans through the upper, middle, and lower lungs from a patient with symptomatic and untreated DIP for 3 years show less of the typical patchy ground-glass opacities but more of a diffuse fibrotic appearance, as would be expected for the natural course of this disease (courtesy of Steve Kirtland, M.D., Seattle, WA).

Desquamative interstitial pneumonia *(continued)*

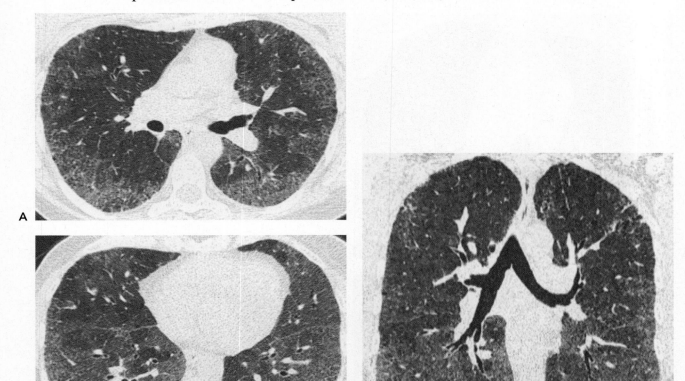

FIGURE 9-27 A–C: Transverse and coronal HRCT images of patient with DIP resulting from heavy smoking show peripheral and basal predominant ground-glass opacity with superimposed reticulation. The costophrenic sulci are relatively spared. DIP is a rare disorder that most commonly occurs in very heavy smokers. It is in the spectrum of macrophage-mediated smoking-related interstitial lung disease that also includes RB and respiratory bronchiolitis-interstitial lung disease (RB-ILD). Histologically, DIP is characterized by the accumulation of pigmented macrophages in the alveoli. A mild interstitial fibrosis may be present and, in smokers, bronchiolitis is nearly universal. Occasionally, a DIP-type reaction may develop secondary to drug toxicity or an underlying connective tissue disease.

Respiratory bronchiolitis

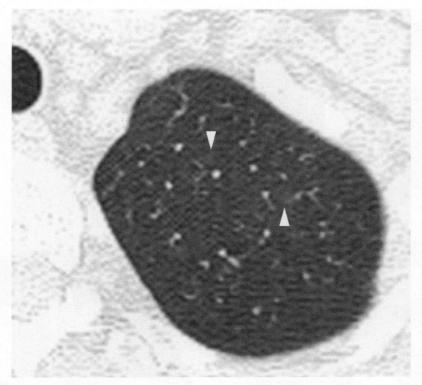

FIGURE 9-28 Coned-down HRCT image of the left lung apex in a smoker shows scattered poorly defined ground-glass attenuation centrilobular nodules. Respiratory bronchiolitis, by definition, does not cause symptoms or functional impairment and is universal in smokers. Scattered poorly defined nodules in the upper lobes characterize the condition. RB is the mildest form of the macrophage-mediated smoking-related interstitial lung diseases.

Respiratory bronchiolitis *(continued)*

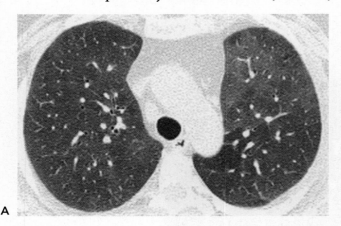

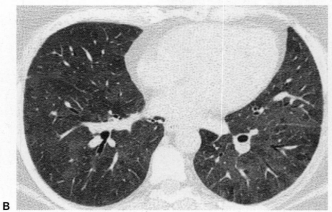

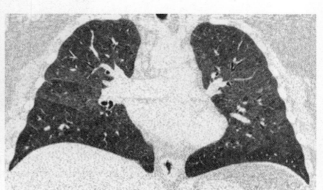

FIGURE 9-29 A–C: Transverse and coronal HRCT images in a smoker with RB-ILD diagnosed at surgical lung biopsy show patchy ground-glass opacity in both lungs with foci of lobular sparing. Patients with RB-ILD usually are heavy smokers and present with dyspnea and mild restrictive physiology. The typical HRCT finding is patchy ground-glass opacity, which usually has a mid and upper lung zone predominance. However, more extensive RB-ILD can be more diffuse as it approaches the degree of intra-alveolar macrophages encountered in DIP.

Respiratory bronchiolitis–associated interstitial lung disease

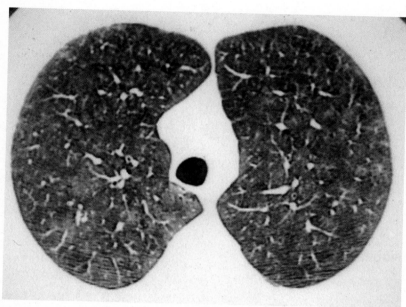

FIGURE 9-30 HRCT scan through the upper lobes shows multiple, subtle, ill-defined centrilobular micronodules distributed throughout the parenchyma. These were limited to the upper lobes in this patient. These findings, along with multifocal regions of ground-glass opacity in an appropriate clinical setting, are typical of RB–associated interstitial lung disease.

Respiratory bronchiolitis–associated interstitial lung disease is a condition usually associated with cigarette smoking that causes a nonspecific inflammatory reaction at the level of the respiratory bronchioles to inhaled irritants. Pathologically, there is a mild inflammatory reaction involving the membranous and respiratory bronchioles. Tan-brown pigmented macrophages within respiratory bronchioles, alveolar ducts, and alveoli (smoker's alveolitis) dominate the pathologic findings.

The HRCT scan features are similar to those of hypersensitivity pneumonitis and include multiple ill-defined 2- to 3-mm intralobular or subpleural micronodules, multifocal ground-glass opacities with a centrilobular distribution, and thickening of bronchial walls and septal lines. Centrilobular branching opacities [the "tree-in-bud" appearance] are absent in RB. Air trapping can be seen on expiratory CT scans.

Respiratory bronchiolitis–associated interstitial lung disease *(continued)*

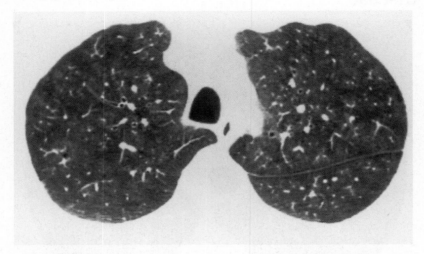

FIGURE 9-31

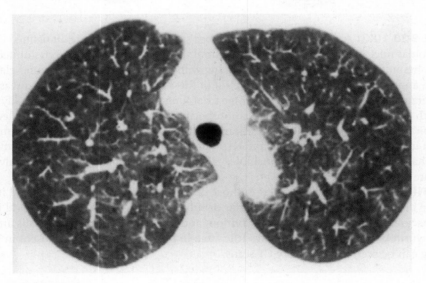

FIGURE 9-32

FIGURES 9-31, 9-32, and 9-33 HRCT scans from three patients with smoking-related respiratory bronchiolitis–associated interstitial lung disease show multiple ill-defined, sublobular, nodular opacities along with regions of ground-glass opacity. There is no evidence of emphysema.

Pathologic studies have revealed that cigarette smoking leads to the accumulation of pigmented macrophages and mucus in the alveolar spaces, mild interstitial inflammation or fibrosis, and bronchiolectasis with peribronchiolar fibrosis.

(continued)

Respiratory bronchiolitis–associated interstitial lung disease *(continued)*

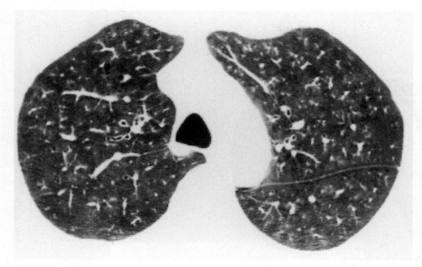

FIGURE 9-33

FIGURES 9-31, 9-32, and 9-33 *(continued)*

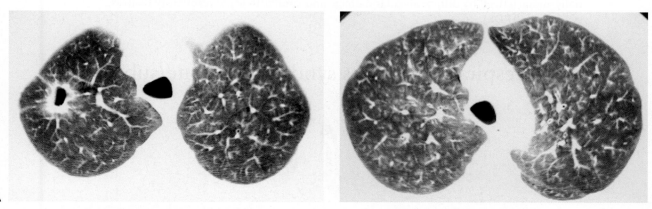

A   B

FIGURE 9-34 A,B: HRCT scans through the upper lobes show multiple subtle, ill-defined centrilobular micronodules and patchy regions of ground-glass opacity distributed throughout the parenchyma. Again, these findings, in the appropriate clinical setting, are typical of respiratory bronchiolitis–associated interstitial lung disease. In this case, note cavitary squamous cell carcinoma **(B)**, also associated with cigarette smoking.

Acute interstitial pneumonia

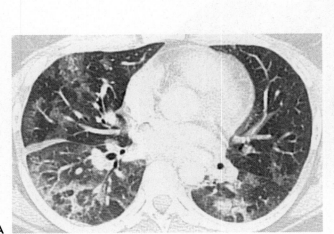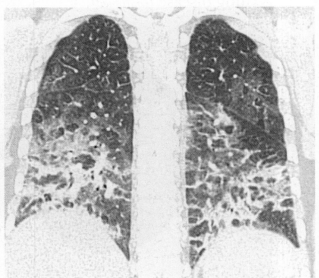

A   B

FIGURE 9-35 **A,B:** Transverse and coronal HRCT images of a young woman with acute interstitial pneumonia show bilateral patchy ground-glass opacity and consolidation with a mid and lower lung zone predominance. Histopathologically, acute interstitial pneumonia is initially characterized by diffuse alveolar damage and similar to acute respiratory distress syndrome (ARDS).

Acute respiratory distress syndrome—acute/subacute phase

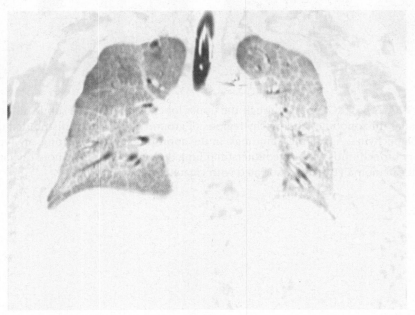

FIGURE 9-36 Coronal HRCT through the mid chest shows extensive diffuse ground-glass opacities with thickening of the interlobular and intralobular septa consistent with the clinical syndrome of ARDS. Imaging distinction between the clinical syndromes of acute lung injury and ARDS is not possible; this distinction is based on the degree of hypoxia, which does not correlate with imaging.

Acute respiratory distress syndrome—pulmonary fibrosis

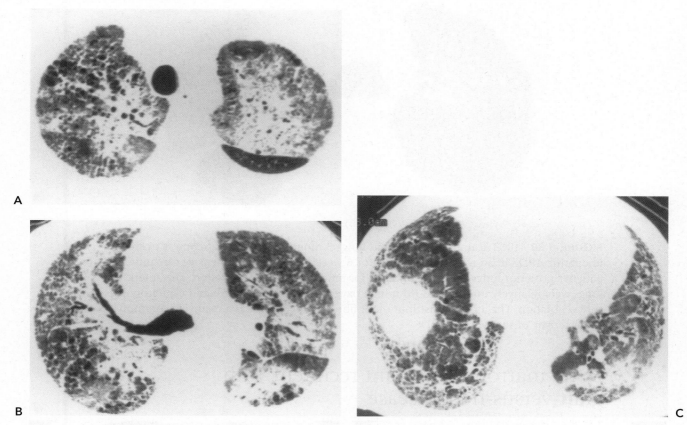

FIGURE 9-37 **A–C:** HRCT scans from a patient with prior ARDS (6 months after acute respiratory failure) show diffuse and extensive honeycombing (lung fibrosis) in the upper and lower, central, and peripheral lung zones. ARDS is a syndrome of diffuse alveolar damage that results in acute respiratory failure and profound hypoxemia. The lungs in survivors of ARDS frequently progress to a chronic phase (more than 2 weeks) of alveolar cell hyperplasia, fibroblast proliferation, interstitial collagen deposition, and architectural remodeling. The lung heals with a variable amount of residual fibrosis, severe in this case, over a 6- to 12-month period.

Acute respiratory distress syndrome—pulmonary fibrosis *(continued)*

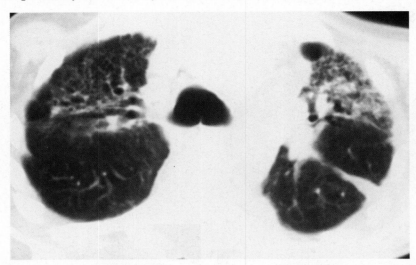

FIGURE 9-38 HRCT scan through the mid lungs 5 months after this patient was treated for idiopathic ARDS in an intensive care unit for 6 weeks. While in the intensive care unit, the patient's posterior lungs were consolidated for much of the hospitalization. The anterior lungs were relatively unprotected from high oxygen levels with positive-end expiratory pressure ventilation. The anterior distribution of fibrotic lung disease is a relatively common characteristic of survivors of ARDS.

Bone marrow transplant recipient with graft-versus-host disease

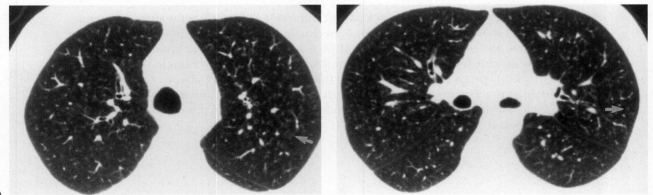

A   B

FIGURE 9-39 A-B: HRCT scans from a patient with graft-versus-host disease show diffuse small, ill-defined nodules (*arrows*). These parenchymal micronodules, arising in peribronchiolar locations, are related to inflammation and dilatation of the bronchioles (bronchiolitis/bronchiolectasis) and associated peribronchiolar fibrosis. The nodular opacities are very similar in appearance to the RB seen in cigarette smokers.

Patients with acute and chronic graft-versus-host disease after allogeneic bone marrow transplantation can uncommonly manifest small airway damage as one of the facets of graft-versus-host disease. The spectrum of small airway pathology can vary from early bronchiolar wall damage to bronchiolitis obliterans. The diagnosis is made in the proper clinical setting in the absence of other identifiable pathogens of bronchiolitis obliterans.

Cryptogenic organizing pneumonia

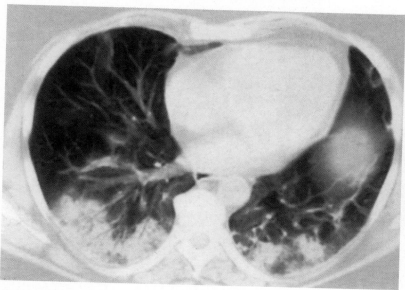

FIGURE 9-40

FIGURES 9-40, 9-41, and 9-42 A,B: HRCT scans from three patients with cryptogenic organizing pneumonia (COP) show multiple peripheral, nonspecific areas of consolidated lung parenchyma. Although some of these areas are well-defined with a nodular or masslike appearance, others are less well demarcated and amorphous in character. Note the very different appearance of COP from constrictive bronchiolitis (see Figs. 5-1 to 5-8), which is an airways disease (not airspace disease) characterized by areas of hyperlucent parenchyma and vasoconstriction.

COP is characterized by the presence of granulation tissue within small airways and areas of organizing pneumonia. It is the organizing pneumonia that makes COP clinically and pathologically different from constrictive bronchiolitis.

The HRCT findings of idiopathic COP are numerous and nonspecific. They include patchy, usually bilateral airspace opacification of a ground-glass or soft tissue density, small nodular opacities, irregular linear opacities, bronchial wall thickening and dilatation, solitary masses, and small pleural effusions. The nodules and parenchymal opacification represent different degrees of the same nonspecific inflammatory process that involves the bronchioles, alveolar ducts, and alveoli. The findings are very similar to those of chronic eosinophilic pneumonia, although COP is slightly more likely to have a peripheral and basilar distribution. HRCT scans better depict the anatomic distribution and extent of COP more accurately than chest radiographs.

(continued)

Cryptogenic organizing pneumonia *(continued)*

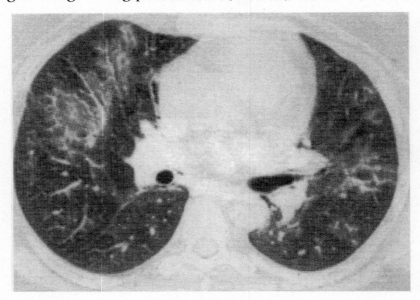

FIGURE 9-41

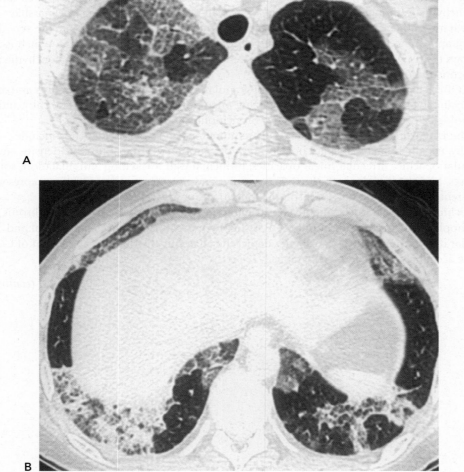

FIGURE 9-42

FIGURES 9-40, 9-41, and 9-42 A,B *(continued)*

Cryptogenic organizing pneumonia *(continued)*

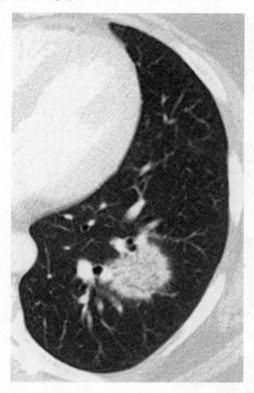

FIGURE 9-43 HRCT image from a patient with cryptogenic organizing pneumonia shows a masslike area of consolidation with central, less dense, ground-glass opacity (the so-called reverse halo sign) in the left lower lobe. Initially thought to be specific for organizing pneumonia, the reverse halo sign has also been described in zygomycosis, tuberculosis, paracoccidioidomycosis (South American blastomycosis), lymphomatoid granulomatosis, and small vessel vasculitis. It can also be present in subacute pulmonary hemorrhage with the peripheral consolidation thought to represent organizing pneumonia around the clearing hemorrhage.

Bronchioloalveolar cell carcinoma in scleroderma

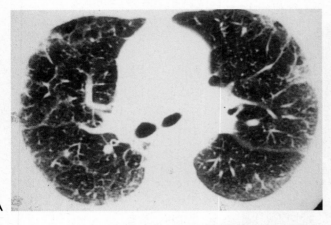

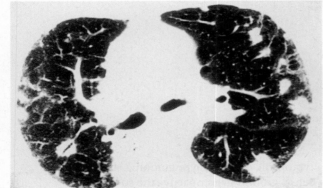

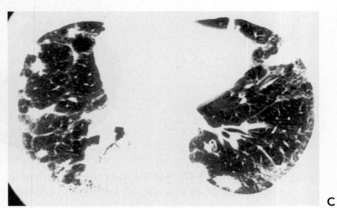

FIGURE 9-44 A–C: HRCT scan through the mid lung from a 69-year-old woman with scleroderma shows a predominantly subpleural distribution of irregular linear opacities with associated architectural distortion. Focal areas of ground-glass attenuation are also noted. This distribution is characteristic of interstitial lung disease associated with collagen vascular disease. In HRCT scans obtained 3 years later, note the development of multifocal bronchioloalveolar cell carcinoma **(B,C)**, with multiple new peripheral masses in both lungs. Note the presence of air-bronchogram in some of the masses. Patients with lung fibrosis have an increased incidence of lung cancer.

Hard metal pneumoconiosis

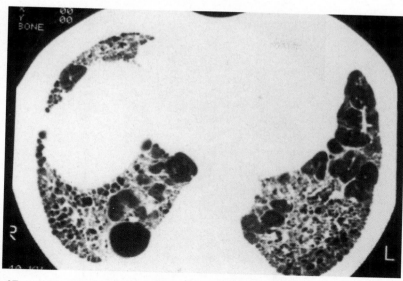

FIGURE 9-45 HRCT scan shows typical end-stage pulmonary fibrosis; in this case caused by giant cell interstitial pneumonia (GIP). GIP is a distinctive and uncommon form of interstitial pneumonia distinguished by the prominence of large, actively phagocytic alveolar giant cells of histiocytic origin in the presence of chronic interstitial pneumonia. The multi-nucleated cells lack viral intranuclear inclusions of the type seen in measles pneumonia. GIP can result from occupational exposure to hard metals or cobalt. Hard metal is a mixture of tungsten carbide and cobalt, to which small amounts of other metals may be added. It is widely used for industrial purposes whenever extreme hardness and high-temperature resistance are needed, such as for cutting tools, oil well drilling bits, and jet engine exhaust ports. Cobalt is the component of hard metal that can be hazardous. Adverse pulmonary reactions include asthma, hypersensitivity pneumonitis, and interstitial fibrosis.

Primary systemic amyloidosis

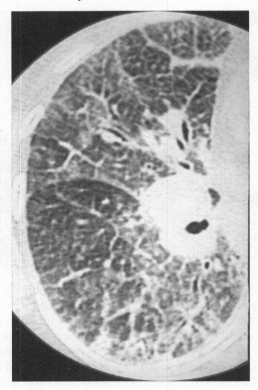

FIGURE 9-46

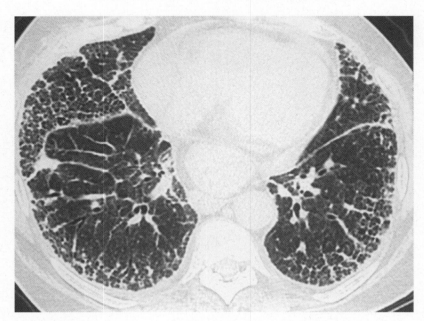

FIGURE 9-47

FIGURES 9-46 and 9-47 HRCT scans from two patients with primary systemic amyloidosis show diffuse interlobular septal thickening in Figure 9-46 and a reticular pattern with honeycombing and traction bronchiectasis in Figure 9-47.

Cyclophosphamide (Cytoxan) drug toxicity

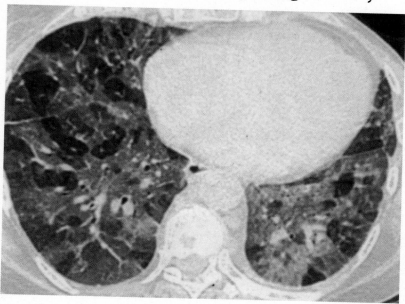

FIGURE 9-48 HRCT scan from a patient with cyclophosphamide drug toxicity shows patchy ground-glass opacities predominantly at the lung bases.

Cyclophosphamide, like numerous antineoplastic drugs, has been linked to toxic pulmonary side effects. Mechanisms include direct pulmonary toxicity and indirect effects through inflammatory reactions. Clinical features are similar for most agents, chronic pneumonitis, and fibrosis. The number of drugs known or suspected of causing pulmonary toxicity is steadily increasing and includes bleomycin, procainamide, nitrofurantoin, cyclophosphamide, penicillamine, busulfan, carmustine, amiodarone, mitomycin, and methotrexate, among others.

HRCT may show a variety of findings in patients with pulmonary drug toxicity. They include (a) fibrosis with or without airspace consolidation, (b) ground-glass opacities, (c) widespread bilateral airspace consolidation, or (d) bronchial wall thickening with distal areas of decreased lung attenuation—that is, reflecting air trapping in obliterative bronchiolitis.

Amiodarone toxicity

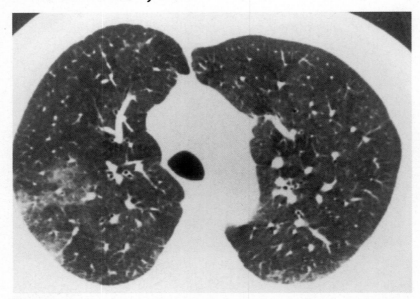

FIGURE 9-49

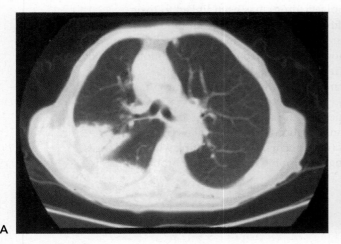

A

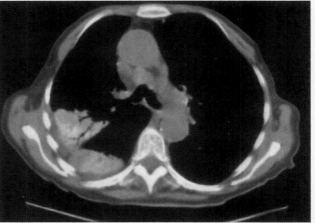

B

FIGURE 9-50

FIGURES 9-49 and 50 A,B: CT scans from two patients with amiodarone pulmonary toxicity show patchy areas of ground-glass opacification distributed diffusely throughout both lungs (Fig. 9-49).

In the patient in Figure 9-50, there also exist airless regions in the posterior segment of the right upper lobe and superior segment of the right lower lobe: These consolidated regions show considerable attenuation or "enhancement" in the absence of any intravenous contrast administration.

Amiodarone is an antiarrhythmic agent that contains iodine. Pulmonary toxicity can occur and likely reflects direct toxic effects, as well as indirect inflammatory and immunologic processes. In other patients with amiodarone toxicity, CT has demonstrated intralobular septal thickening and visceral pleural thickening.

Pulmonary drug toxicity

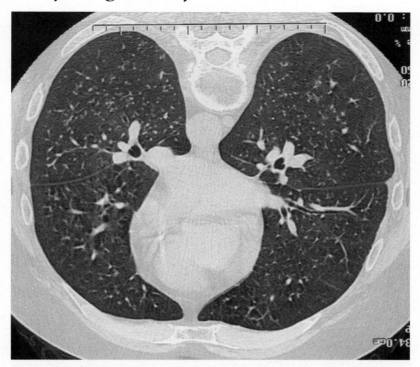

FIGURE 9-51 HRCT scan from a patient with a diagnosis of acute myelogenous leukemia who developed a diffuse erythematous rash over his entire body, with persistent cough and fever, shows a diffuse pattern of 1- to 2-mm nodules in a random distribution. Bronchoalveolar lavage and bronchoscopic biopsies were all negative for infection or malignancy. The patient had been taking the antibiotic ciprofloxacin before development of symptoms and the CT scan abnormalities. The patient's symptoms and CT scan abnormalities resolved after discontinuation of antibiotic therapy. Drug toxicity is often a diagnosis of exclusion and must show the appropriate temporal relationship to drug administration.

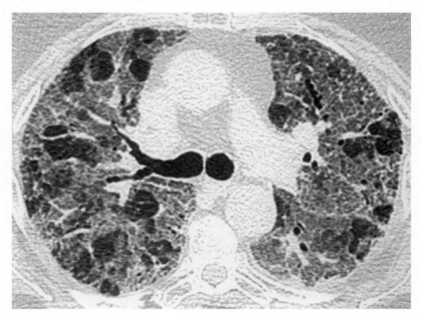

FIGURE 9-52 HRCT scan through the mid lungs from a patient with severe pulmonary drug toxicity from l-tryptophan. Note the mosaic pattern of lung attenuation and regions of traction bronchiectasis.

Acute eosinophilic pneumonia

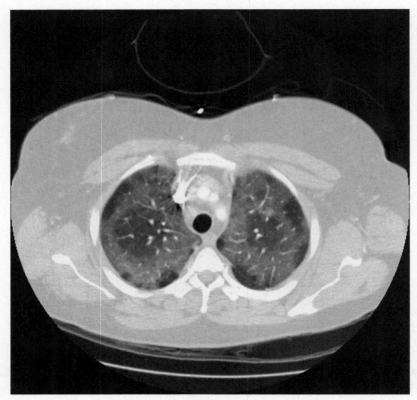

FIGURE 9-53 Transverse HRCT scan through the upper chest from a patient with acute eosinophilic pneumonia shows nonspecific ground-glass opacities, here with a somewhat peripheral distribution. Typical findings of acute eosinophilic ammonia are generally nonspecific, with bilateral areas of ground-glass attenuation, interlobular septal thickening, and occasionally denser parenchymal consolidation similar to those of other etiologies of pulmonary edema, but consideration should also be given to other etiologies for nonspecific diffuse lung opacities such as viral or atypical bacterial pneumonia and pulmonary hemorrhage, depending upon the clinical scenario.

Chronic eosinophilic pneumonia

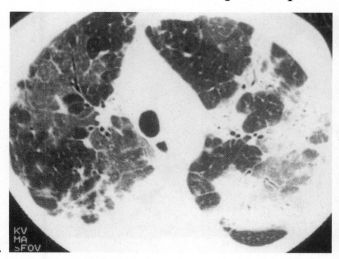
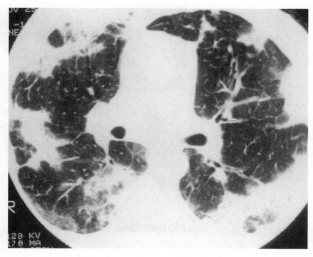

A   B

FIGURE 9-54 A,B: HRCT scans from a patient with chronic eosinophilic pneumonia show nonspecific diffuse, but patchy, bilateral regions of opacification.

The classic radiographic pattern of chronic eosinophilic pneumonia is opacification of the airspace in the peripheral third of the lungs, often with upper lung zone distribution. However, this classic pattern is seen in only a minority of patients with this disease; more often the areas of opacification are distributed diffusely. The CT pattern, although helpful, is not sufficiently specific for diagnosis and must be correlated with the clinical scenario. A similar nonspecific peripheral pattern of airspace opacification can be seen with other inflammatory processes of the airways or pulmonary vasculature, including such diverse etiologies as bacterial pneumonia or pulmonary vasculitides; the clinical scenario is useful in limiting the differential diagnosis.

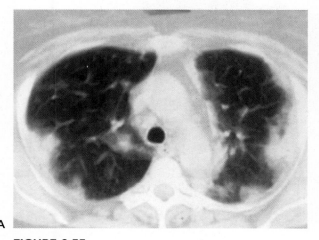
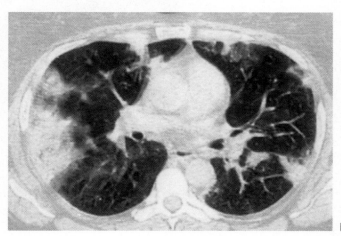

A   B

FIGURE 9-55

FIGURES 9-55 A,B, 9-56, and 9-57 HRCT scans from three patients with chronic eosinophilic pneumonia show multiple diffuse, bilateral, peripheral patchy regions of opacification, some with a nodular appearance (*arrowheads*). There is often an upper lung distribution. Differential diagnostic considerations include COP and, in certain situations, even reactivation tuberculosis.

When peripheral airspace disease is present in chronic eosinophilic pneumonia, it is often better detected with CT than with chest radiographs because of the improved ability to resolve for overlapping structures. Indeed, using CT, and, in particular, HRCT, this peripheral pattern can be identified in patients whose chest radiographs show more of a "diffuse" process.

(continued)

Chronic eosinophilic pneumonia *(continued)*

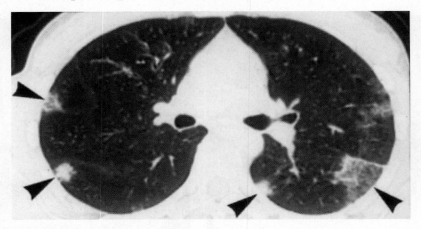

FIGURE 9-56

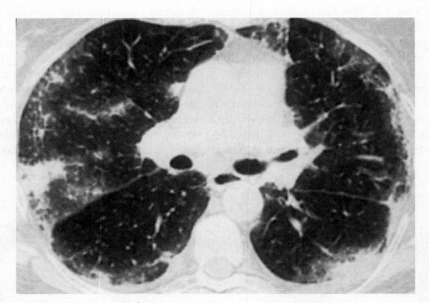

FIGURE 9-57

FIGURES 9-55 A,B, 9-56, and 9-57 *(continued)*

Chronic eosinophilic pneumonia *(continued)*

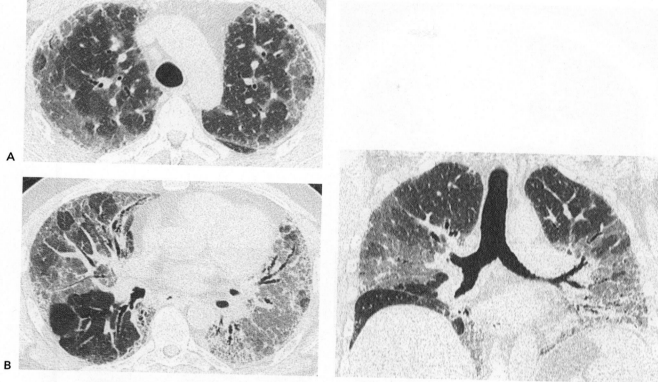

A

B

C

FIGURE 9-58 A–C: Transverse and coronal HRCT images from a patient with chronic eosinophilic pneumonia demonstrate peripheral ground-glass opacity and reticulation in the upper lobes that is more extensive in the lower lobes. Mild fibrosis is characterized by traction bronchiectasis in the lower lungs.

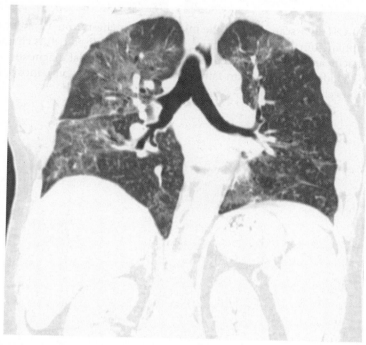

FIGURE 9-59 Coronal reformatted HRCT scan through the mid chest from a patient with chronic eosinophilic pneumonia shows nonspecific diffuse, but patchy, bilateral regions of ground-glass opacity.

Pulmonary lymphangiomatosis

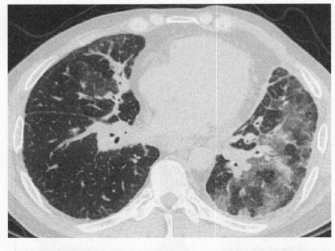

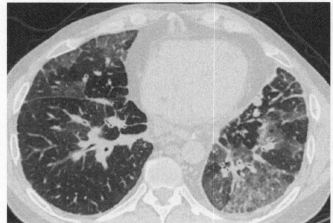

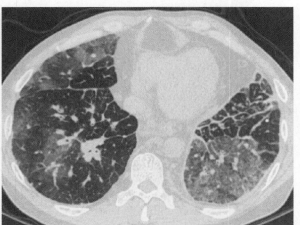

FIGURE 9-60 A–C: HRCT scan through the mid and lower chest from a patient with diffuse pulmonary lymphangiomatosis shows diffuse infiltrative lung disease. It is characterized by ground-glass opacity and interlobular septal thickening. Differential diagnostic considerations include congestive heart failure, pulmonary alveolar proteinosis, and pulmonary veno-occlusive disease.

Sarcoidosis

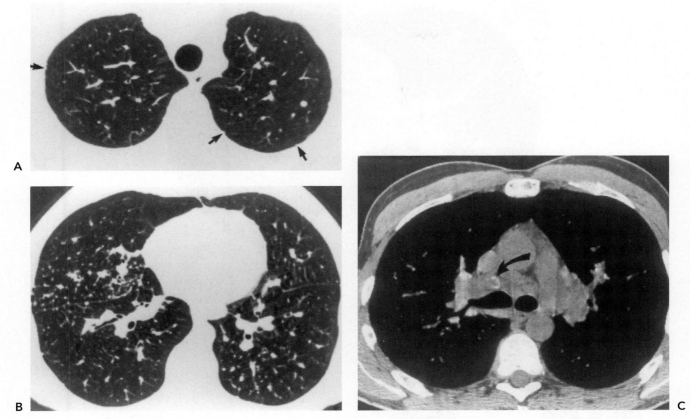

FIGURE 9-61 A–C: HRCT scans show a spectrum of findings in this patient with sarcoidosis. Note the small subpleural nodules in upper zone (*arrows*), peribronchovascular nodular thickening in middle zone, and adenopathy with eggshell hilar lymph node calcification (*curved arrow*).

Sarcoidosis is a systemic disorder characterized by widespread development of nonspecific, noncaseating granulomas. The etiology is unknown. Pulmonary disease associated with sarcoidosis may resolve spontaneously or progress to fibrosis. Because lymphadenopathy is the most common intrathoracic manifestation of sarcoidosis, the chest radiograph is abnormal in 90% to 95% of patients at some point, although 5% to 15% present with a normal chest radiograph.

Sarcoidosis *(continued)*

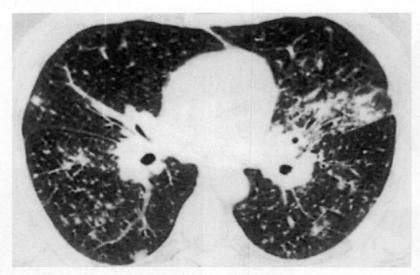

FIGURE 9-62

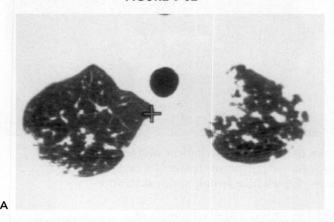

A

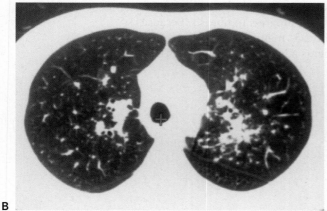

B

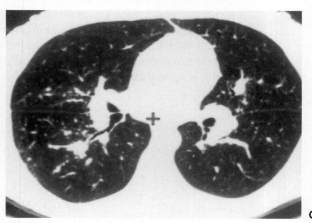

C

FIGURE 9-63

FIGURES 9-62 and 9-63 A–C: HRCT scans from two patients with sarcoidosis show relatively symmetric nodular infiltration along peribronchovascular bundles. Subpleural nodules and hilar adenopathy are also noted.

In the lung, sarcoid granulomas are distributed primarily along the lymphatics, and, therefore, the peribronchovascular interstitial space, the interlobular septa, and subpleural interstitial space are involved. Nodules represent coalescent granulomas, usually have irregular margins, and are typically 2 to 10 mm in diameter. Parenchymal opacities commonly involve the upper and middle lung zones but can also involve the lower lung zones.

Sarcoidosis *(continued)*

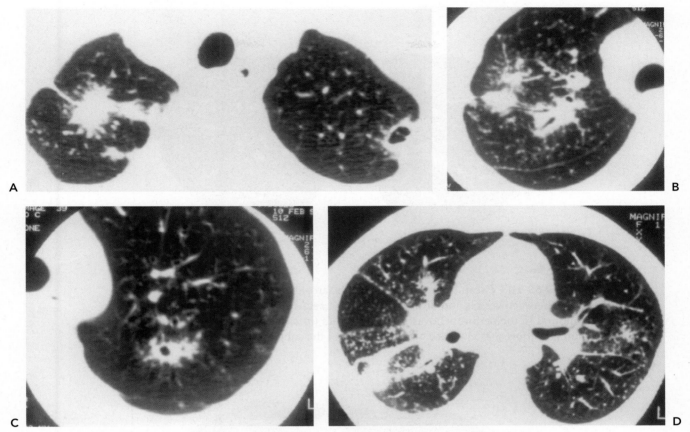

FIGURE 9-64 A–D: HRCT scans from a patient with sarcoidosis show many of the HRCT features of sarcoidosis and include nodules, masslike confluent nodules, fibrosis with lung architectural distortion and traction bronchiectasis, thickening of the pleural surfaces, ground-glass opacities, and air-filled cavities or cysts. In other words, sarcoidosis can have many different appearances, even within the same patient.

Sarcoidosis *(continued)*

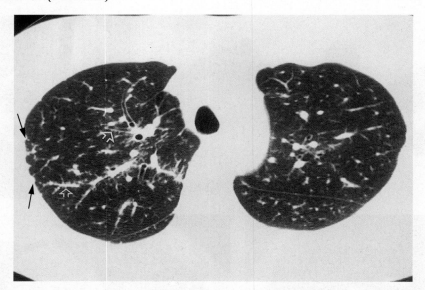

FIGURE 9-65 HRCT scan from this patient with sarcoidosis shows nodularity of the interface between vessels and bronchial walls and aerated lung, secondary to noncaseating granulomas in the peribronchovascular lymphatics (*arrowheads*). Note studding of the pleural surface (*arrows*), as evidence of involvement of the subpleural lymphatics.

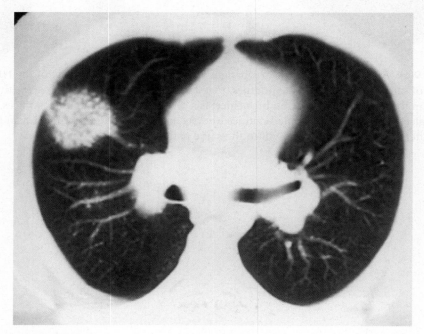

FIGURE 9-66

FIGURES 9-66, 9-67, 9-68 A–C, and 9-69 A,B: HRCT scans from four patients with sarcoidosis show focal regions of masslike consolidation. All these patients had associated hilar adenopathy. On careful inspection, many of these "masses" appear to be areas of confluent micronodules. This is an unusual manifestation of sarcoidosis, occurring in less than 5% of cases. Differential diagnostic considerations include lymphoma, Wegener's granulomatosis, bronchioloalveolar carcinoma, and COP. The clinical presentation can help distinguish among these diseases (Fig. 9-69 courtesy of R. Eisenberg, M.D., Boston, MA).

(continued)

Sarcoidosis *(continued)*

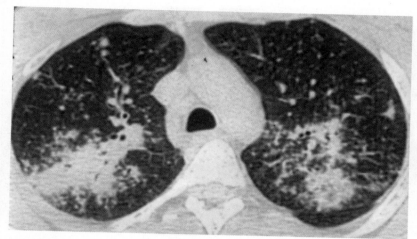

FIGURE 9-67

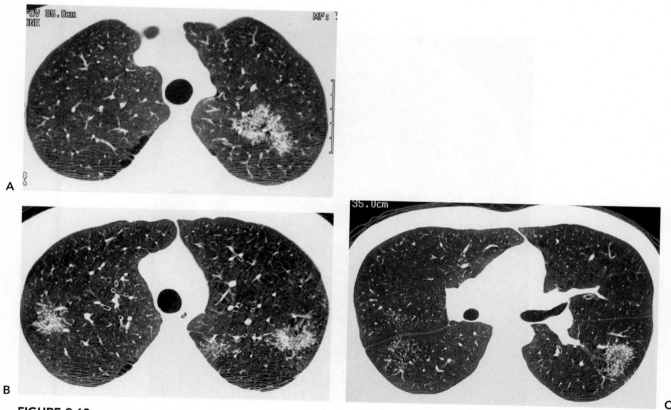

A

B

FIGURE 9-68

FIGURES 9-66, 9-67, 9-68 A–C, and 9-69 A,B *(continued)*

C

Sarcoidosis *(continued)*

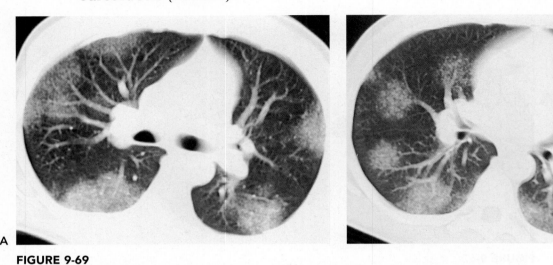

A   B

FIGURE 9-69

FIGURES 9-66, 9-67, 9-68 A–C, and 9-69 A,B *(continued)*

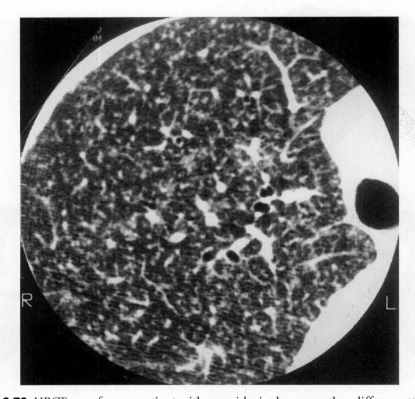

FIGURE 9-70 HRCT scan from a patient with sarcoidosis shows a rather diffuse pattern of 2- to 3-mm micronodules in a characteristic perilymphatic distribution. Subpleural nodules, beaded interlobular septa, and nodular vascular interfaces are caused by granuloma formation in the perilymphatic interstitium. Also note an unusual degree of nodular interlobular septal thickening.

Sarcoidosis *(continued)*

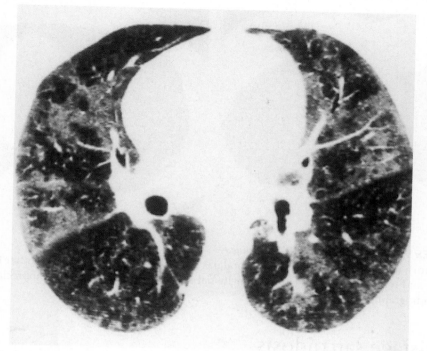

FIGURE 9-71 HRCT scan from a patient with sarcoidosis, is addition to perilymphatic nodules, also shows a ground-glass pattern of attenuation that is occasionally seen in sarcoidosis. The ground-glass attenuation is caused by alveolar granulomas and inflammation beyond the resolution limits of the CT scanner. Rarely, this appearance resembles alveolar proteinosis.

Lofgren's syndrome

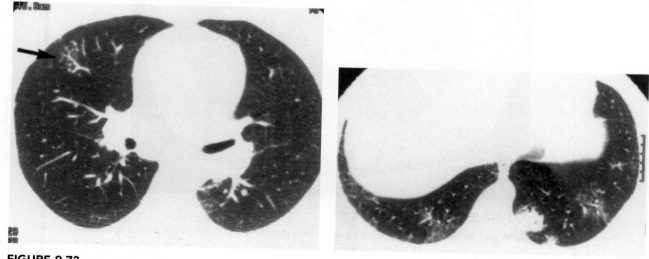

FIGURE 9-72

FIGURES 9-72 A,B and 9-73 A,B: HRCT scans from two patients with a specific presentation of acute sarcoidosis, called *Lofgren's syndrome*, show subtle focal nodular infiltrates and ground-glass opacity (Fig. 9-72B) within the lungs. Note a "tree-in-bud" appearance (Fig. 9-72A) *(arrow)* similar to that seen in another active granulomatous process—tuberculosis. Patients with Lofgren's syndrome usually have fevers, skin lesions (usually erythema

(continued)

Lofgren's syndrome *(continued)*

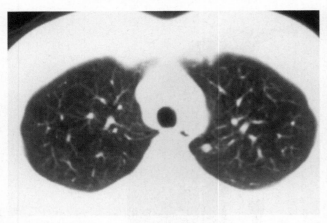
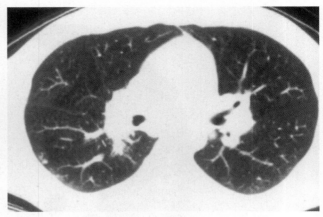

A   B

FIGURE 9-73

FIGURES 9-72 A,B and 9-73 A,B *(continued)*
nodosum), uveitis, arthralgias or polyarthralgias (usually of the foot, ankle, or other large joints), and hilar adenopathy. Lung parenchymal sarcoidosis is not generally appreciated by chest radiograph, as in these cases.

End-stage sarcoidosis

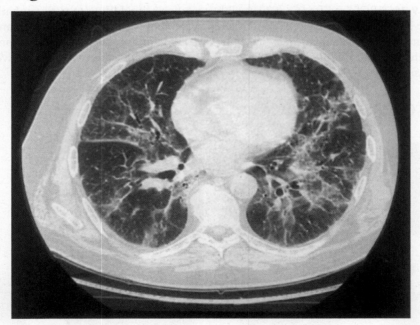

FIGURE 9-74

FIGURES 9-74 and 9-75 A–C: HRCT scans from two patients with end-stage sarcoidosis show extensive lung fibrosis. The fibrotic infiltrative changes have resulted in architectural distortion, including traction bronchiectasis. There is still a relatively central distribution of the fibrotic process that is characteristic of sarcoidosis.

Many of the parenchymal findings on HRCT scans can be considered representations of both reversible and irreversible disease. Nodules, irregularly marginated nodules, and alveolar or pseudoalveolar consolidation are inflammatory lesions that may be reversible with or without therapy, whereas septal thickening, parenchymal bands, and lung distortion are usually fibrotic lesions that are irreversible.

(continued)

End-stage sarcoidosis *(continued)*

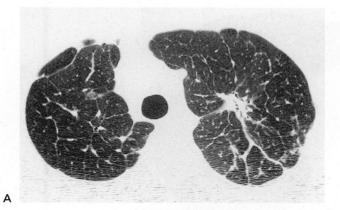

A

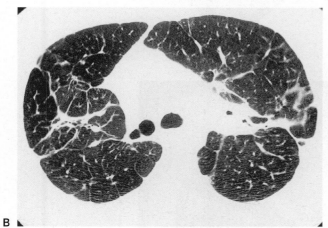

B

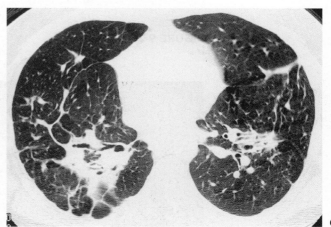

C

FIGURE 9-75

FIGURES 9-74 and 9-75 A–C *(continued)*

End-stage sarcoidosis *(continued)*

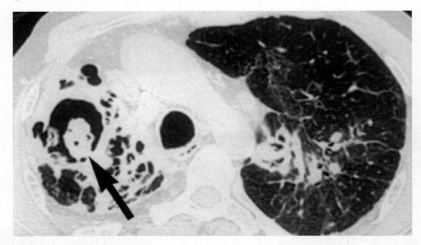

FIGURE 9-76

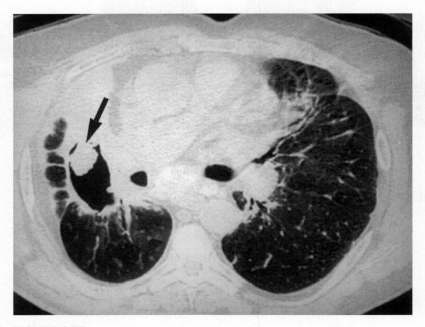

FIGURE 9-77

FIGURES 9-76, 9-77, and 9-78 HRCT scans from three patients with cavitary/cystic sarcoidosis each show aspergillomas in the upper lobe cavities *(arrows)*. There are extensive regions of traction bronchiectasis and architectural distortion, most marked in the upper lobes in these patients with end-stage sarcoidosis. Associated pleural thickening is a common finding with an aspergilloma. Note that Figure 9-77 is an HRCT scan performed in the prone position and shows a mobile mycetoma within this preexisting cavity.

(continued)

End-stage sarcoidosis *(continued)*

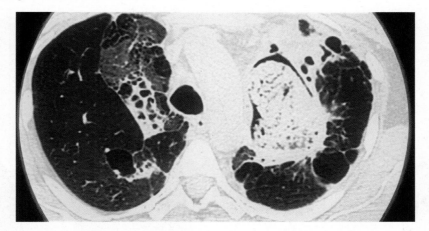

FIGURE 9-78

FIGURES 9-76, 9-77, and 9-78 *(continued)*

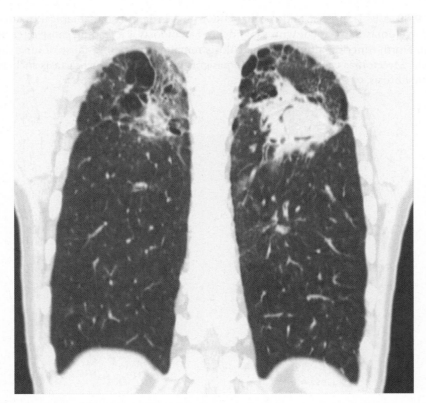

FIGURE 9-79 Coronal HRCT scan from a patient with end-stage sarcoidosis shows typical extensive fibrotic and cystic destruction in both upper lobes with a fungus ball noted within a large cavity in the left upper lobe.

End-stage sarcoidosis *(continued)*

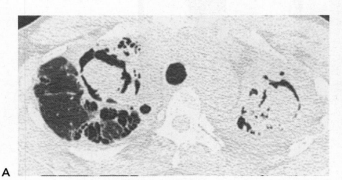

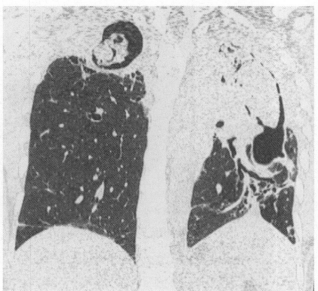

FIGURE 9-80 A,B: Transverse and coronal HRCT images demonstrate biapical cavities containing mycetomas in a patient with sarcoidosis. Sarcoidosis is a leading cause of cavitary disease in North America, although tuberculosis remains the leading cause of lung cavities worldwide. Mycetomas can also develop in patients with severe bronchiectasis such as those with cystic fibrosis.

Sarcoidosis and air trapping

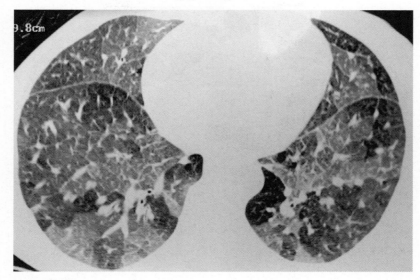

FIGURE 9-81

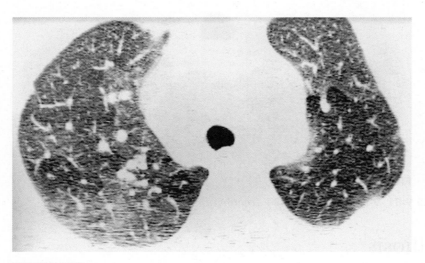

FIGURE 9-82

FIGURES 9-81, 9-82, 9-83, and 9-84 Expiratory HRCT scans from four patients with varying degrees of parenchymal involvement by sarcoidosis show air trapping at the lobular, subsegmental, and segmental airway levels.

Expiratory HRCT is a useful method to assess areas of lung parenchymal air trapping in a variety of lung diseases involving the small and large airways. The cause of the air trapping in patients with sarcoidosis is likely multifactorial, including bronchostenosis, endobronchial granulomas, accumulation of secretions in larger and smaller airways, bronchial hyperreactivity, and associated pulmonary fibrosis.

The air trapping is not specific for a given stage of sarcoidosis or to a specific level of airway obstruction, occurring not only at the level of the secondary lobule but also in smaller and larger airways, at the sublobular, subsegmental, and segmental levels. Air trapping as evidenced by expiratory HRCT is a supportive diagnostic finding of sarcoidosis.

(continued)

Sarcoidosis and air trapping *(continued)*

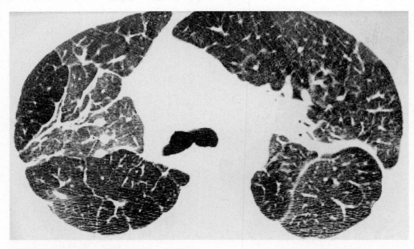

FIGURE 9-83

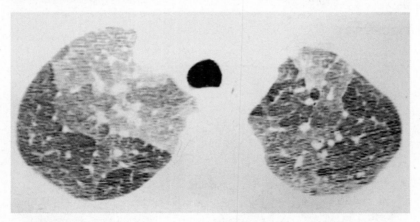

FIGURE 9-84

FIGURES 9-81, 9-82, 9-83, and 9-84 *(continued)*

Berylliosis

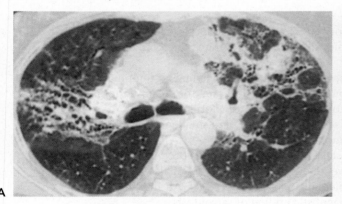

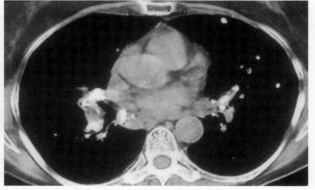

A   B

FIGURE 9-85 A,B: HRCT scan from a patient with berylliosis shows a bilateral, predominantly perihilar, fibrotic, infiltrative process with honeycombing and architectural distortion, including traction bronchiectasis. There are calcified nodules within the parenchymal process as well as calcified hilar and mediastinal nodes.

(continued)

Berylliosis (continued)

FIGURE 9-85 A,B *(continued)*

Berylliosis, in its chronic form, occurs after the chronic inhalation of metal dust that contains beryllium alloys. The major sources of exposure now occur primarily in beryllium-processing plants and the aerospace and nuclear power industries. The findings in berylliosis are indistinguishable from sarcoidosis both radiologically and pathologically. Berylliosis is a systemic disorder that, in its chronic form, produces nonnecrotizing granulomatous and fibrotic disease in the lungs, lymph nodes, pleura, skin, and elsewhere.

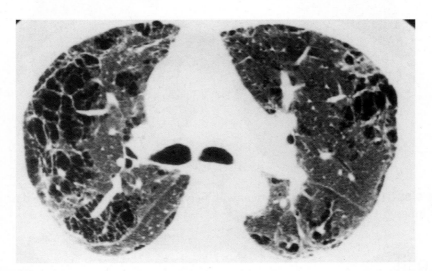

FIGURE 9-86 HRCT scan from a patient in the advanced stage of berylliosis shows a nonspecific, fibrotic, end-stage lung appearance.

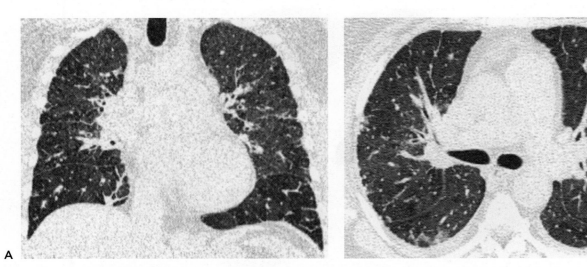

A   B

FIGURE 9-87 A,B: Transverse and coronal HRCT images show multiple discrete tiny nodules predominantly in a perilymphatic distribution in addition to extensive ground-glass opacity. Mild interlobular septal thickening is present, particularly in the mid and lower lung zones.

Berylliosis *(continued)*

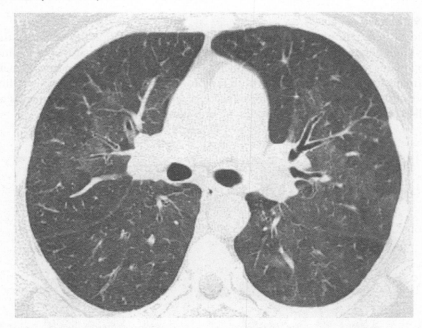

FIGURE 9-88 HRCT image from a patient with berylliosis shows pachy ground-glass opacity in both lungs.

Silicosis

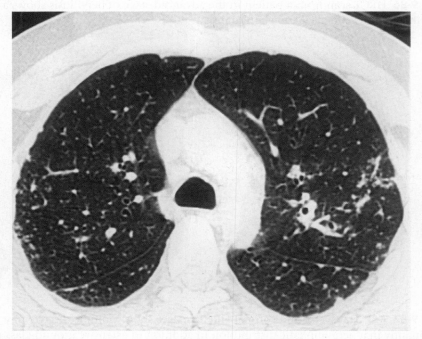

FIGURE 9-89 HRCT scans from a patient with silicosis show characteristic findings of multiple, small, well-circumscribed, rounded nodules in the lung parenchyma that have a predilection for the upper and posterior lung. Some of the nodules are calcified.

Silicosis is caused by inhalation of dust containing high concentrations of crystallized silicon dioxide of or silica dust. Sandblasting and hard rock mining are most frequently

(continued)

Silicosis *(continued)*

FIGURE 8-89 *(continued)*

associated with silicosis. Coal workers' pneumoconiosis results from inhalation of coal dust. The radiographic and CT abnormalities are the same for these two pneumoconioses and are characterized by the presence of small, rounded nodules in the lung parenchyma, predominantly in the upper lobes, especially with milder disease. Nodules are typically centrilobular or subpleural in location, rarely calcified, sharply circumscribed, and usually measure 2 to 5 mm in diameter, although they may be as much as 10 mm in diameter. Eggshell calcification may occur in mediastinal or hilar lymph nodes. These pneumoconioses can progress and be complicated by the development of large massive areas of fibrosis in the upper lung zones. Dyspnea in these patients is usually caused by superimposed pulmonary emphysema rather than the silicotic nodules; the emphysema is easily detected on HRCT.

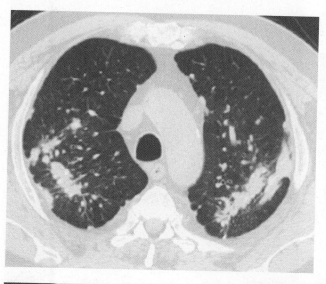

A

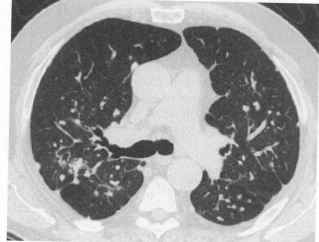

B

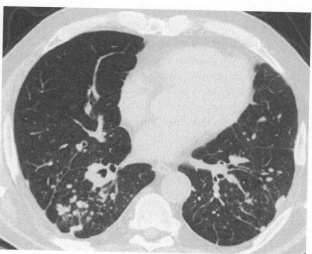

C

FIGURE 9-90 A–C: HRCT scan through the upper mid and lower chest from a patient with silicosis shows characteristic findings of innumerable diffuse small well-circumscribed nodules. The nodules have a predilection for the mid and posterior lung. Some of the nodules are calcified. There are conglomerate masses in the dorsal aspect of the upper lobes. Silicosis results from exposure to high concentrations of silicon dioxide or silica dust. Sandblasting and hard rock mining are most frequently associated with silicosis.

Silicosis *(continued)*

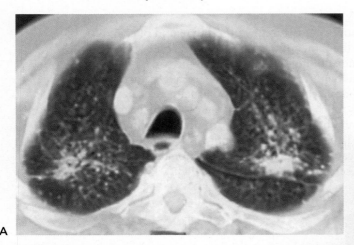

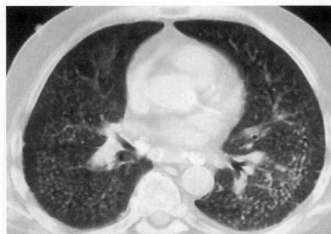

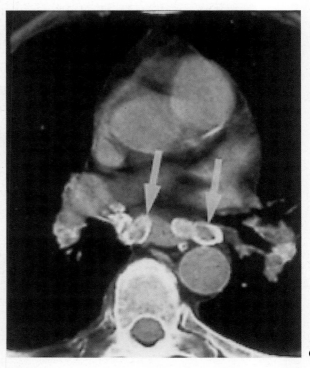

FIGURE 9-91

FIGURES 9-91 A–C and 9-92 A,B: HRCT scans from two patients with silicosis show conglomerate masses, also called *progressive massive fibrosis*, in the upper lungs, indicating complicated silicosis. (Coal worker's pneumoconiosis has a similar appearance.) Conglomerate masses arise from a coalescence of silicotic nodules and tend to develop in the midportion or periphery of the upper lobes and migrate toward the hila. Paracicatricial emphysema usually develops between the conglomerate mass and the pleura. Also, note the typical eggshell calcification of mediastinal nodes (*arrows*). Eggshell calcification may also be seen in sarcoidosis.

(continued)

Silicosis *(continued)*

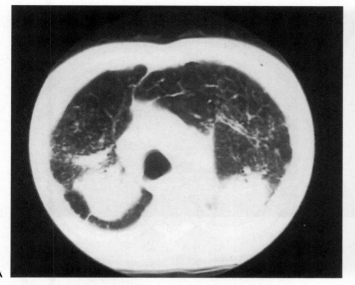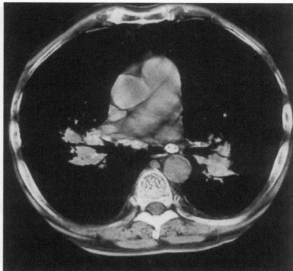

A

B

FIGURE 9-92

FIGURES 9-91 A–C and 9-92 A,B *(continued)*

Alveolar microlithiasis

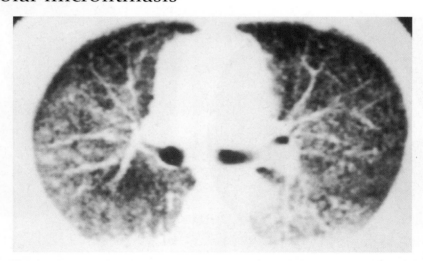

FIGURE 9-93 CT scan from a patient with alveolar microlithiasis shows diffuse, bilateral, tiny, calcified nodules. Differential diagnostic considerations include metastatic calcification, aspiration of barium, talcosis, silicosis, and so forth. Alveolar microlithiasis is a rare disease of unknown etiology characterized by the accumulation of intra-alveolar microliths. Most patients with alveolar microlithiasis are asymptomatic until late in the disease, when pulmonary fibrosis can develop.

Metastatic calcification

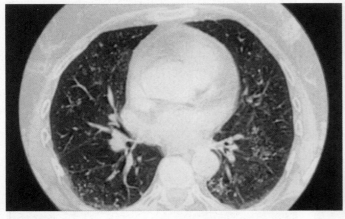

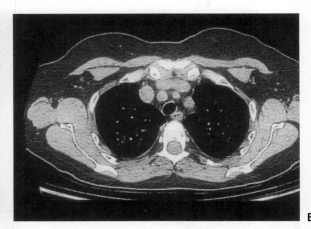

A   B

FIGURE 9-94

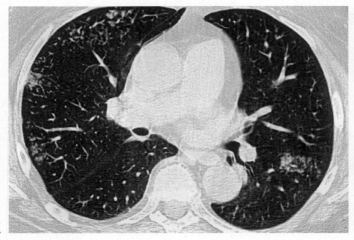

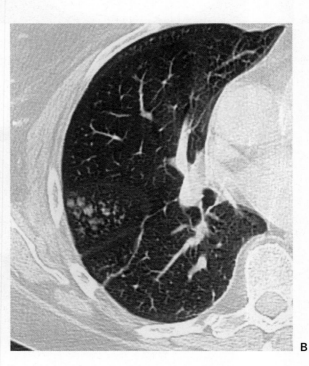

A   B

FIGURE 9-95

FIGURES 9-94 A,B and 9-95 A,B: HRCT scans from two patients with chronic renal failure and secondary hyperparathyroidism show bilateral ill-defined lung nodules, calcified on the soft tissue window settings.

The characteristic appearance of metastatic calcification is multifocal regions of ill-defined, 3- to 10-mm calcified nodules. These nodules, occurring as a precipitation of calcium salts within the lung, are found in patients with hypercalcemia and are usually clinically asymptomatic.

Lymphangitic carcinomatosis

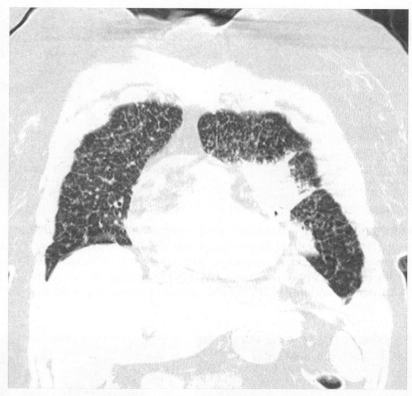

FIGURE 9-96 Coronal HRCT scan through the anterior chest from a 59-year-old woman with a large lingular lung cancer shows diffuse micronodules throughout the lungs, with a particular lymphatic distribution consistent with diffuse lymphangitic carcinomatosis. These nodules are not randomly distributed; note the pattern of nodular, beaded thickening of the many prominent interlobular septa indicating tumor infiltration within the lymphatics.

Erdheim-Chester disease

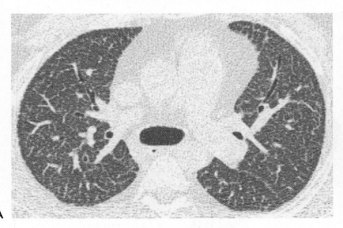
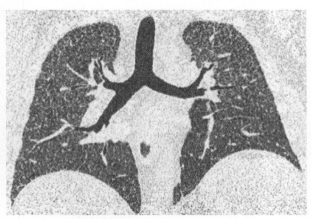

A   B

FIGURE 9-97 **A,B:** Transverse and coronal HRCT images from a patient with Erdheim-Chester disease (ECD) show intralobular reticulation and subpleural nodules. ECD is a non-Langerhans histiocytosis that most commonly affects the bone. Pulmonary involvement is rare and usually portends a poor prognosis. Histiocytes aggregate in the pulmonary lymphatics and HRCT findings can mimic lymphangitic spread of tumor or sarcoidosis.

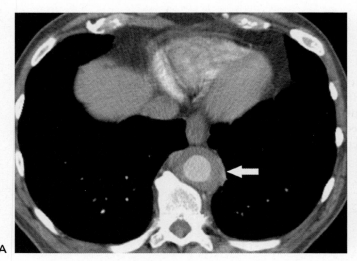
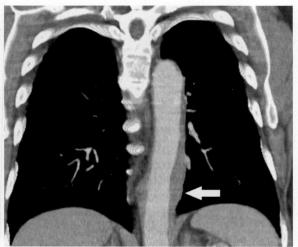

A   B

FIGURE 9-98 **A,B:** Transverse contrast-enhanced CT image and coronal oblique thin-slab volume rendered CT image from a patient with ECD demonstrate infiltrative soft tissue surrounding the descending aorta (*arrows*). Unlike retroperitoneal fibrosis and fibrosing mediastinitis, the infiltrative soft tissue does not compress encased structures. Lymphoma can have a similar appearance.

Idiopathic pulmonary hemosiderosis

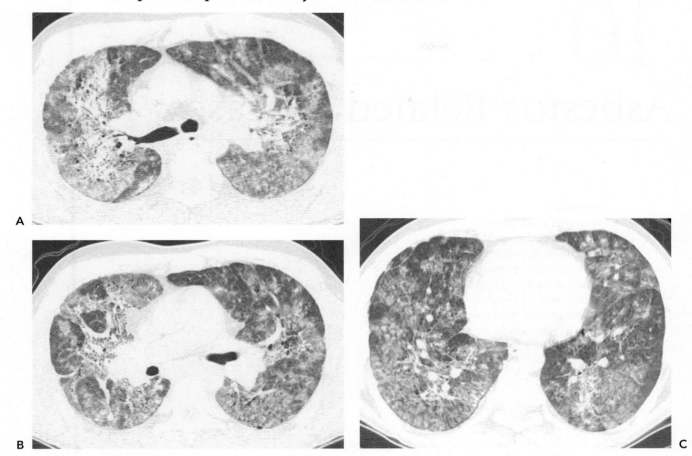

FIGURE 9-99 A–C: HRCT scans through the mid and lower chest from a 27-year-old man with an acute exacerbation of chronic idiopathic pulmonary hemosiderosis show evidence of perihilar lung fibrosis with some retraction and distortion of the central airways as well as areas of more ill-defined confluent acinar/centrilobular nodules reflecting areas of presumed acute pulmonary hemorrhage in the lower lungs. This rare disease is characterized by microcytic iron deficiency anemia and hypoxia resulting from chronic pulmonary hemorrhage of unknown etiology or pathogenesis. CT scanning may show areas of confluent airspace consolidation in the acute setting and a more nonspecific reticulonodular pattern in patients with recurrent or chronic disease.

10

Asbestos-Related Diseases

Asbestosis
Asymmetric asbestosis
Thin, calcified pleural plaques
Thin, noncalcified plaques
Thick, calcified pleural plaques
Pleural plaques
Cardiac surface plaque
Diffuse pleural thickening
Rounded atelectasis
Mesothelioma

Asbestosis

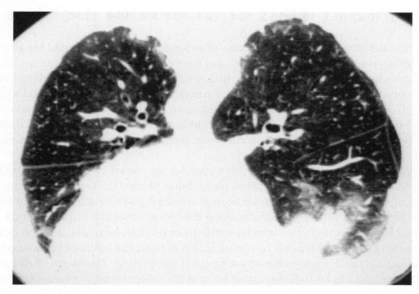

FIGURE 10-1

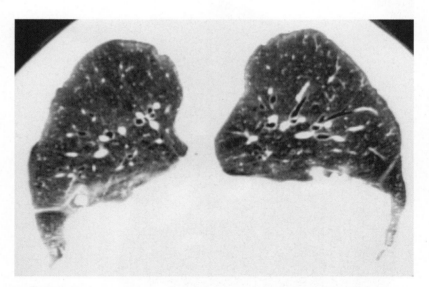

FIGURE 10-2

FIGURES 10-1, 10-2, 10-3, 10-4, 10-5, 10-6, 10-7, 10-8, 10-9, 10-10, 10-11, AND 10-12
Multiple HRCT scans, all from patients with occupational asbestos exposure, show varying degrees of lung fibrosis, from mild to severe, typical of the spectrum of asbestosis evident with HRCT scanning.

Early or mild fibrotic changes are often most evident in the dorsum of the lung, in which case-prone images are useful to distinguish from the normal gravity-dependent opacity that can be present. Many patients with asbestosis will have pleural plaques (*arrows* in Fig. 10-8), which serve as a biomarker of exposure to asbestos particles.

(continued)

Asbestosis *(continued)*

FIGURES 10-1, 10-2, 10-3, 10-4, 10-5, 10-6, 10-7, 10-8 A,B, 10-9, 10-10, 10-11, 10-12 *(continued)*

The earliest detectable HRCT scan features of asbestosis include thickened intralobular core structures, ground-glass lung opacities, and thickened interlobular septa—all with mild lobular architectural distortion (Figs. 10-1, 10-2, 10-3). As fibrosis progresses, larger areas of scarring become evident, with the formation of parenchymal bands (Fig. 10-4) and subpleural lines (Fig. 10-5) with increased architectural distortion. As the fibrosis becomes severe, there is traction bronchiectasis (Figs. 10-6 and 10-7) and honeycombing (Figs. 10-8 to 10-10), often involving more and more lung parenchyma, including the anterior lung as well (Figs. 10-11 and 10-12).

Pathologically, thickened intralobular core structures are caused by peribronchiolar fibrosis. Thickened interlobular septa are a result of interlobular fibrotic thickening or edema. The confluence of subpleural peribronchiolar fibrosis creates the subpleural curvilinear line. Subpleural fibrosis can extend proximally along the bronchovascular bundle to form parenchymal bands. Ground-glass opacities arise from mild alveolar wall and interlobular septal thickening caused by fibrosis or edema that is beyond the limits of resolution of HRCT, causing a generalized increase in background attenuation. Asbestosis often has a UIP-like pattern and can be indistinguishable from IPF except when plagues are present.

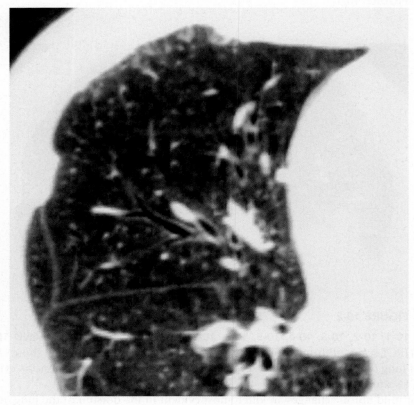

FIGURE 10-3

Asbestosis *(continued)*

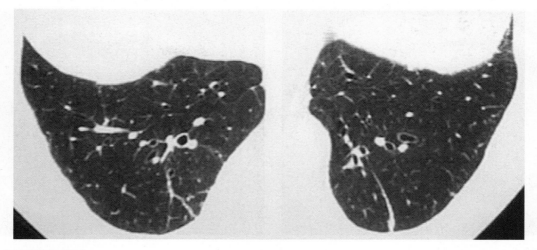

FIGURE 10-4

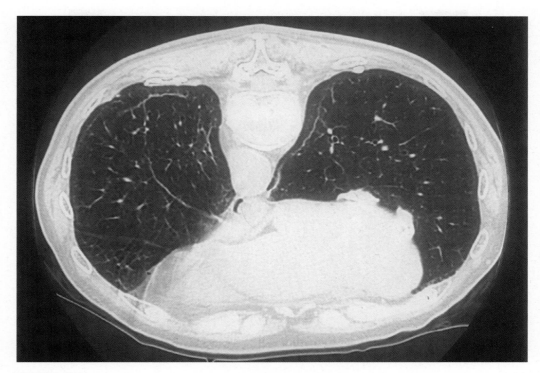

FIGURE 10-5
FIGURES 10-1, 10-2, 10-3, 10-4, 10-5, 10-6 A,B, 10-7, 10-8, 10-9, 10-10, 10-11, and 10-12 *(continued)*

Asbestosis *(continued)*

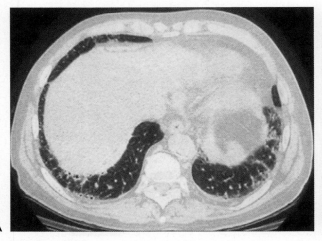

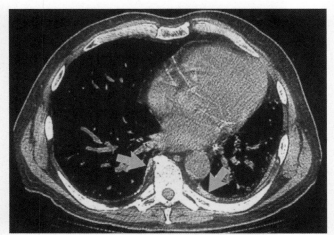

A

B

FIGURE 10-6

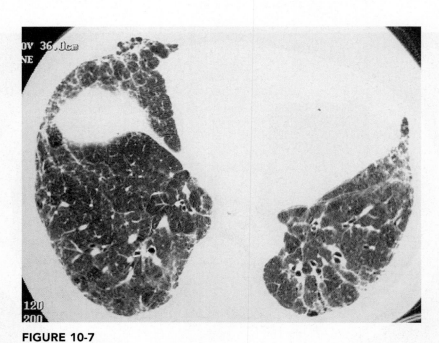

FIGURE 10-7

FIGURES 10-1, 10-2, 10-3, 10-4, 10-5, 10-6 A,B, 10-7, 10-8, 10-9, 10-10, 10-11, and 10-12 *(continued)*

Asbestosis *(continued)*

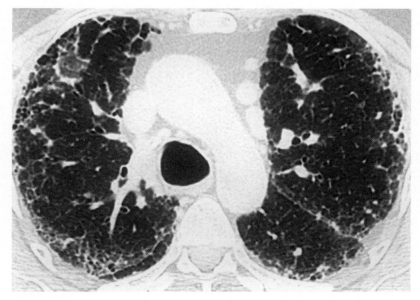

FIGURE 10-8

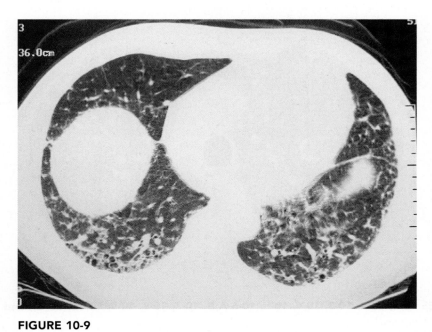

FIGURE 10-9

FIGURES 10-1, 10-2, 10-3, 10-4, 10-5, 10-6 A,B, 10-7, 10-8, 10-9, 10-10, 10-11, and 10-12 *(continued)*

Asbestosis *(continued)*

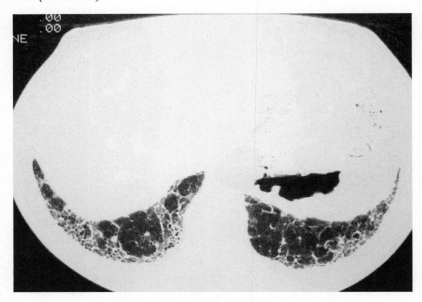

FIGURE 10-10

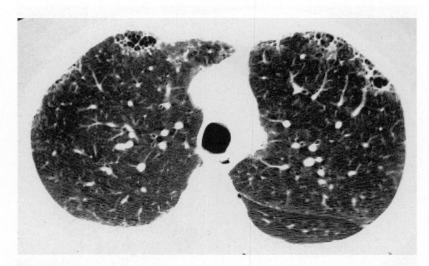

FIGURE 10-11

FIGURES 10-1, 10-2, 10-3, 10-4, 10-5, 10-6 A,B, 10-7, 10-8, 10-9, 10-10, 10-11, and 10-12 *(continued)*

Asbestosis *(continued)*

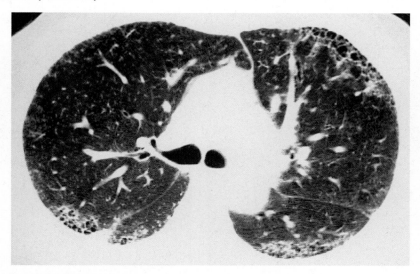

FIGURE 10-12

FIGURES 10-1, 10-2, 10-3, 10-4, 10-5, 10-6 A,B, 10-7, 10-8, 10-9, 10-10, 10-11, and 10-12 *(continued)*

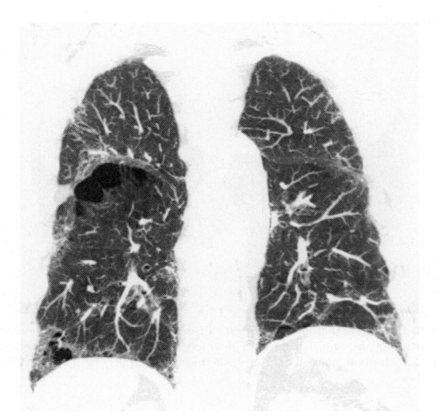

FIGURE 10-13 Coronal reformat HRCT through the posterior chest from a patient with mild asbestosis shows a typical posterior and basilar predominant pattern of lung fibrosis, though not completely sparing the upper lobes. Paraseptal emphysema in the right lower lobe marginates with the upper portion of the right major fissure.

Asbestosis *(continued)*

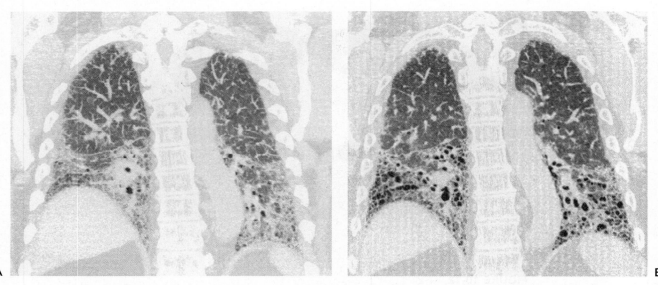

A   **B**

FIGURE 10-14 A,B: Coronal reformat HRCT scans through the posterior chest from a patient with severe asbestosis show the typical basilar predominant pattern of lung fibrosis, in this case much more severe, with areas of end-stage honeycombing involving the majority of the lower lobes and milder interstitial fibrosis involving the peripheral lung up to the lung apices.

Asymmetric asbestosis

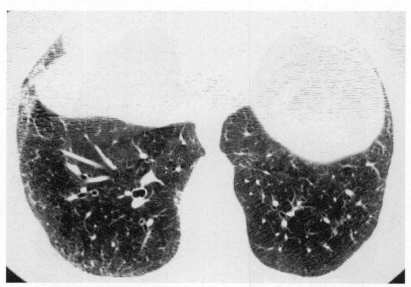

FIGURE 10-15 HRCT scan from a patient with asbestosis shows asymmetric pulmonary fibrosis, involving predominately the right lower lobe, with milder fibrotic changes on the opposite side. This is an unusual pattern of asbestosis.

Thin, calcified pleural plaques

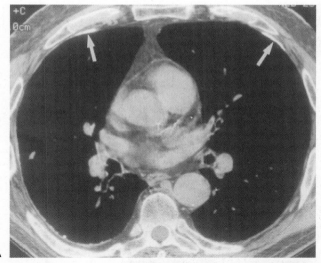

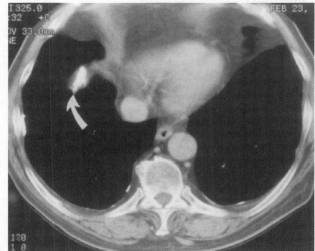

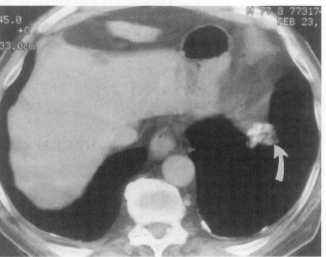

FIGURE 10-16 A–C: HRCT scans show bilateral, thin, partially calcified pleural plaques in typical locations (*arrows*) in this patient with occupational exposure to asbestos. Note the plaques atop each hemidiaphragm (*curved arrows*). Also, note that the plaques are evident inside the normal intercostal fat. This can help distinguish plaques from intercostal vessels.

The plaques are in typical locations. Pleural plaques seen in these typical locations (posterior/paravertebral, anterolateral, and diaphragmatic pleural surfaces) are caused by asbestos exposure; these plaques usually involve the parietal pleura. Approximately 30 years from the time of first exposure to asbestos fibers are needed for a 50% chance of forming pleural plaques. Calcification within plaques suggests a heavier fiber burden. Visceral pleural thickening, best seen in the pleural fissures, can also occur in patients with asbestos exposure and is also related to the years since first asbestos exposure. Pleural plaques are not predictive of asbestosis.

There are five asbestos-related pleural diseases: mesothelioma and four benign pleural reactions—(i) pleural effusions, (ii) calcified or noncalcified pleural plaques, (iii) diffuse pleural thickening, and (iv) rounded atelectasis.

Thin, noncalcified plaques

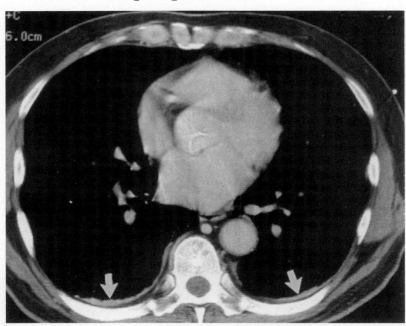

FIGURE 10-17 HRCT scan from this patient with occupational exposure to asbestos shows typical but less extensive bilateral, thin, noncalcified pleural plaques (*arrows*). Note that the plaques are evident inside the normal intercostal fat.

Thick, calcified pleural plaques

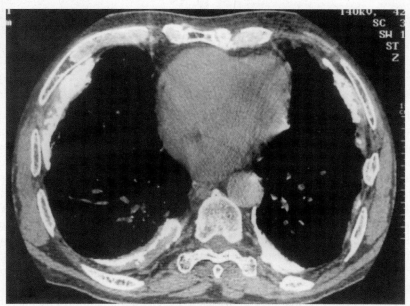

FIGURE 10-18 HRCT scan from a patient with occupational exposure to asbestos shows bilateral extensive, thick, calcified pleural plaques. Again, note that the plaques occur in typical locations: posterior/paravertebral and anterolateral pleural surfaces. Extensive calcified diaphragmatic plaques were also present (not shown).

Thick, calcified pleural plaques *(continued)*

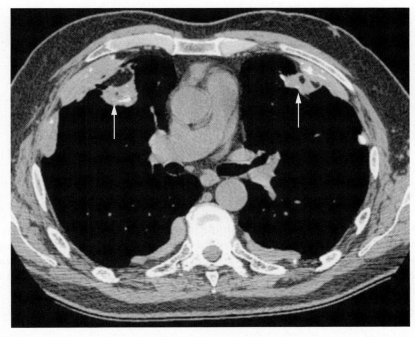

FIGURE 10-19 HRCT scan from a patient with occupational exposure to asbestos again shows bilateral extensive, thick, calcified pleural plaques occurring in typical locations: posterior/paravertebral and anterolateral pleural surfaces. Also note rounded atelatasis bilaterally (*arrows*).

Pleural plaques

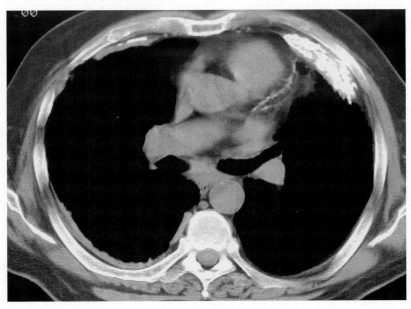

FIGURE 10-20 HRCT scan from a patient with occupational exposure to asbestos shows the variety of pleural plaques that can be evident, even within a single patient. Note both thick and thin, as well as calcified and noncalcified pleural plaques, all evident at the same scan level.

Pleural plaques *(continued)*

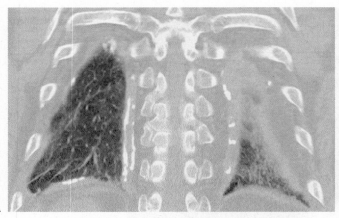
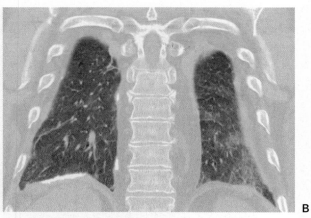

A

B

FIGURE 10-21 A,B: Coronal HRCT scans through the posterior chest from a patient with occupational exposure to asbestos show **(A)** typical calcified pleural plaque over the top of the right hemidiaphragm and noncalcified diffuse pleural thickening in the left hemithorax, again highlighting the occasional variety of appearances within the same patient. In **B**, note the typical calcified pleural plaque in the paravertebral region.

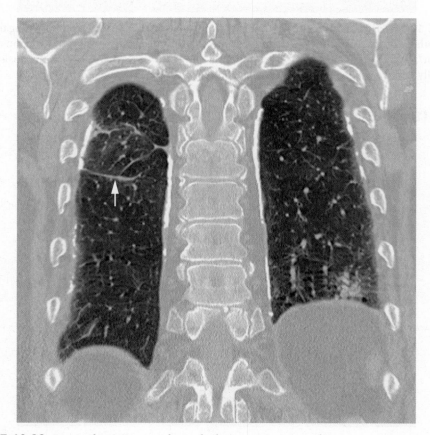

FIGURE 10-22 Coronal HRCT scan through the posterior chest from a patient with occupational exposure to asbestos shows typical calcified pleural plaque, in this case in the paravertebral region of the thorax. Note the associated parenchymal band in the right lung (*arrow*).

Cardiac surface plaque

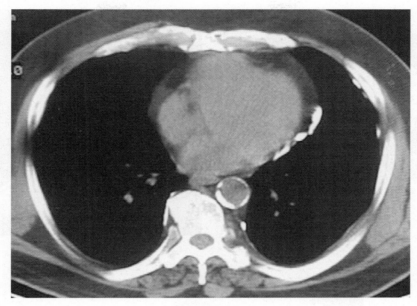

FIGURE 10-23 HRCT scan from a patient with occupational exposure to asbestos shows, in addition to the typical plaque locations, a calcified pleural plaque on the cardiac parietal pleural surface. These plaques are less common.

Diffuse pleural thickening

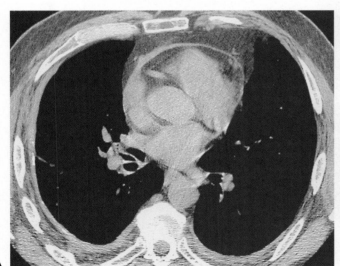 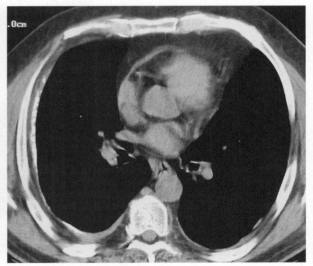

A   B

FIGURE 10-24 A,B: In A, an HRCT scan from a patient with occupational exposure to asbestos shows an area of diffuse pleural thickening with minimal calcification. **B:** A repeat HRCT scan, obtained at the same anatomic level as in **A** 3 years later, shows progressive calcification of the diffuse pleural thickening.

Diffuse pleural thickening is defined as a smooth, noninterrupted pleural opacity extending over at least one fourth of the chest wall. Diffuse pleural thickening is usually caused by the residua of a benign asbestos-related pleuritis with pleural effusion or confluent pleural plaques. As pleural plaques or areas of diffuse pleural thickening become progressively thicker and larger, they can cause varying degrees of restrictive pulmonary function. Associated pulmonary fibrosis is infrequent.

Rounded atelectasis

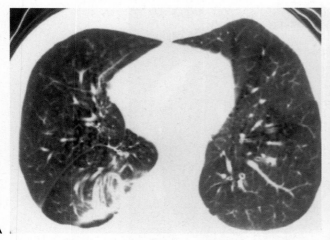
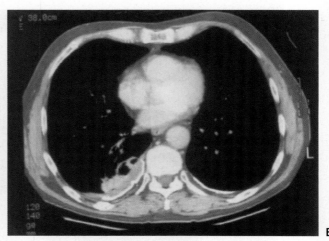

A   B

FIGURE 10-25

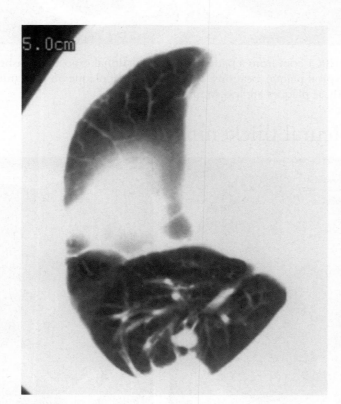

FIGURE 10-26

FIGURES 10-25 A,B, 10-26, and 10-27 HRCT scans from three different patients with rounded atelectasis show the typical wedge-shaped, pleural-based pulmonary opacity with vessels sweeping into the center. Asbestos-related rounded atelectasis is a nonmalignant radiographic consequence of asbestos exposure that can mimic lung cancer. It occurs in the lung periphery; is due to pleural adhesions and fibrosis causing deformation of the lung; and can occur after any insult that causes pleural scarring, including surgery or trauma, as well as asbestos-related pleural disease.

(continued)

Rounded atelectasis *(continued)*

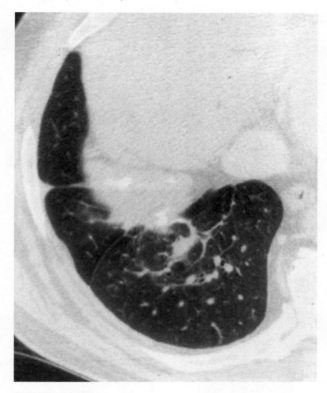

FIGURE 10-27

FIGURES 10-25 A,B, 10-26, and 10-27 *(continued)*

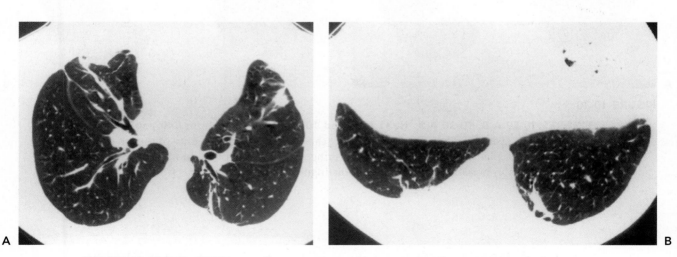

A   B

FIGURE 10-28 A,B: HRCT scans from a patient with occupational exposure to asbestos show four separate and distinct areas of rounded atelectasis, two anteriorly and two posteriorly. Rounded atelectasis is usually a solitary finding, although it may be multiple, as in this case, and can involve any lobe of the lung, although the posterior lung bases are the most common sites.

Rounded atelectasis *(continued)*

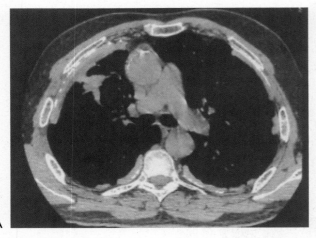
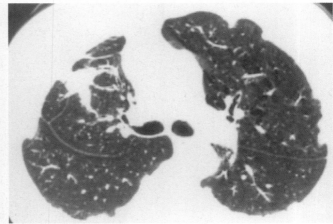

FIGURE 10-29

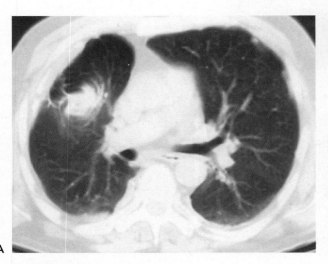
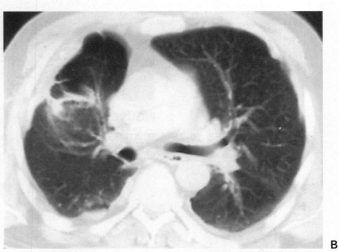

FIGURE 10-30

FIGURES 10-29 A,B, 10-30 A,B, 10-31 A–C, and 10-32 HRCT scans from four patients with rounded atelectasis all show a similarity to lung cancers. Note the contiguity of the "mass," with large, thick pleural plaques as a distinguishing, although not pathognomonic, feature. Sometimes it is impossible to radiologically distinguish rounded atelectasis from a lung cancer.

(continued)

Rounded atelectasis *(continued)*

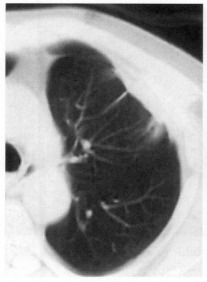
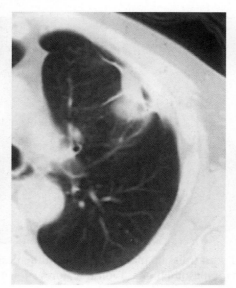
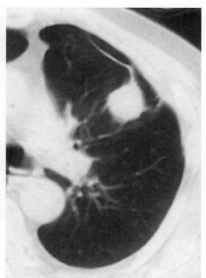

A,B   C

FIGURE 10-31

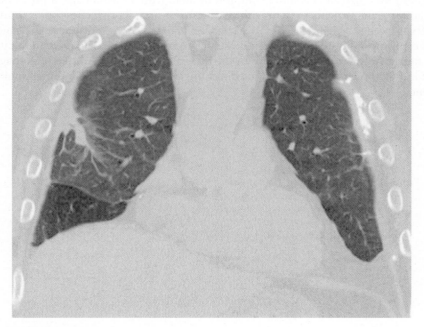

FIGURE 10-32

FIGURES 10-29 A,B, 10-30 A,B, 10-31 A–C, and 10-32 *(continued)*

Mesothelioma

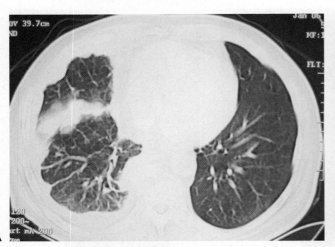
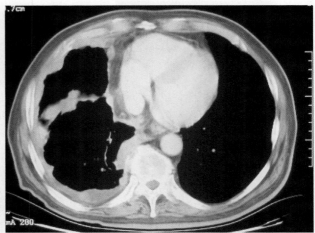

A

B

FIGURE 10-33 A,B: HRCT scan from a patient with occupational exposure to asbestos and right-sided diffuse malignant mesothelioma. Typical features shown here include lobular circumferential thickening of the tumor around the lung, in **A**. In **B**, note the nodular thickening by tumor of the visceral pleural, along the major fissure. Other features that can be seen include pleural effusions, lung parenchyma, mediastinum, or chest wall invasion.

Malignant mesothelioma is more common in men, with a median age at presentation of more than 60 years. Patients present with symptoms of nonpleuritic chest pain, shortness of breath, fever, sweats, weight loss, or fatigability. As many as 80% of cases are associated with asbestos exposure, and the latency period usually exceeds 20 years. The median duration of survival ranges from 4 to 18 months from the time of diagnosis. The differential diagnosis includes indolent pleural granulomatous infections and mesenchymal and metastatic pleural malignancy.

11

Masses

Bronchioloalveolar cell carcinoma
Adenocarcinoma
Carcinoma with eccentric calcification
Carcinoma with dystrophic calcification
Enhancing carcinoma
Adenocarcinoma with hematogenous metastases
Metastases
Mucosa-associated lymphoid tissue lymphoma
Mucosa-associated lymphoid tissue hyperplasia
Non-Hodgkin's lymphoma
Cavitary squamous cell carcinoma
Bilateral adenocarcinomas
Pulmonary hamartoma
Carcinoid tumor
Bronchocele
Focal mucus impaction from endobronchial lesion
Wegener granulomatosis
Sarcoidosis
Silicosis with progressive massive fibrosis
Primary pulmonary amyloidosis

Bronchioloalveolar cell carcinoma

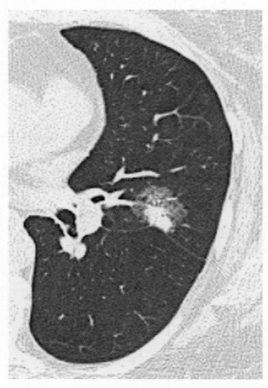

FIGURE 11-1 HRCT image of the left lung shows a mixed attenuation subpleural nodule in the left upper lobe with a halo of ground-glass opacity. Notice slight retraction on the major fissure from the solid component and that the pulmonary vessels pass through the ground-glass component uninterrupted.

Bronchioloalveolar cell carcinoma *(continued)*

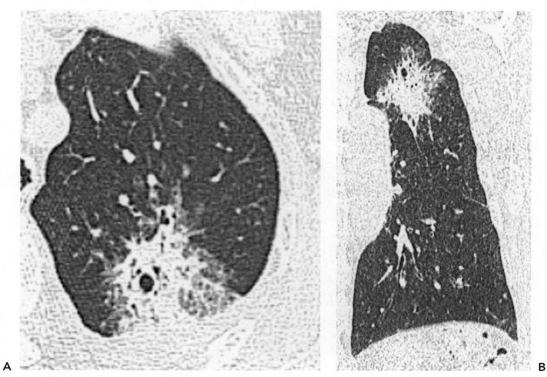

FIGURE 11-2 Transverse **(A)** and coronal **(B)** HRCT images of the left lung show mixed attenuation left upper lobe mass with a solid central component and periphery of ground-glass opacity. In the center of the mass are several "bubble lucencies" or foci of pseudocavitation, a phenomenon that may result from distal airway obstruction from lepidic growth of tumor.

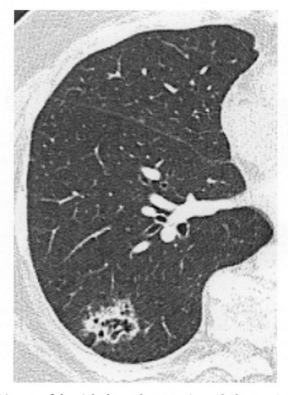

FIGURE 11-3 HRCT image of the right lung shows an irregularly marginated right lower lobe nodule with multiple central pseudocavitations.

Bronchioloalveolar cell carcinoma *(continued)*

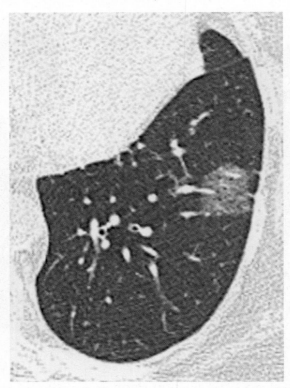

FIGURE 11-4 HRCT image of the left lung shows a pure ground-glass attenuation nodule in the left lower lobe, proven to be bronchioloalveolar carcinoma (BAC) on resection. Ground-glass attenuation BACs may either slowly enlarge or gradually become more solid over time. As these neoplasms may have slower growth rates, long-term follow-up may be required.

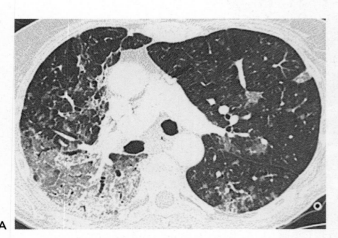
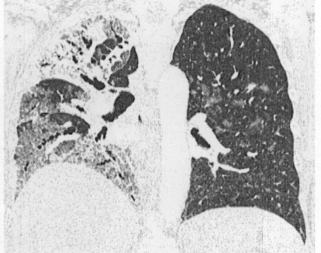

A   B

FIGURE 11-5 Transverse **(A)** and coronal **(B)** HRCT images from a patient with disseminated bronchioloalveolar carcinoma show patchy ground-glass opacity, more extensive in the right lung, and patchy right lung consolidation. There is right upper lobe volume loss with central varicoid bronchiectasis.

Bronchioloalveolar cell carcinoma *(continued)*

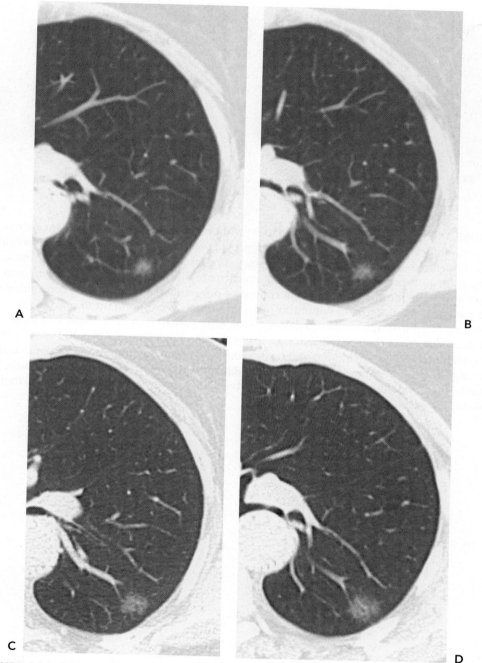

FIGURE 11-6 A–D: Sequential HRCT images each approximately 1 year apart show slow growth of the left lower lobe ground-glass attenuation nodule. Bronchioloalveolar carcinoma can demonstrate growth on HRCT by enlargement, increasing attenuation, or both.

Bronchioloalveolar cell carcinoma *(continued)*

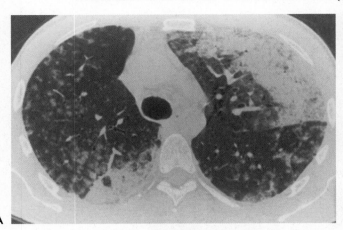
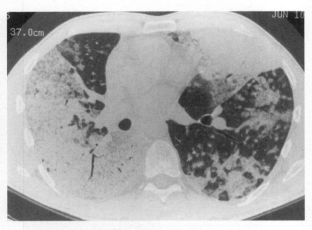

A   B

FIGURE 11-7 A,B: HRCT scans from a patient with multifocal bronchioloalveolar carcinoma show multifocal regions of consolidated parenchyma with air bronchograms as well as multiple, ill-defined, small, rounded opacities, suggesting endobronchial dissemination. These features are nonspecific and may represent any airspace-filling process, such as pneumonia or pulmonary hemorrhage. The clinical context of nonresolving or progressive consolidation in a patient lacking signs and symptoms of an infection is very important in making the diagnosis of bronchioloalveolar carcinoma. Also, note a small area in the right mid lung **(B)** that even shows the nonspecific "crazy paving" appearance. Approximately 15% to 25% of bronchioloalveolar carcinomas will be disseminated at presentation; when disseminated, as above, the tumor is unresectable and the prognosis is very poor. Differential diagnostic considerations would include lymphoproliferative disease, cryptogenic organizing pneumonia and chronic eosinophilic pneumonia.

Bronchioloalveolar cell carcinoma *(continued)*

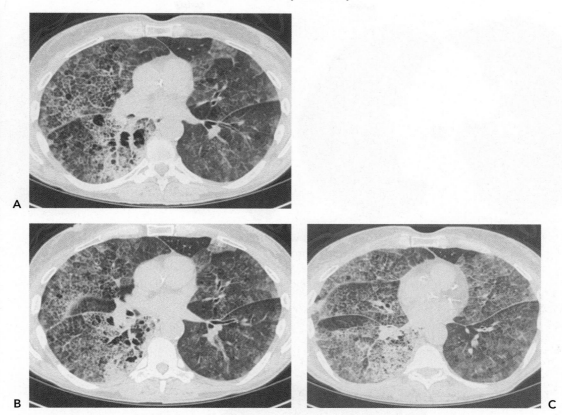

FIGURE 11-8 A–C: Bronchioloalveolar carcinoma is a distinct form of adenocarcinoma. Its CT appearance may be a focal nodule, segmental or lobar consolidation, or a diffuse pattern. This high-resolution CT scan shows diffuse infiltrative bronchioloalveolar carcinoma. Note diffuse ground-glass opacity superimposed on interlobular septal thickening. Differential diagnosis would include pulmonary alveolar proteinosis, congestive heart failure and pulmonary veno-occlusive disease. Note relative sparing of anatomic lobular and multilobular regions.

Bronchioloalveolar cell carcinoma *(continued)*

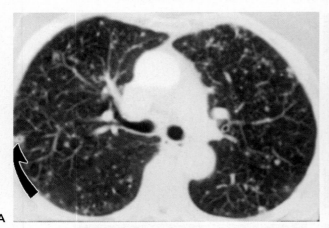
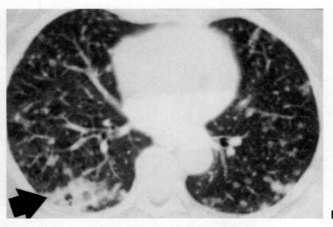

A   B

FIGURE 11-9 A,B: CT scans from a patient with multifocal bronchioloalveolar carcinoma show a diffuse, small, nodular infiltrative process throughout both lungs with no basilar, apical, central, or peripheral predominance. Some of the nodules were cavitated (*curved arrow*). There was a focal region of masslike consolidation in the posterior and lateral basal segments of the right lower lobe (*arrow*).

Adenocarcinoma

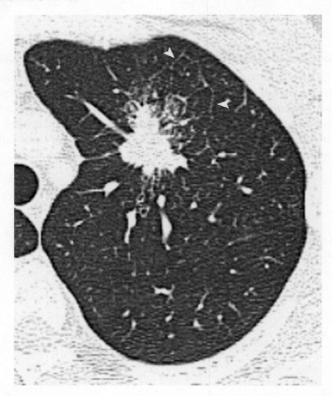

FIGURE 11-10 HRCT image of the left lung shows a spiculated upper lobe mass with surrounding ground-glass attenuation. Adjacent interlobular septal thickening represents local lymphangitic spread of carcinoma. Adenocarcinomas can induce a desmoplastic reaction in lung, leading to their spiculated appearances.

Adenocarcinoma *(continued)*

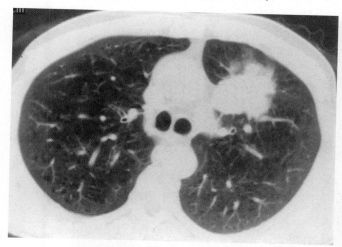
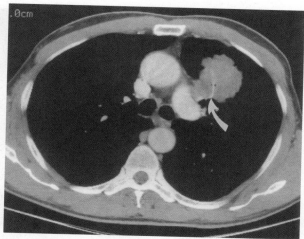

FIGURE 11-11 A,B: CT scan from a patient with a left upper lobe adenocarcinoma **(A)** shows enhancing pulmonary vessels *(arrow)* **(B)** within the low-density (water) mass (the CT angiogram sign). This is a nonspecific sign that is suggestive of malignancy but can be seen in other etiologies of lung consolidation.

Carcinoma with eccentric calcification

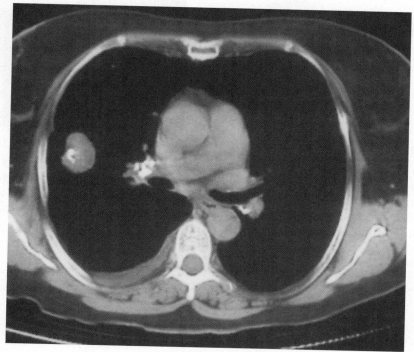

FIGURE 11-12 CT scan shows a 2.5-cm nodule in the right upper lobe that contains eccentric calcification and calcified hilar lymph nodes. Because eccentric calcification is an indeterminate indicator of benignity, the lung nodule was resected and proved to be an adenocarcinoma. The calcification was a granuloma that had been engulfed by the bronchogenic carcinoma. This lung cancer may have developed as a "scar carcinoma." To be considered benign, calcification must be central, diffuse, laminated, or chondroid ("popcorn").

Carcinoma with dystrophic calcification

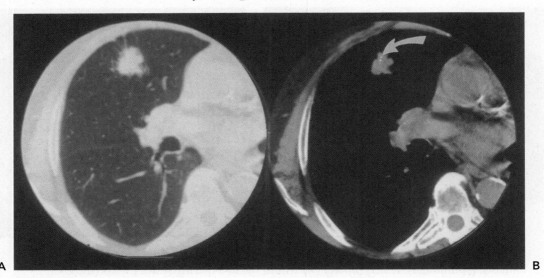

A   B

FIGURE 11-13

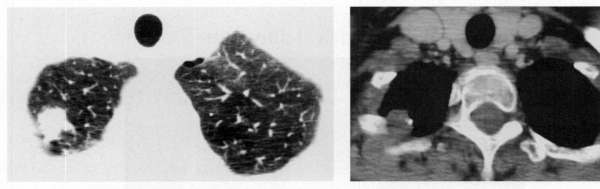

A   B

FIGURE 11-14

FIGURES 11-13 A,B and 11-14 A,B: HRCT scans from two different patients show a small amount of eccentric calcification (*arrow*) within lobulated, spiculated mass in the right upper lobe. Eccentric calcification is not indicative of benignity. There is no evidence of fat within the mass to suggest a diagnosis of hamartoma, as in Figure 11-26. After surgical resection, these were both shown to be squamous cell carcinomas with dystrophic calcification.

Enhancing carcinoma

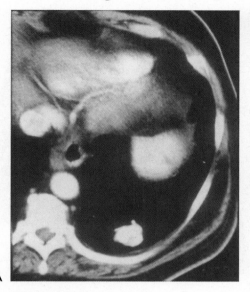
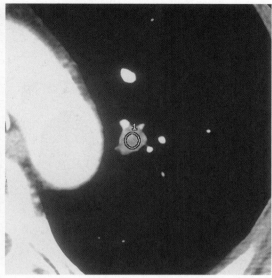

A

B

FIGURE 11-15 A,B: Contrast-enhanced CT scan shows a 2.5-cm homogeneously dense nodule in the left lower lobe. It appears to be "calcified" in a benign pattern. Thin sections through this nodule 5 minutes after this image was obtained showed no evidence of calcification. The apparent calcification was caused by intense enhancement of this vascular primary adenocarcinoma of the lung. This is a pitfall that one needs to be aware of, particularly with fast CT scanners. Lung nodule enhancement can be an indication of malignancy.

Measurement of lung nodule enhancement at CT may be helpful in distinguishing benign from malignant lesions. Nodules that enhance less than 15 Hounsfield units over a 4-minute period after injection of contrast material are highly likely to be benign. Nodules that enhance more than 15 Hounsfield units are slightly more likely to be malignant than benign. In a large multicenter study, nodule enhancement at CT was evaluated and found to have a sensitivity of 98% and a specificity of 58%. Nodule in **B** is a 1.5-cm radiologically indeterminate nodule. It did not enhance after intravenous administration of iodine and contrast material. It has been stable for a period of 4 years and should be benign. This is most likely a granuloma.

Adenocarcinoma with hematogenous metastases

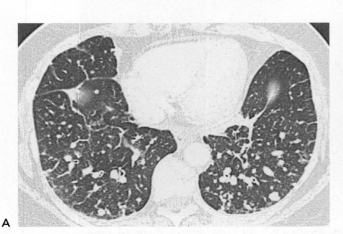

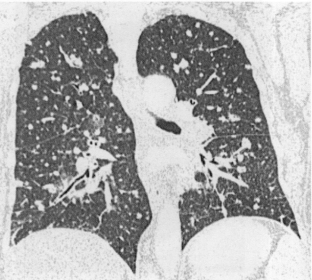

A

B

FIGURE 11-16 A,B: Transverse and coronal HRCT images from a patient with metastatic adenocarcinoma of unknown primary show innumerable nodules present throughout the lungs. Foci of interlobular septal thickening, most pronounced in the lower lobes, represent lymphangitic spread of tumor. Septal thickening in lymphangitic carcinomatosis can be smooth or nodular.

Metastases

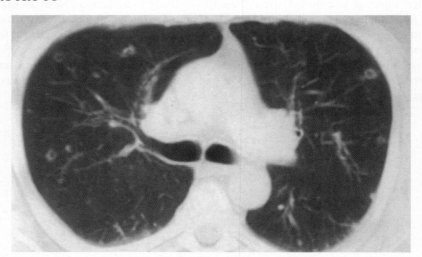

FIGURE 11-17 CT scan from a patient with metastatic pancreatic adenocarcinoma shows multiple, bilateral, small pulmonary nodules, many of which are cavitated. Other differential diagnostic possibilities include disseminated granulomatous infection, lymphoproliferative disorder, and, less commonly, Wegener granulomatosis.

Metastases *(continued)*

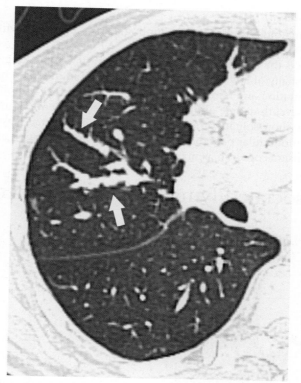

FIGURE 11-18 HRCT image from a patient with metastatic renal cell carcinoma shows dilated right upper lobe pulmonary vessels, which have a beaded appearance.

Mucosa-associated lymphoid tissue lymphoma

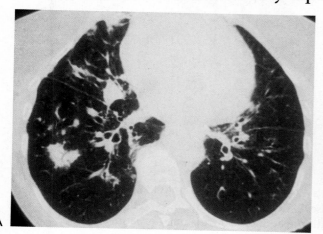
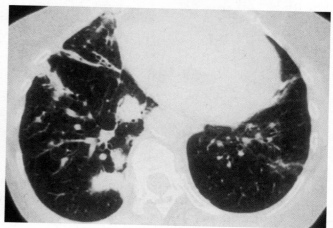

A   B

FIGURE 11-19 **A,B:** HRCT scans from a 59-year-old woman with Sjögren's syndrome show multiple areas of dense opacification in the right middle and lower lobe with prominent air bronchograms. Biopsy showed a low-grade B-cell lymphoma [mucosa-associated lymphoid tissue (MALT) type].

This tissue is a component of the much more extensive mucosa-associated lymphoid tissue (MALT) present in the gastrointestinal tract, lung, thyroid, breast, bladder, skin, and salivary glands. MALT is not prominent in normal lungs but is acquired under conditions of chronic pulmonary infections or in the setting of collagen vascular diseases, such as Sjögren's

Mucosa-associated lymphoid tissue lymphoma *(continued)*

FIGURE 11-19 *(continued)*

syndrome and rheumatoid arthritis. MALT lymphoma arises from cells within these lymphoid follicles.

MALT lymphoma is the most common primary lymphoma of the lung, present in 74% to 78% of cases. It is usually of low histologic grade and B-cell immunophenotype. Most are stage I or II at presentation and remain localized to the lung. MALT lymphoma typically occurs in the sixth or seventh decade of life and has an equal incidence in men and women.

CT scans typically show solitary or multiple nodules, parenchymal masses with air bronchograms, or a reticulonodular pattern. Hilar adenopathy and cavitation are uncommon findings. Pleural effusions occur in as many as 25% of patients.

Mucosa-associated lymphoid tissue hyperplasia

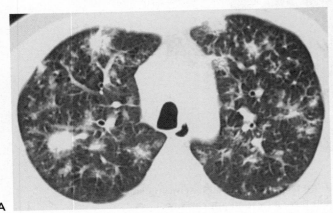

A

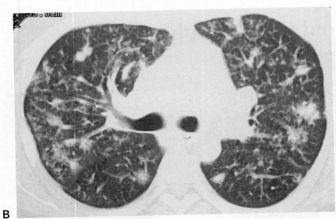

B

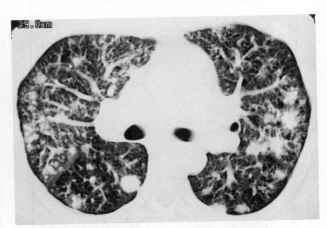

C

FIGURE 11-20 A–C: Multiple HRCT scans from a 42-year-old man with polyclonal MALT hyperplasia show multiple bilateral areas of dense, ill-defined opacification, as well as more discrete mass formation. Tissue is necessary for diagnosis and distinguishing polyclonal disease from monoclonal disease.

Non-Hodgkin's lymphoma

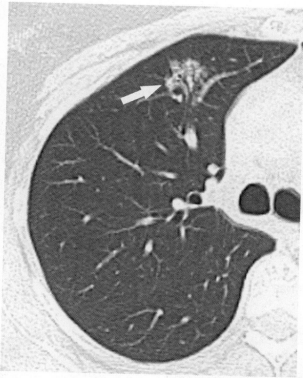

FIGURE 11-21 HRCT image of the right lung demonstrates a mixed-attenuation nodule in the anterior segment of the right upper lobe (*arrow*), shown to be non-Hodgkin's lymphoma arising in the MALT. MALTomas are usually low-grade lymphomas, which usually grow around airways. Air bronchograms may be present.

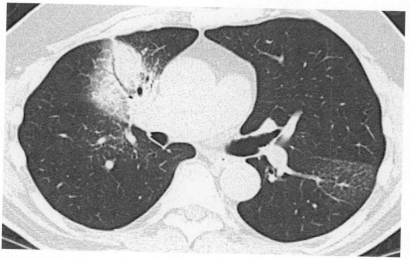

FIGURE 11-22 HRCT image from a patient with primary pulmonary extramarginal B-cell non-Hodgkin's lymphoma shows masslike consolidation in the anterior segment of the right upper lobe with air bronchograms, ground-glass opacity, and interlobular septal thickening in the periphery. In the left lower lobe is a more subtle focus of ground-glass opacity with superimposed interlobular septal thickening. Primary pulmonary lymphoma is uncommon, occurring far less frequently than secondary lymphomatous involvement of the lung. Round pneumonia, cryptogenic organizing pneumonia, bronchioloalveolar carcinoma, and even sarcoidosis can have a similar appearance.

Cavitary squamous cell carcinoma

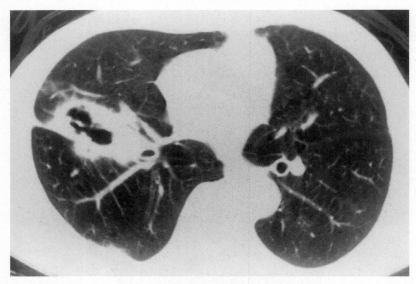

FIGURE 11-23

A 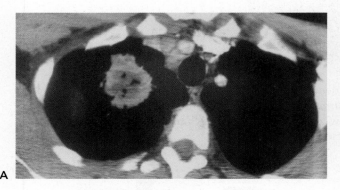 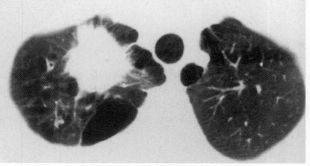 B

FIGURE 11-24

FIGURES 11-23 and 11-24 A,B: CT scans from two patients with squamous cell carcinoma of the lung show large lung masses with central necrosis and cavitation. Squamous cell carcinomas, closely associated with cigarette smoking, are the most common lung malignancies to cavitate, especially with increasing size.

Bilateral adenocarcinomas

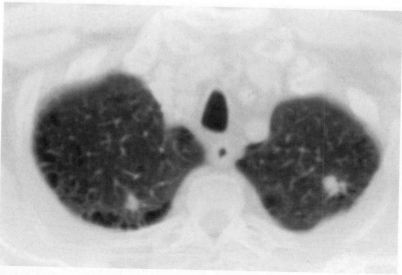

FIGURE 11-25 CT scan shows bilateral apical spiculated lung masses surgically proved to be synchronous lung cancers. The incidence of detection of multiple primary bronchogenic carcinomas has increased with the advent of CT; incidence is generally considered to be 1% of lung cancers. Most patients are heavy smokers. Multiple primary bronchogenic carcinomas may be bilateral, synchronous, or metachronous. Mild paraseptal emphysema is present.

Pulmonary hamartoma

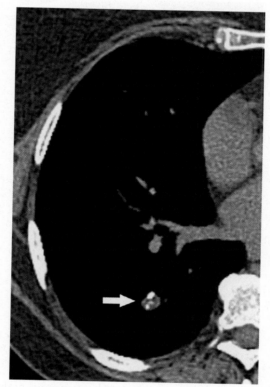

FIGURE 11-26 CT image of right lung shows heterogeneous lower lobe nodule (*arrow*) with coarse calcification and foci of macroscopic fat. The presence of macroscopic fat is essentially diagnostic for pulmonary hamartoma.

Pulmonary hamartoma *(continued)*

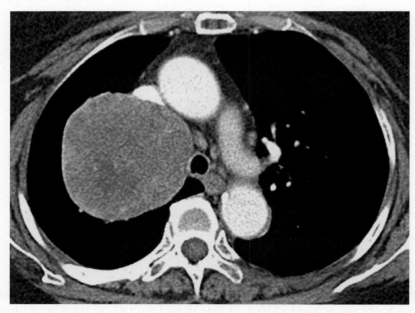

FIGURE 11-27 Contrast-enhanced CT image demonstrates a large, heterogeneous mass in the right lung compressing the superior vena cava and mediastinum. This was proven to be a hamartoma at resection. The majority of hamartomas are smaller than 4 cm, and, because of their peripheral predominance, most do not cause symptoms.

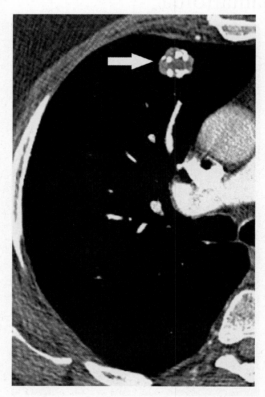

FIGURE 11-28 Contrast-enhanced CT image shows a heterogenous nodule in the right middle lobe (*arrow*) that contains coarse "popcorn" calcification and several foci of macroscopic fat. The presence of either macroscopic fat or "popcorn" calcification is nearly pathognomonic for pulmonary hamartomas.

Pulmonary hamartoma *(continued)*

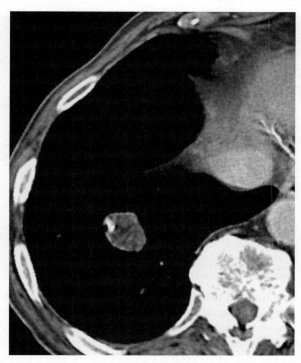

FIGURE 11-29 Contrast-enhanced CT image demonstrates a heterogenous right lower lobe nodule with a single coarse calcification and multiple foci of macroscopic fat. Pulmonary hamartomas are not true hamartomas and are more likely benign neoplasms or "mesenchymomas", as they develop later in life and can slowly grow over time.

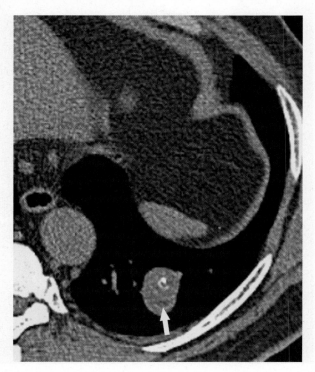

FIGURE 11-30 Unenhanced CT image shows a heterogeneous left lower lobe nodule with a focal coarse calcification and a tiny focus of macroscopic fat (*arrow*). Pulmonary hamartomas demonstrate little to no 18-fluoro-deoxyglucose (FDG) uptake on positron emission tomography (PET) imaging. If necessary, the diagnosis can often be confirmed on transthoracic core needle biopsy.

Carcinoid tumor

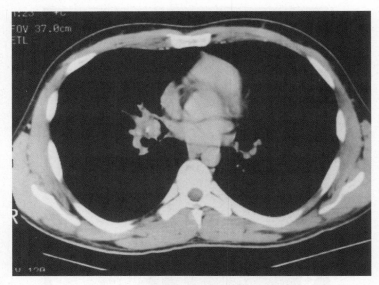

FIGURE 11-31 CT scan through the right hilum shows a 2-cm mass with central calcification, in this case, a carcinoid tumor. CT detection of calcification within carcinoid tumors is not uncommon and was seen in approximately 40% of central carcinoid tumors in one series. Ossification, by one of the bioactive secretions of the tumor, is induced in the surrounding bronchial cartilage. This explains two features: the chunky nature of the "calcifications" and the predominance of this finding in central carcinoid tumors versus the relative lack of calcification in peripheral carcinoid tumors, where the bronchial cartilage is not present.

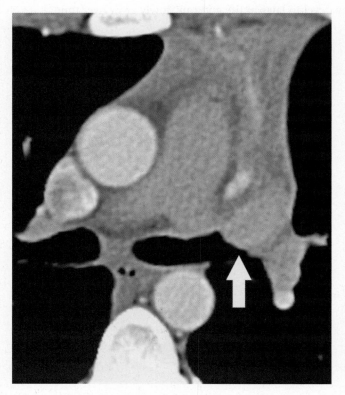

FIGURE 11-32 Contrast-enhanced CT image shows a smooth, ovoid nodule in the left upper lobe bronchus (*arrow*) resulting in left upper lobe collapse. Endobronchial carcinoids usually have smooth borders, enhance homogenously, and grow along the long axis of the airway. Carcinoids are low-grade malignant neoplasms, which are a part of the neuroendocrine tumors of the lung that also include large cell neuroendocrine tumor and small cell lung carcinoma.

Carcinoid tumor *(continued)*

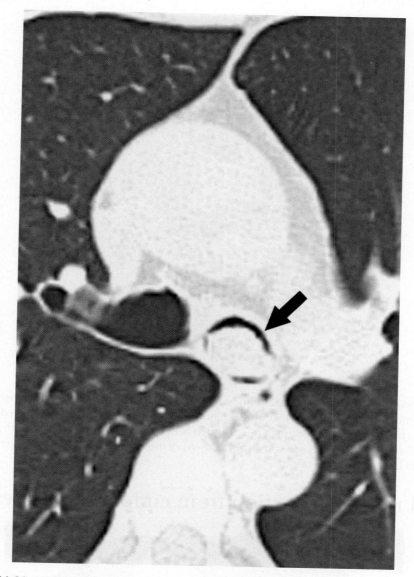

FIGURE 11-33 HRCT image at the level of the tracheal carina shows a soft tissue nodule in the left main bronchus. Patients with endobronchial carcinoids may present with signs and symptoms of large airway obstruction including cough, wheezing, lobar collapse, and recurrent pneumonia.

Bronchocele

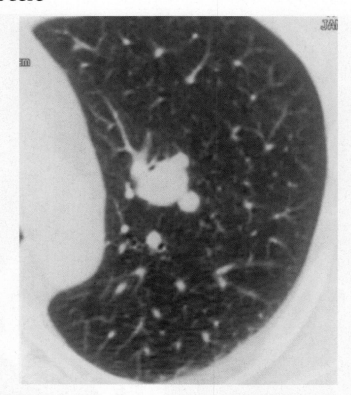

FIGURE 11-34 HRCT scan shows a rounded mass in the left upper lobe, closely associated with the bronchovascular bundle of the anterior segment. Contiguous scans showed this "mass" to be tubular, representing a mucus-filled bronchocele distal to an atretic airway of bronchial atresia. Expiratory CT scans (not shown) demonstrated air trapping in the anterior segmental bronchus distribution.

Focal mucus impaction from endobronchial lesion

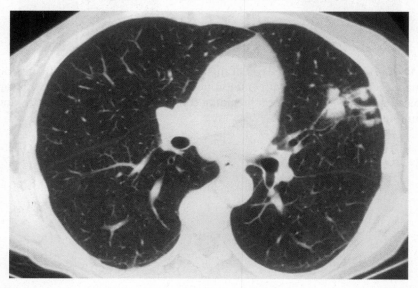

FIGURE 11-35 HRCT scan shows focal, dilatated, impacted bronchi in a segmental distribution, peripheral to a nodular mass. This mucus retention was secondary to an endobronchial non–small cell carcinoma. Focal mucus impaction, particularly in the absence of other signs of inflammatory small airway disease, should raise concern for neoplastic endobronchial obstruction.

Wegener granulomatosis

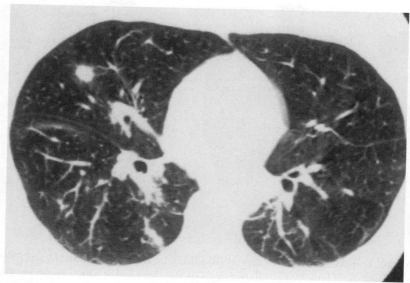

FIGURE 11-36 CT scan from a patient with Wegener granulomatosis shows multiple pulmonary nodules with irregular margins.

   Wegener granulomatosis is characterized on CT scans as multiple nodules or masses with irregular margins, often with cavitation, and peripheral pulmonary consolidations resembling pulmonary infarcts. Angiocentric forms of granulomatous vasculitis of the lung, as opposed to bronchocentric granulomatosis, include Wegener granulomatosis, allergic angiitis, lymphomatoid granulomatosis, and necrotizing sarcoid granulomatosis. Wegener granulomatosis is a well-defined syndrome characterized by necrotizing granulomatous vasculitis of the upper and lower respiratory tracts, segmental necrotizing glomerulonephritis, and systemic small vessel vasculitis. In Wegener granulomatosis, improvement occasionally occurs in one area while disease progresses elsewhere in the lung.

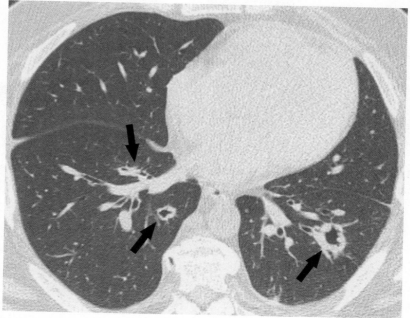

FIGURE 11-37 HRCT image from a patient with active Wegener granulomatosis shows scattered small cavitary nodules in both lungs (*arrows*). The cavities have irregular thick walls and vary in size.

Wegener granulomatosis *(continued)*

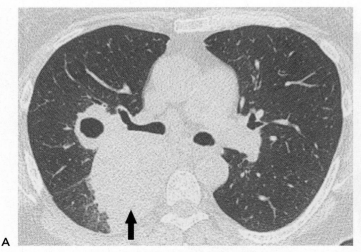
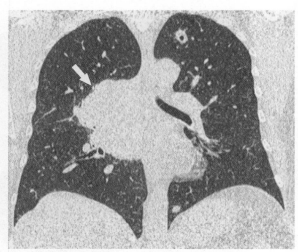

A   B

FIGURE 11-38 Transverse **(A)** and coronal **(B)** HRCT images from a patient with Wegener granulomatosis show a large consolidated mass in the right lower lobe (*arrows*) and a cavitary left upper lobe nodule. Nodules and masses in active Wegener granulomatosis usually vary in size and degree of cavitation, although cavitation is more common in larger masses. Lung masses of Wegener granulomatosis often cavitate when the diameter is more than 2 cm. Differential diagnostic considerations include bronchioloalveolar carcinoma, lymphoma, metastasis, disseminated granulomatous infection, sarcoidosis, and Wegener granulomatosis.

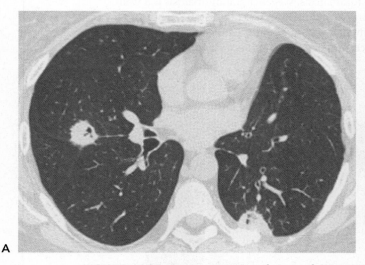
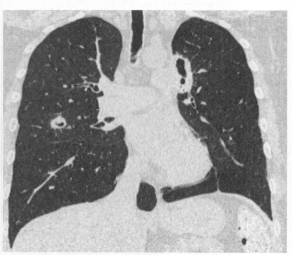

A   B

FIGURE 11-39 Transverse **(A)** and coronal **(B)** HRCT images from a patient with Wegener granulomatosis show scattered nodules in both lungs with varying degrees of cavitation.

Wegener granulomatosis *(continued)*

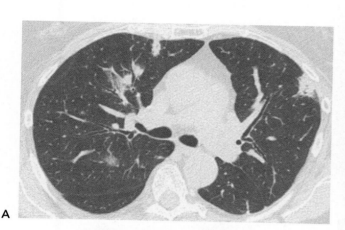

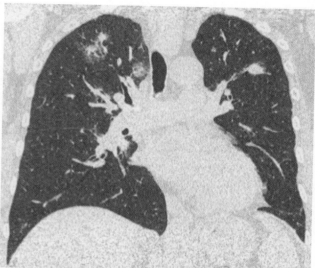

FIGURE 11-40 A Transverse and **B** coronal HRCT images from a patient with Wegener granulomatosis demonstrate multiple foci of nodular consolidation and ground-glass opacity. Hemorrhage is often present in active Wegener granulomatosis and may manifest as ground-glass opacity, consolidation, or both.

Sarcoidosis

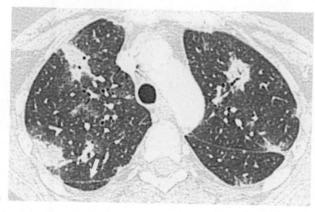

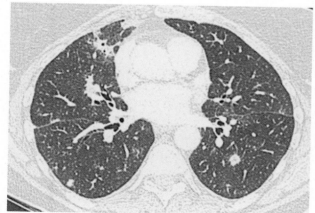

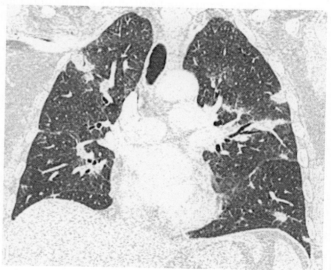

FIGURE 11-41 A–C: Transverse and coronal HRCT images from a patient with sarcoidosis show multiple nodular and masslike foci of peribronchial consolidation. Note the similarity to Wegener granulomatosis. Small perilymphatic nodules are also present along the right major fissure.

Silicosis with progressive massive fibrosis

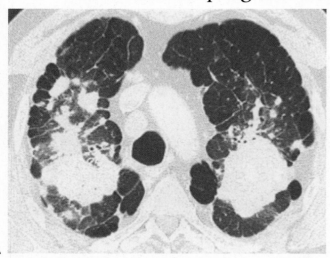

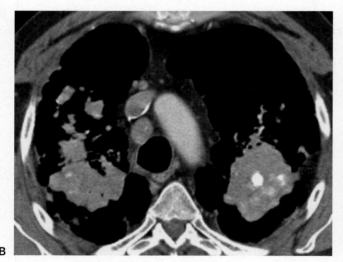

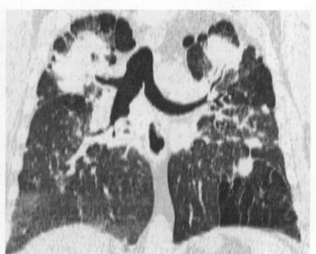

FIGURE 11-42 A,B: Transverse HRCT images (lung and mediastinal window settings) show heterogenous soft tissue masses in the upper lobes with adjacent smaller nodules, architectural distortion, and paracicatricial emphysema. An enlarged right paratracheal lymph node is present. **C:** Coronal reformation shows bilateral upper lobe volume loss with upward retraction of both hila.

Primary pulmonary amyloidosis

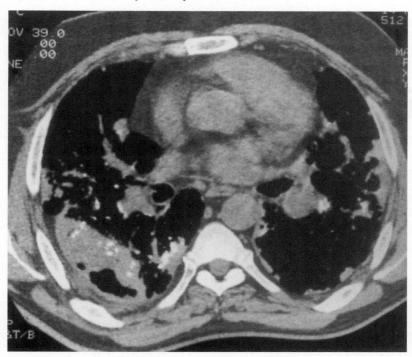

FIGURE 11-43 HRCT scan through the mid lung from a patient with primary pulmonary amyloidosis shows confluent subpleural opacities containing several calcific foci. Primary pulmonary amyloidosis is a rare disease that occurs in three forms: (i) tracheobronchial, (ii) nodular parenchymal, and (iii) the least common but most clinically significant, diffuse parenchymal or alveolar septal amyloidosis, as in this case. In the alveolar septal form, amyloid deposition in the lung is often widespread, involving small blood vessels and the parenchymal interstitium, and multifocal small nodules of amyloid may be present. The diffuse parenchymal or alveolar septal form of amyloidosis is least common but is most significant clinically. Patients with diffuse parenchymal amyloidosis are more likely to die of respiratory failure than are patients with the two other forms of the disease. Radiologically, alveolar septal amyloidosis appears as nonspecific diffuse interstitial or alveolar opacities that, once established, change very little over time. The abnormal areas can calcify or, rarely, show frank ossification. Calcification of small interstitial nodules may also be seen in silicosis, coal worker's pneumoconiosis, and usual interstitial pneumonia.

12

Infectious Pneumonia

Tuberculosis
Tuberculous lymphadenopathy
Mycetoma
Thoracoplasty and plombage
Mycobacterium avium-intracellulare complex
Adenovirus pneumonia
Coccidioidomycosis
Histoplasmosis
Nocardiosis
Septic pulmonary emboli
Early pneumonia
Invasive aspergillosis
Actinomycosis
Blastomycosis

Tuberculosis

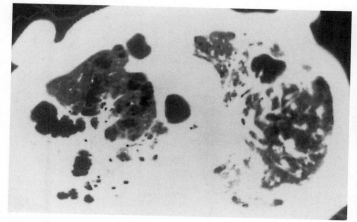 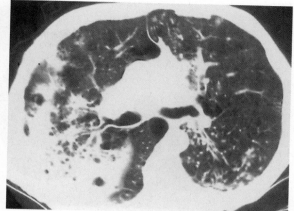

FIGURE 12-1

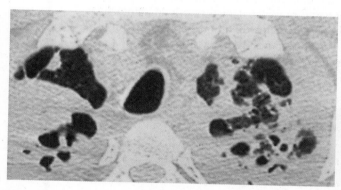 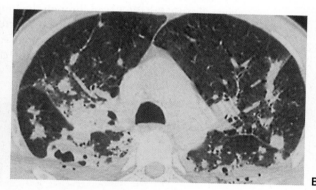

FIGURE 12-2

FIGURES 12-1 A,B and 12-2 A,B: HRCT scans from two patients show typical manifestations of reactivation tuberculosis. There are extensive fibrocavitary changes in the apices of these patients. Multiple cavities with extensive cicatricial changes are common features that result in upper lobe volume loss, often with shift of the trachea to the ipsilateral side. Lymphadenopathy is not a common feature of reactivation tuberculosis. The organisms spread hematogenously to the lung apices during the primary tuberculous infection, where they can remain dormant for years before reactivating. Because *Mycobacterium tuberculosis* is an obligate aerobe, the high oxygen tensions in the upper lungs offer an ideal environment for them to thrive. The presence of cavitation in reactivation tuberculosis is not in and of itself indicative of activity but should be considered indeterminate for activity. Comparison with old radiographs or CT scans is essential to determine disease stability.

Tuberculosis *(continued)*

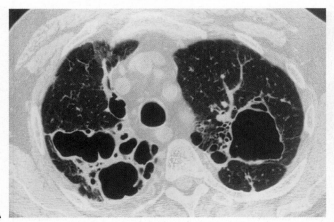
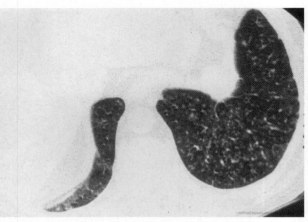

A

B

FIGURE 12-3 A: HRCT scan through the upper lung from a patient with reactivation tuberculosis and cough shows considerable fibrosis, architectural distortion, bronchiectasis, and cavitary changes as postinflammatory sequelae of the infection. There are no CT signs to support active disease. **B:** HRCT scan through the lung bases, however, depicts poorly marginated branching and V-shaped centrilobular structures, consistent with an infectious bronchiolitis, the so-called "tree-in-bud" (TIB) appearance. The appearance in this setting was suspicious for active endobronchial tuberculosis; sputum cultures were positive for tuberculosis.

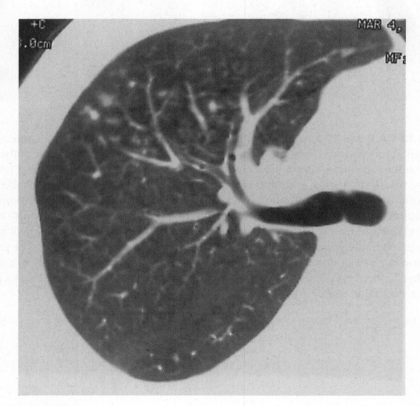

FIGURE 12-4

FIGURES 12-4 and 12-5 CT scans from two patients with sputum-positive tuberculosis show small, ill-defined, peripheral acinar nodules grouped around small bronchovascular bundles; the grouping of these nodules suggests multiple, abnormally filled acini within several secondary pulmonary lobules.

(continued)

Tuberculosis *(continued)*

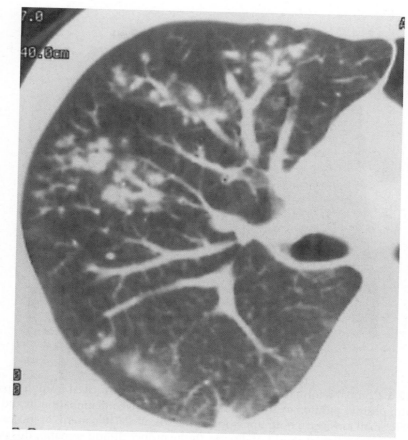

FIGURE 12-5

FIGURES 12-4 and 12-5 *(continued)*

Bronchiolitis and bronchiolectasis are nonspecific inflammatory processes of the small airways caused by many different insults. The TIB pattern is a direct CT scan finding of bronchiolar disease for the CT scan findings of endobronchial spread of *M. tuberculosis*. This pattern is analogous to the larger airway "finger-in-glove" appearance of bronchial impaction but on a much smaller scale. The *TIB pattern* has become a popular descriptive term for many bronchiolar disease processes all with similar appearances, although it is still often used inappropriately to imply a pathognomonic finding for tuberculosis. The list of diseases associated with the bronchioles that can potentially produce a TIB pattern at CT scanning is extensive. The more common disease processes can be grouped as follows: (i) infection, (ii) immunologic disorders, (iii) congenital disorders, (iv) aspiration, and (v) idiopathic condition.

Therefore, this TIB appearance of active tuberculosis with endobronchial spread is characteristic (but not pathognomonic) of active tuberculosis. In the proper clinical setting, it is thought to be a reliable criterion for disease activity, distinct from old fibrotic lesions. With appropriate medical therapy, these lesions will often clear without residua.

Tuberculosis *(continued)*

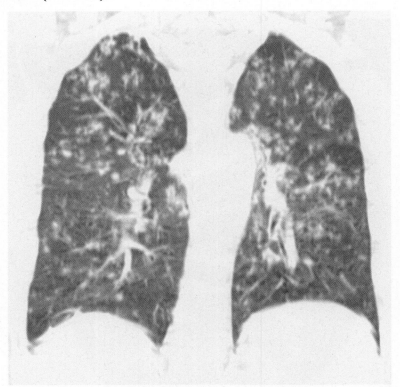

FIGURE 12-6 Coronal reformat HRCT scan through the posterior chest from this patient with sputum positive pulmonary tuberculosis shows extensive inflammation in and around innumerable small airways in both upper lobes, the so-called TIB pattern, in this case indicative of active endobronchial spread of disease. In the proper clinical scenario, this pattern often reflects a high degree of contagion.

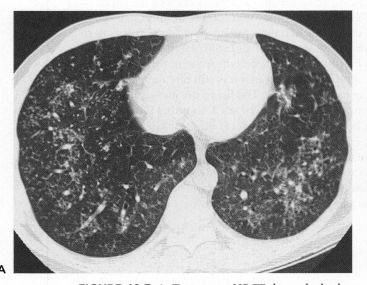

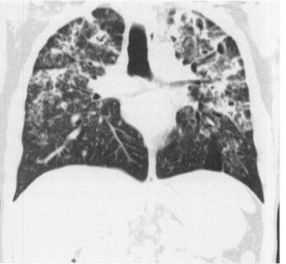

A   B

FIGURE 12-7 **A:** Transverse HRCT through the lower chest from a patient with active tuberculosis shows innumerable diffuse, 1- to 2-mm, sharply defined nodules in the lower lobes, a distribution pattern consistent with lymphohematogenous dissemination

(continued)

Tuberculosis *(continued)*

FIGURE 12-7 *(continued)*
(miliary tuberculosis). In the same patient in **B**, coronal HRCT through the mid chest shows mid and upper lung fibrocystic inflammatory tuberculosis with associated "tree-in-bud" opacities typical for endobronchial spread of infection. Miliary tuberculosis is usually a complication of primary tuberculosis, although it may result from reactivation of latent infection. It represents hematogenous spread from the primary focus of infection. A similar miliary pattern may also be seen with silicosis; fungal infections, such as histoplasmosis coccidioidomycosis; and rheumatoid lung disease.

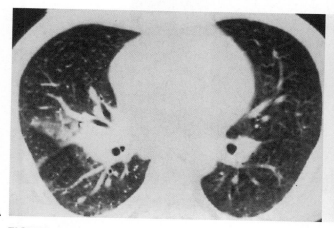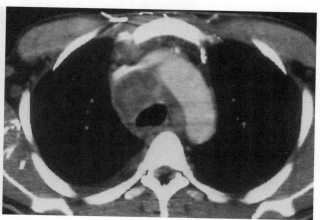

A   B

FIGURE 12-8

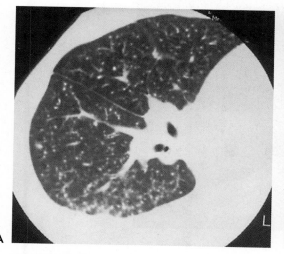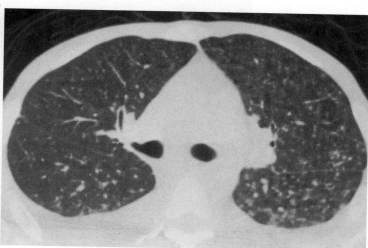

A   B

FIGURE 12-9

FIGURES 12-8 A,B and 12-9 A,B: HRCT scans from two immunocompromised patients with human immunodeficiency virus (HIV) infection show parenchymal consolidation and lymphadenopathy (Fig. 12-8 **A,B**), miliary nodules, and pleural effusions from disseminated infection (Fig. 12-9 **A,B**). The presentation of tuberculosis in patients with HIV infection depends on the extent of immune compromise. With a relatively normal immune system, tuberculous infection resembles that in the non–HIV-infected individual. As the immune system is compromised, tuberculous infection resembles that of primary tuberculosis, with consolidation and lymphadenopathy or hematogenous dissemination, even though the disease is usually reactivation of latent organisms.

Tuberculous lymphadenopathy

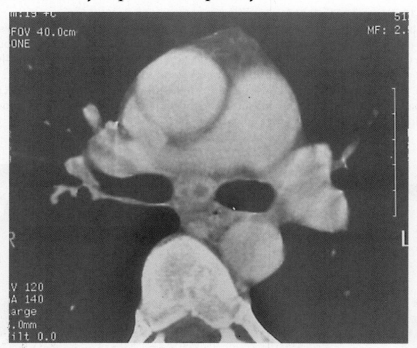

FIGURE 12-10

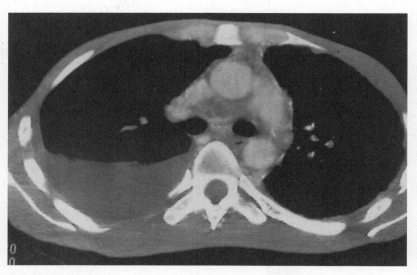

FIGURE 12-11

FIGURES 12-10, 12-11, 12-12, and 12-13 HRCT scans from four immunocompromised patients with HIV-related tuberculosis show both peripheral enhancing necrotic lymph nodes and diffusely enhancing lymph nodes as part of the spectrum of lymphadenopathy seen in HIV-related tuberculosis. This finding may also be seen in histoplasmosis or cryptococcosis but is less common with lymphoma or Kaposi sarcoma.

(continued)

Tuberculous lymphadenopathy *(continued)*

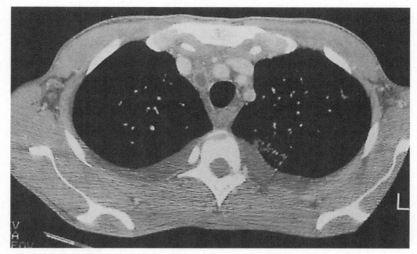

FIGURE 12-12

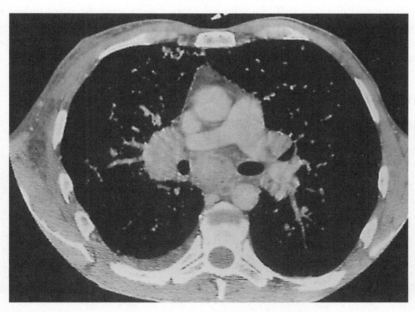

FIGURE 12-13

FIGURES 12-10, 12-11, 12-12, and 12-13 *(continued)*

Mycetoma

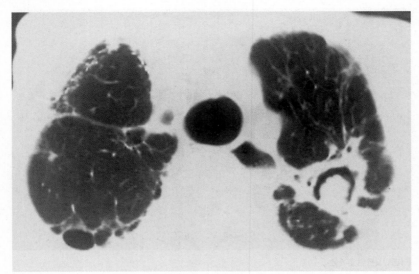

FIGURE 12-14 HRCT scan from a patient with fibrocavitary tuberculosis shows a rounded mass in a dependent position within a left upper lobe cavity. Note the surrounding fibrotic changes. Cavities of any etiology, but particularly tuberculous cavities, may become secondarily involved with saprophytic fungi, usually an *Aspergillus* species, resulting in mycetoma formation.

Thoracoplasty and plombage

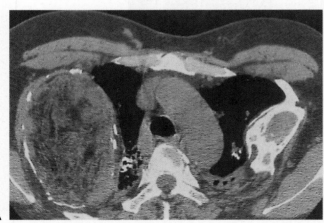
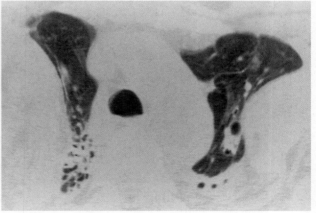

A   B

FIGURE 12-15 **A,B:** HRCT scan from a patient with prior tuberculosis and current hemoptysis shows a plombage with wax in the right hemithorax (oleothorax) and a thoracoplasty of the left hemithorax. Before the use of antituberculous antibiotics, several different methods of therapy were used to treat tuberculosis. Most of these therapies revolved around putting the lung at rest, including serial iatrogenic pneumothoraces, thoracoplasty, and plombage, in which different materials, such as Lucite balls or wax, were placed into the hemithorax. Note the extensive upper lobe scarring and bronchiectasis as residua of tuberculous infection, likely the source of hemoptysis. This appearance is radiographically indeterminate for tuberculous activity.

Mycobacterium avium-intracellulare complex

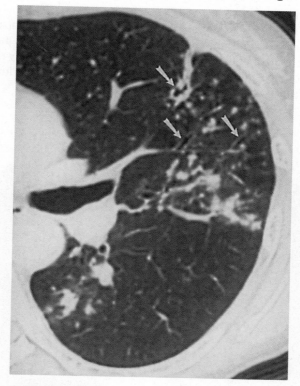

FIGURE 12-16

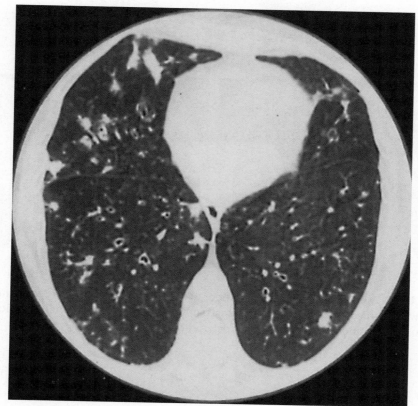

FIGURE 12-17

FIGURES 12-16, 12-17, and 12-18 HRCT scans from three patients with *Mycobacterium avium-intracellulare* complex show bronchiectasis with associated small, nodular opacities (*arrows*).

(continued)

Mycobacterium avium-intracellulare complex *(continued)*

FIGURES 12-16, 12-17, and 12-18 *(continued)*
This combination of findings is a common manifestation of nontuberculous mycobacterial infection, often *M. avium-intracellulare* complex. Among immunocompetent patients, this disease appears to be more prevalent in the lower lungs of older women especially right middle lobe and lingula. Other nontuberculous *Mycobacteria* that can also rarely cause lung infection in humans include *M. gordonae, M. kansasii,* and *M. xenopi.*

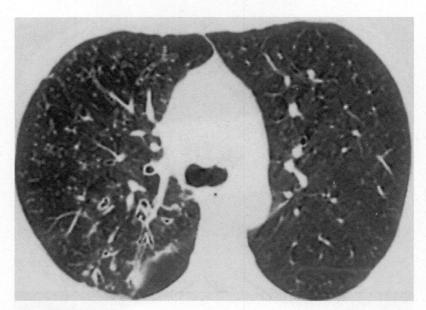

FIGURE 12-18

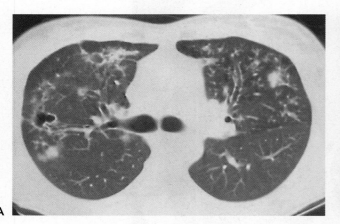

A

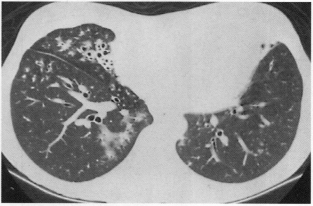

B

FIGURE 12-19 A,B: HRCT scans from a patient with AIDS and *M. avium-intracellulare* complex show bronchiectasis with associated small, nodular opacities; these manifestations are similar to those found in the immunocompetent host.

Mycobacterium avium-intracellulare complex *(continued)*

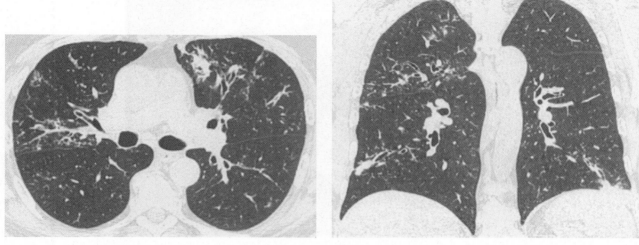

A   B

FIGURE 12-20 Transverse (**A**) and coronal (**B**) HRCT images from a patient with *M. avium-intracellulare* infection demonstrate mild bronchiectasis with associated bronchial wall thickening and bronchial mucoid impaction. Patchy consolidation and ground-glass opacity surround some of the abnormal airways. *M. avium-intracellulare* has a predilection for the anterior segments of the upper lobes, the right middle lobe, and lingula.

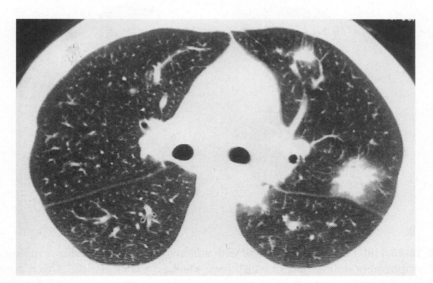

FIGURE 12-21 HRCT scan from a patient with AIDS, obtained at the level of the carina, shows scattered irregularly marginated nodules in the left lung. Nodules, cavities, consolidation, lymphadenopathy, and airways disease are all typical of this infection in the setting of AIDS. The pattern, therefore, may be indistinguishable from *M. tuberculosis*. The disease is usually disseminated by the time it affects the lungs and is seen in patients with advanced AIDS.

Mycobacterium avium-intracellulare complex *(continued)*

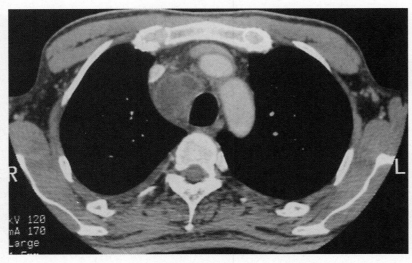

FIGURE 12-22 CT scan from a patient with AIDS and *M. avium-intracellulare* complex shows an enlarged, necrotic, peripherally enhancing lymph node that suggests a mycobacterial infection, such as tuberculosis or *M. avium-intracellulare* complex, as in this case.

Adenovirus pneumonia

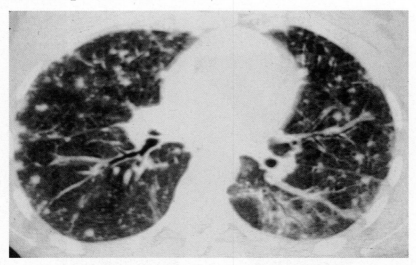

FIGURE 12-23 HRCT scan from a patient with adenovirus pneumonia shows multiple, ill-defined peripheral nodules, some of which have small associated "halos." This is a nonspecific pattern of infection that can be seen with disseminated granulomatous infections, such as tuberculosis, histoplasmosis (see Figs. 12-31 to 12-33), coccidioidomycosis, or even metastatic disease.

Coccidioidomycosis

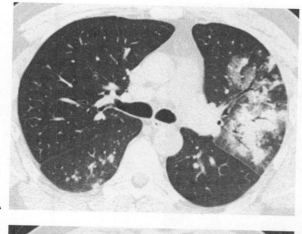

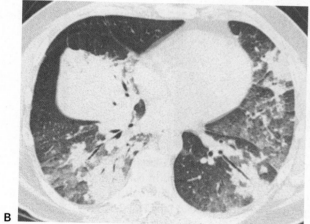

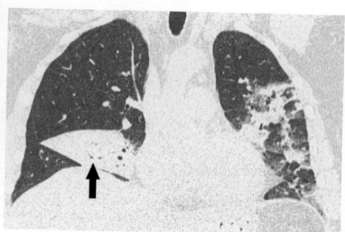

FIGURE 12-24 A–C: Transverse and coronal HRCT images from a patient who developed coccidioidomycosis after a golfing trip in Arizona show multifocal lung consolidation and ground-glass opacity predominantly in a peribronchial distribution. The right middle lobe has also collapsed (*arrow*).

Coccidioidomycosis *(continued)*

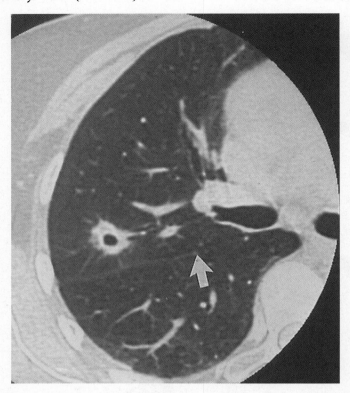

FIGURE 12-25 HRCT scan from a patient with coccidioidomycosis shows a 2.5-cm spiculated and cavitated nodule in the posterior segment of the right upper lobe. Spiculation is a sign that is usually more indicative of malignancy, but it can occur secondary to inflammatory processes, as in this case. Also note an incomplete right major fissure (*arrow*) (see Fig. 2-10).

Histoplasmosis

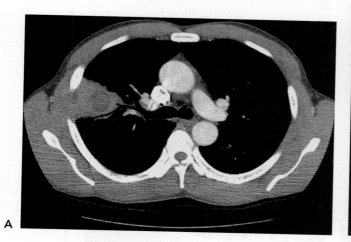

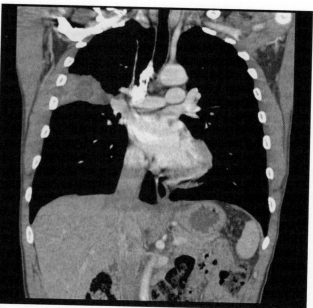

FIGURE 12-26 A,B: Transverse and coronal HRCT from an immunocompetent patient with acute histoplasmosis pneumonia shows a wedge-shaped area of dense consolidation in the right upper lobe with a spherical area of low-attenuation within. No lymphadenopathy was present. As the patient was symptomatic, there was likely a large organism inoculum. Found worldwide, including in parts of central and South America and parts of Africa, *Histoplasma capsulatum* is endemic to the Ohio, Missouri, and Mississippi River valleys in the United States. It can infect both immunocompetent and immunocompromised hosts.

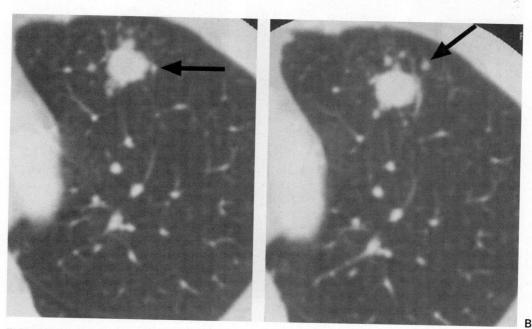

FIGURE 12-27 A,B: CT scans show a 1.5-cm uncalcified nodule in the left upper lobe. Closer inspection shows multiple, tiny "satellite" nodules (*arrows*). Although nonspecific, this finding is usually indicative of a granulomatous as opposed to a neoplastic process, in this case caused by *Histoplasma* granuloma.

Histoplasmosis *(continued)*

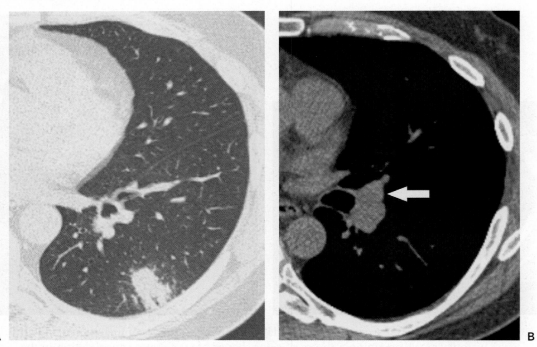

FIGURE 12-28 A,B: A. HRCT image of the left lung shows a large subpleural nodule surrounded by ground-glass opacity in the left lower lobe. **B.** HRCT image (mediastinal window settings) demonstrates left hilar lymphadenopathy (*arrow*).

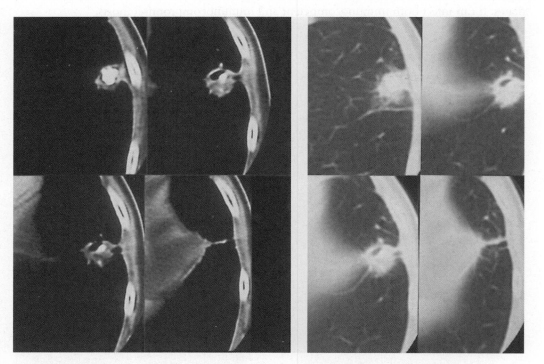

FIGURE 12-29 CT scans show a 2.5-cm spiculated cavitary nodule with eccentric calcification. There is a pleural tail. CT findings are indeterminate but worrisome for scar carcinoma arising adjacent to a calcified granuloma. Videothoracoscopic biopsy showed the nodule to be a histoplasmosis caseating granuloma.

Histoplasmosis *(continued)*

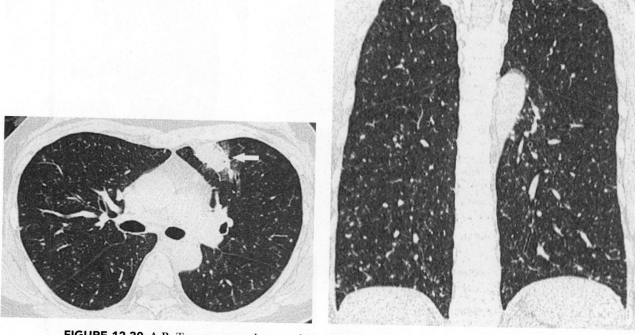

FIGURE 12-30 A,B: Transverse and coronal HRCT images from a patient treated with inflix-imab for rheumatoid arthritis who developed histoplasmosis show scattered small nodules in both lungs. A larger nodular focus of consolidation is present in the lingula *(arrow)*.

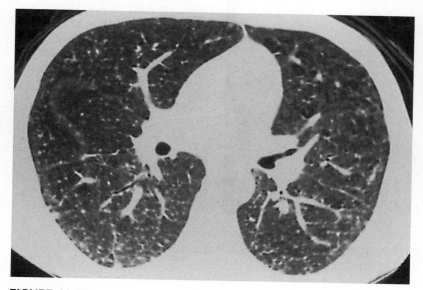

FIGURE 12-31

FIGURES 12-31, 12-32 A,B, and 12-33 A,B: HRCT scans from three patients with AIDS and histoplasmosis show the typical miliary nodules throughout the lungs. In AIDS patients, histoplasmosis nearly always presents with disseminated disease.

(continued)

Histoplasmosis *(continued)*

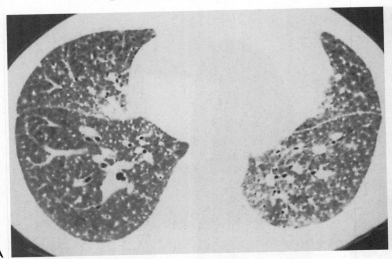

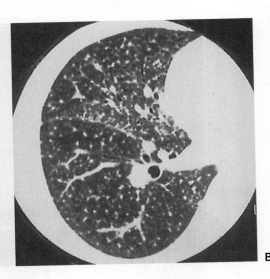

A

B

FIGURE 12-32

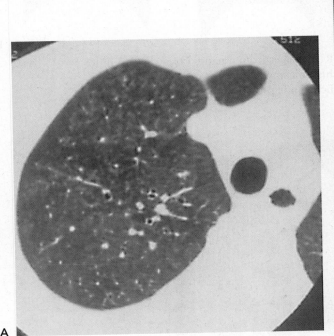

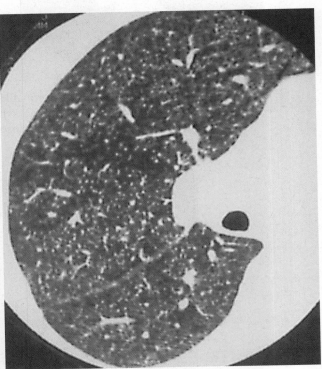

A

B

FIGURE 12-33

FIGURES 12-31, 12-32 A,B, and 12-33 A,B *(continued)*

Nocardiosis

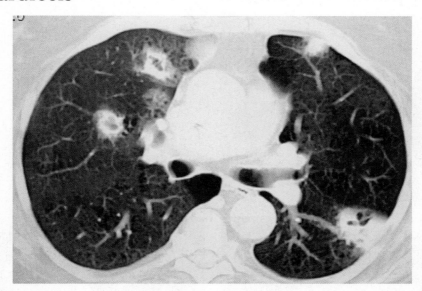

FIGURE 12-34 CT scan through the mid lungs from an immunocompromised patient with nocardiosis shows multiple, predominantly peripheral, ill-defined cavitary masses. This is one of the more typical appearances for pulmonary *Nocardia* infection, although it is nonspecific. Other disease processes that can have a similar appearance include septic thromboembolic disease, cavitary metastases, Wegener granulomatosis, and fungal infections.

Nocardia species are gram-positive filamentous branching rods found worldwide in soil and decaying organic matter. Humans are most commonly infected by inhalation through the respiratory tract. Extrapulmonary involvement, either as the primary or the secondary site, occurs in 20% to 40% of cases. The three *Nocardia* species that are pathogenic in humans are *N. asteroides* (most common), *N. brasiliensis*, and *N. caviae*.

Nocardial infections are rare but increasing in frequency in immunocompromised hosts, especially with defects in cellular immunity, such as those receiving intensive corticosteroid or other immunosuppressive therapy (solid organ transplant recipients; those with malignancies; those with connective tissue disease, especially systemic lupus erythematosus; those with inflammatory bowel disease; and those with pemphigus). The infection is also seen in patients with a variety of chronic disorders, such as tuberculosis, pulmonary emphysema, dysgammaglobulinemia, diabetes mellitus, AIDS, chronic granulomatous disease of childhood, pulmonary alveolar proteinosis, lymphoreticular malignancies, and alcoholism.

Pulmonary presentation can be an acute, subacute, or chronic pneumonitis. Chest radiographic and CT scan findings of nocardiosis are diverse and include single or multiple nodular masslike opacities, patchy bronchopneumonic infiltrates, dense consolidation, thick-walled cavities, diffuse alveolar infiltrates, and reticular-nodular miliary infiltrates. Cavitation is present in one fourth of patients and intrathoracic lymphadenopathy is rare (case courtesy of J. Pluss, M.D., Madigan Army Medical Center, Tacoma, WA).

Septic pulmonary emboli

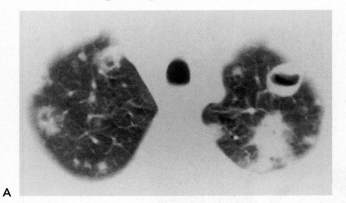

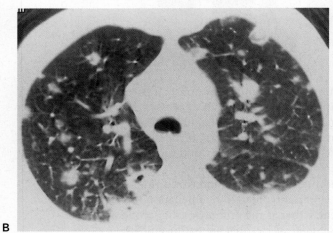

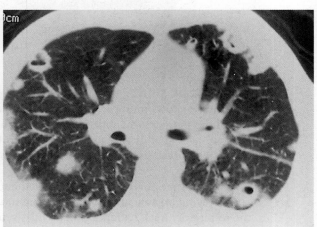

FIGURE 12-35 **A–C:** CT scans through the upper (**A**), middle (**B**), and lower (**C**) lungs from a patient with septic emboli show multiple peripheral nodules and wedge-shaped opacities, many of which have cavities, scattered throughout the lungs. Wegener granulomatosis and cavitary metastases can have a similar appearance, although the clinical presentation is usually quite distinct.

Early pneumonia

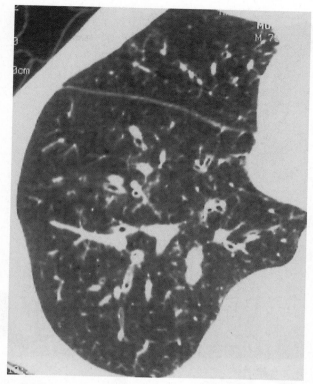

FIGURE 12-36 HRCT scan shows hazy ground-glass opacity around the lower lobe subsegmental bronchovascular bundles. This nonspecific finding not evident on the chest radiograph, in this case, represents an early pneumonia that blossomed into a typical lobar pneumonia the next day.

Invasive aspergillosis

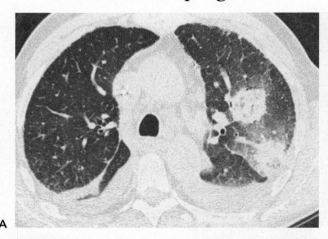

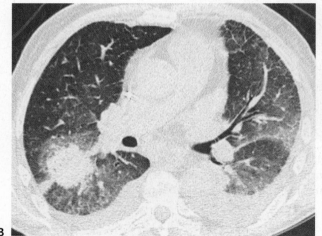

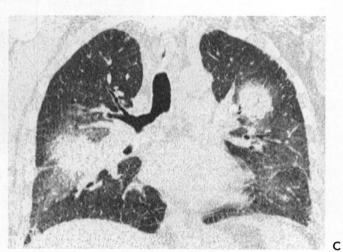

FIGURE 12-37 A–C: Transverse and coronal HRCT images from a patient with angioinvasive aspergillosis who underwent peripheral blood stem cell transplant for leukemia show bilateral masslike areas of consolidation with surrounding ground-glass opacity. Small pleural effusions are present.

Invasive aspergillosis *(continued)*

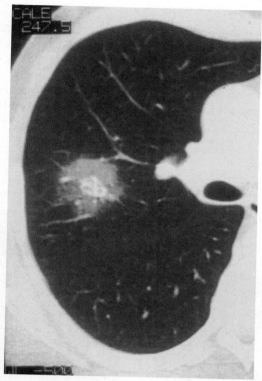

FIGURE 12-38 HRCT scans from an immunocompromised patient after bone marrow transplant show lung nodules with surrounding ground-glass opacities, or "halos." These findings in an immunocompromised host suggest that the most likely diagnosis is a fungal infection, particularly invasive aspergillosis, Wegener granulomatosis, Kaposi sarcoma, an angioinvasive tumor, or even a recent transbronchial lung biopsy could have a similar appearance.

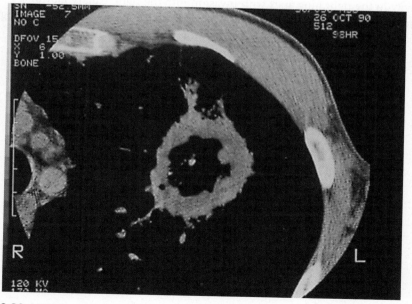

FIGURE 12-39 HRCT scan from an immunocompromised patient with invasive pulmonary aspergillosis shows a cavitary lung mass. Note the thick, irregular wall of the mass. Invasive pulmonary aspergillosis is a relatively frequent abnormality in the immunocompromised host.

(continued)

Invasive aspergillosis *(continued)*

FIGURE 12-39 *(continued)*
Typical HRCT findings of invasive pulmonary aspergillosis early in the course of infection are single or multiple inflammatory nodules or masslike consolidation representing bronchopneumonia. Air crescent formation has been reported to be highly suggestive of invasive pulmonary aspergillosis but this is a late radiographic sign. Also early in the course of infection, a ground-glass–like "halo" around areas of opacity can be seen; this is a nonspecific sign that, in the case of fungal infection, corresponds to a central fungal nodule surrounded by a rim of coagulative necrosis.

Actinomycosis

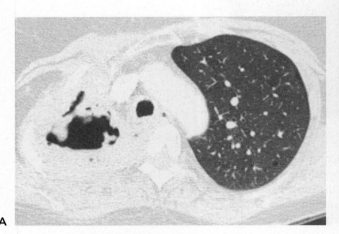

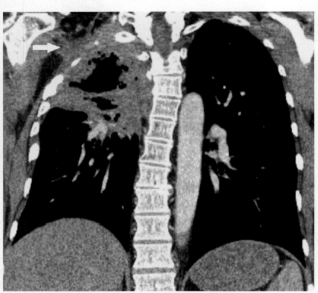

A   B

FIGURE 12-40 A,B: Transverse and coronal contrast-enhanced HRCT images show a thick-walled cavity in the right lung apex with invasion into the right axillary fat (*arrow*). Actinomycosis most commonly develops in patients with poor dentition. Traversing tissue planes is a feature characteristic of actinomycosis as in this case.

Blastomycosis

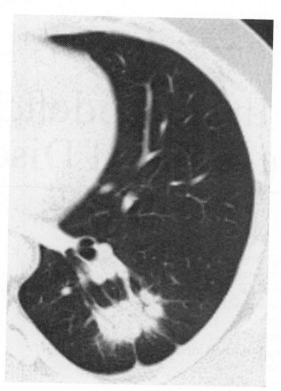

FIGURE 12-41 HRCT image of the left lung from a patient with North American blastomycosis shows a spiculated nodule in the left lower lobe, containing air bronchograms. Blastomycosis can affect the skin, lungs, bone, and prostate gland. In the lungs, focal or multifocal consolidation can develop with occasional caviation. Consolidation can be masslike, as in the case, mimicking lung carcinoma. Pleural effusions and lymphadenopathy are not typical features of blastomycosis. Less commonly, the infection may be disseminated throughout the lungs with either miliary or somewhat larger nodules.

13

Acquired Immunodeficiency Syndrome–Related Diseases

Pneumocystis jiroveci pneumonia
Infectious bronchiolitis
Cytomegalovirus
Varicella pneumonia
Cryptococcosis
Histoplasmosis
Obstructing bronchial aspergillosis
Invasive aspergillosis
Kaposi sarcoma
Lymphoid interstitial pneumonia
Lymphoproliferative disorder
Non-Hodgkin's lymphoma

Pneumocystis jiroveci pneumonia

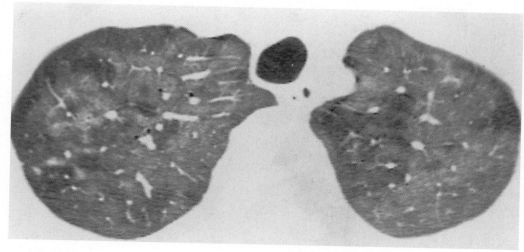

FIGURE 13-1

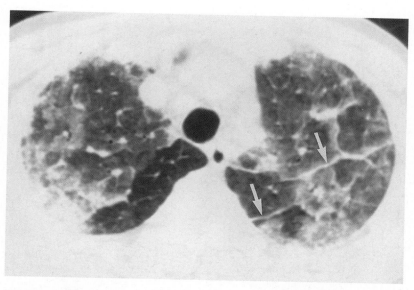

FIGURE 13-2

FIGURES 13-1 and 13-2 HRCT scans from two different patients with acquired immunodeficiency syndrome (AIDS) and *Pneumocystis jiroveci* pneumonia (PCP) show a predominantly ground-glass patchwork pattern of opacity through which the vessels remain visible. This is the most common HRCT pattern of PCP. Ground-glass density is caused by a combination of intra-alveolar exudates as well as some degree of alveolar septal thickening. Variable lobular involvement produces a mosaic pattern; note the presence of uninvolved lobules. Significant interlobular septal thickening (*arrows*) reflects edema or cellular infiltration.

Other less common HRCT scan patterns of PCP are an interstitial pattern, nodules, and upper lobe cavities, and cystic spaces. Occasional associated findings include pneumothorax, adenopathy, and pleural effusions (5% or less); these associated findings may be related to intercurrent disease.

Pneumocystis jiroveci pneumonia *(continued)*

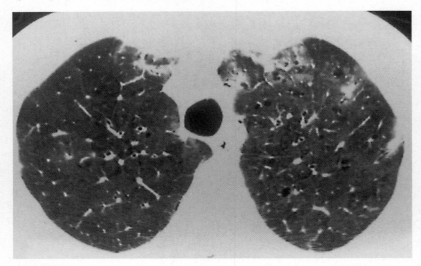

FIGURE 13-3

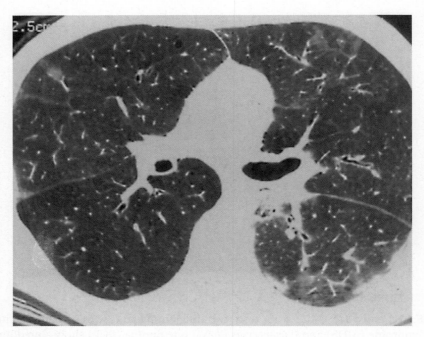

FIGURE 13-4

FIGURES 13-3 and 13-4 HRCT scans from these two patients with AIDS and PCP show typical diffuse but patchy ground-glass opacity of a mild PCP infection.

Pneumocystis jiroveci pneumonia *(continued)*

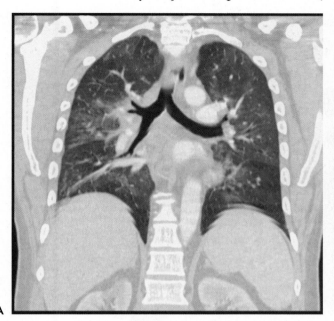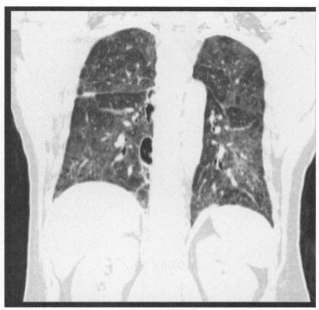

A   B

FIGURE 13-5 **A,B:** Coronal HRCT scans from two patients with AIDS and PCP both show a rather diffuse distribution of ground-glass opacities throughout the lungs.

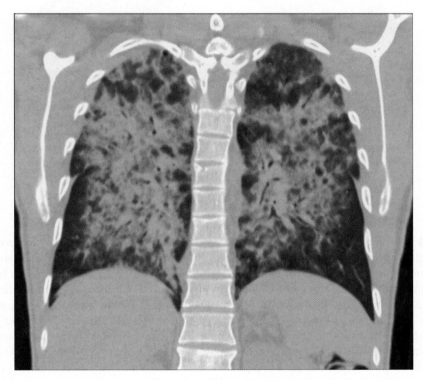

FIGURE 13-6 Coronal HRCT scan from a patient with AIDS and organizing subacute extensive PCP shows a pattern of bilateral coarse linear densities, some in an interlobular or peribronchovascular distribution, in conjunction with architectural distortion, extensive consolidation as well as ground glass opacities.

Pneumocystis jiroveci pneumonia *(continued)*

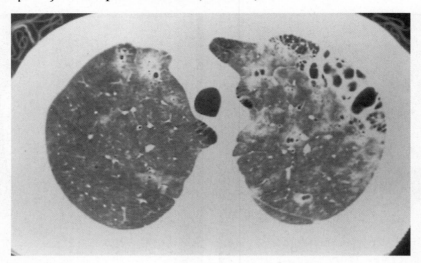

FIGURE 13-7

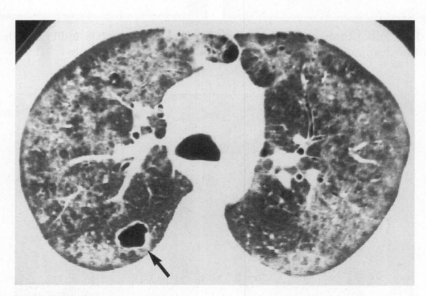

FIGURE 13-8

FIGURES 13-7 and 13-8 HRCT scans from two patients with AIDS and PCP show both ground-glass opacity, areas of ground-glass opacity with superimposed reticulation suggesting organization, and thin-walled cystic lesions (*arrow*). The *P. jiroveci* organism can cause necrotizing, thin-walled, intraparenchymal cavities. Cysts in PCP may arise during the acute inflammatory phase, in which case they typically are surrounded by ground-glass opacity, or they may develop as a later sequela, at a point when much of the ground-glass opacity may have resolved. These cysts are typically apical and subpleural, lined by fibrosis or alveolar parenchyma with little inflammation. Cysts may appear in as many as 40% of cases of PCP. Resolution of CT findings can be incomplete despite clinical recovery after therapy; cystic disease can persist but can also heal with no residua.

Pneumocystis jiroveci pneumonia *(continued)*

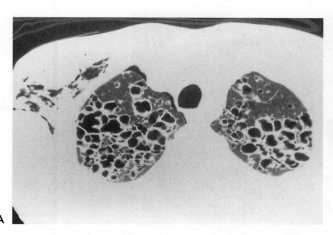
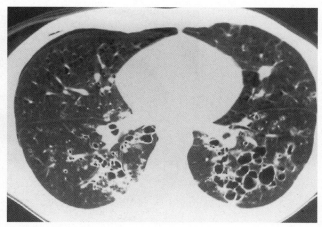

A

B

FIGURE 13-9 A,B: CT scans from patients with AIDS and PCP show thin-walled pulmonary cystic lesions of PCP in both the upper lobes **(A)** and the lower lobes **(B)**. The upper lobe cysts are typical, whereas cystic disease secondary to PCP involving the lower lobes is less common. Also note a focal mass in the lingula. There is also a small right pneumothorax, a complication of cystic PCP.

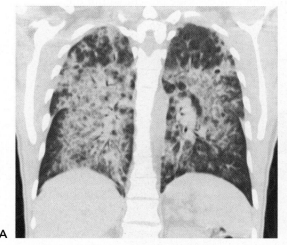
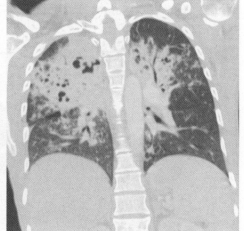

A

B

FIGURE 13-10 A,B: Coronal reformat HRCT scans through the posterior chest from a profoundly immunocompromised patient with AIDS and PCP show the progression of disease in a patient receiving inadequate treatment. In **A**, note the coarse reticular and ground-glass opacities with a peribronchovascular distribution in most of the lungs reflecting a likely combination of chronic inflammation and organization but without cystic disease. In **B**, four months later, note the more confluent mid and upper lung opacities, now showing cavity destruction.

Pneumocystis jiroveci pneumonia *(continued)*

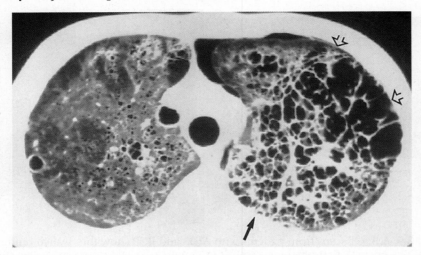

FIGURE 13-11 HRCT scan from a patient with AIDS and advanced cystic PCP shows virtual replacement of the left lung parenchyma by cystic lesions of PCP. When profuse, these cysts may coalesce and enlarge, with only thin fibrotic strands separating them. This appearance may mimic that of orderly end-stage honeycombed lung *(arrow)*. As cysts enlarge, the appearance becomes more disorganized *(open arrows)*. Note the left pneumothorax associated with these subpleural cysts. Innumerable tiny cysts are present within the ground-glass opacity in the right lung.

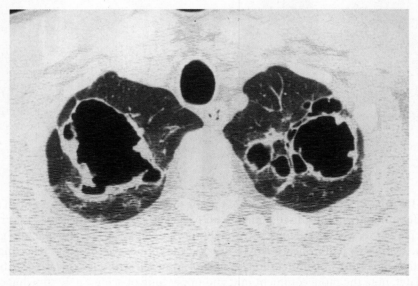

FIGURE 13-12 HRCT scan through the lung apices from a patient with AIDS and chronic cystic PCP shows replacement of much of the lung parenchyma with irregular cysts with nodular walls. These often assume bizarre shapes, with multiple septations that actually represent the walls of coalescent cysts. Note the absence of signs of lung inflammation. With this degree of lung destruction, the appearance is quite nonspecific and is indistinguishable from other cavitary and cystic processes.

Pneumocystis jiroveci pneumonia *(continued)*

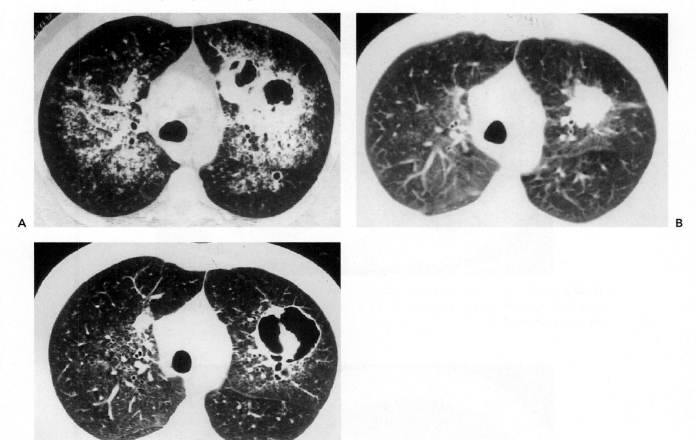

FIGURE 13-13 A–C: Sequential HRCT scans at the level of the aortic arch, obtained over a 7-month period, from a patient with cystic PCP show the evolution of the cysts over time. **A:** During the period of acute pneumonia, ill-defined nodular opacities in a perihilar distribution have produced some areas of confluent consolidation. Irregularly thick-walled cystic lesions have developed in the left lung within an area of dense consolidation. **B:** Image at the same level 3 months after treatment shows regression in the nodules and consolidation, with coarse reticular changes remaining in the affected regions. The cysts have coalesced, with slight enlargement of the central airspace concomitant with thinning of their walls. The intervening wall produces the appearance of a nodular intracystic septum. **C:** Four months later, volume loss in these regions is consistent with further fibrosis. The cystic lesions have collapsed and coalesced, forming a spiculated mass in the left upper lobe. Note retraction and displacement of the oblique fissure. Cysts in PCP may regress and disappear, may remain chronically after resolution of pneumonia, or may collapse and form focal dense scars.

Pneumocystis jiroveci pneumonia *(continued)*

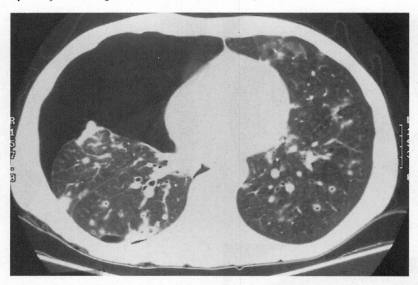

FIGURE 13-14 HRCT scan from this patient with AIDS and PCP show nodules and cavitating nodules in both lungs. Pneumothorax is a common complication resulting from the cystic changes of PCP.

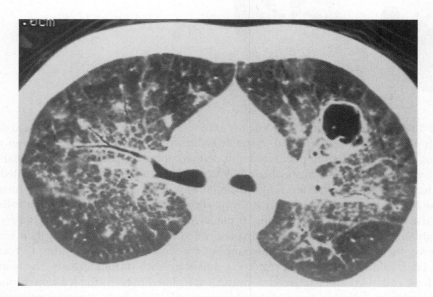

FIGURE 13-15 HRCT scan from a patient with AIDS and PCP shows cystic disease and more of a reticular, "crazy-paving" pattern, than a ground-glass pattern. Note both fine and coarse reticular patterns. The reticular pattern, most apparent in the central perihilar regions, has a similar appearance to that which can be seen with pulmonary alveolar proteinosis pulmonary hemorrhage, acute respiratory distress syndrome, and lipoid pneumonia.

Infectious bronchiolitis

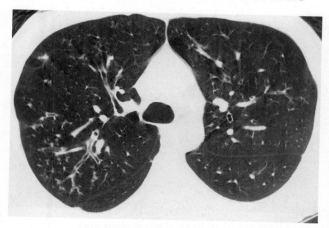

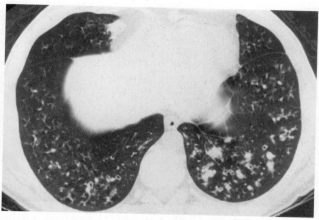

A

B

FIGURE 13-16 **A:** HRCT scan through the upper lungs from a woman with AIDS and a productive cough shows bronchiectasis and bronchial wall thickening in the posterior right upper lobe. Peripherally small centrilobular nodular and branching structures represent bronchioles impacted with inflammatory material. **B:** Thick-walled, dilatated bronchi, with and without impaction, are appreciated at the lung bases. Centrilobular impacted bronchioles with peribronchiolar inflammation are present. Sputum culture was positive for *Streptococcus pneumoniae.*

Bacterial infections have superseded PCP as the most common infection in the lungs of AIDS patients. These may manifest as bacterial pneumonia, but increasingly infectious bronchitis and bronchiolitis are recognized as causes of acute lung symptoms in AIDS.

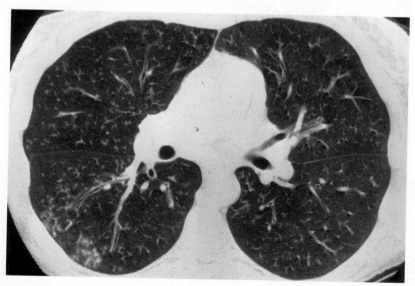

FIGURE 13-17 HRCT scan from a patient with AIDS shows bronchial wall thickening without definite dilatation in the superior segment of the right lower lobe. Peripherally, bronchioles impacted with inflammatory material produce centrilobular densities with a characteristic "tree-in-bud" pattern. Peribronchiolar inflammation likely accounts for the hazy margins of many of these nodules. This nonspecific appearance can be seen in both bacterial and mycobacterial infections.

Infectious bronchiolitis *(continued)*

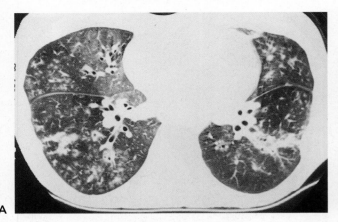

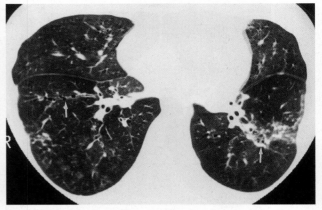

A

B

FIGURE 13-18 A,B: HRCT scans from a patient with AIDS, obtained both pretreatment and posttreatment for bacterial bronchitis, show areas of bronchial and bronchiolar impaction involving all lobes **(A)**. A mosaic opacity pattern, with low-opacity regions corresponding to zones of bronchiolitis, suggests regional hypovascularity and shunting consequent to small airways disease. In **B**, a subtle mosaic opacity pattern remains on the HRCT image at the same level 1 month after antibiotic therapy. Much of the bronchiolar impaction and inflammation have regressed, however. Note that bronchiectasis has developed in the anterior basilar segment of the right lower lobe and lateral basilar segment of the left lower lobe *(arrows)*.

Cytomegalovirus

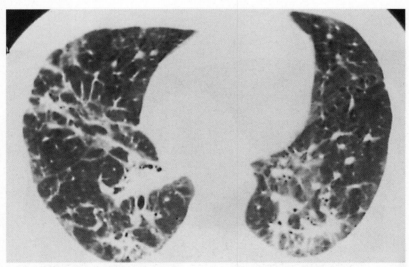

FIGURE 13-19

FIGURES 13-19, 13-20, and 13-21 HRCT scans from three patients with AIDS show part of the spectrum of disease manifested by pulmonary cytomegalovirus infection. The most common CT findings are nodules, consolidation, septal thickening, and ground-glass opacities (Fig. 13-19). Ground-glass opacities (Figs. 13-20), masses, and a miliary pattern (Fig. 13-21) can also be seen, all of which are nonspecific. Biopsy is essential in diagnosis.

(continued)

Cytomegalovirus *(continued)*

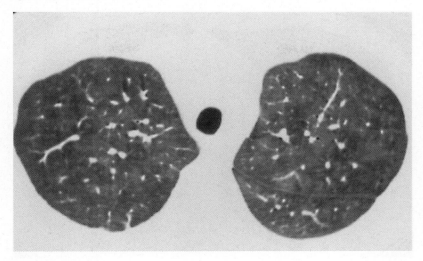

FIGURE 13-20

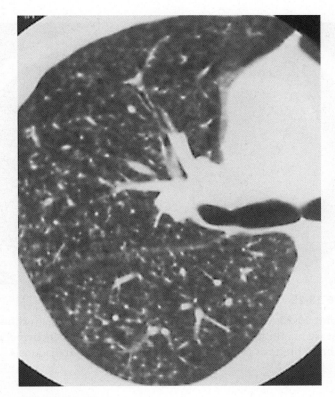

FIGURE 13-21

FIGURES 13-19, 13-20, and 13-21 *(continued)*

Cytomegalovirus *(continued)*

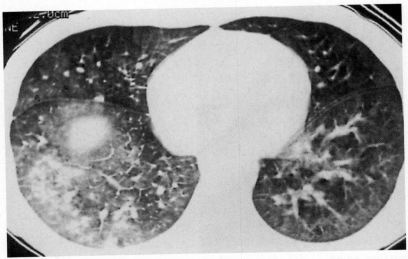

FIGURE 13-22

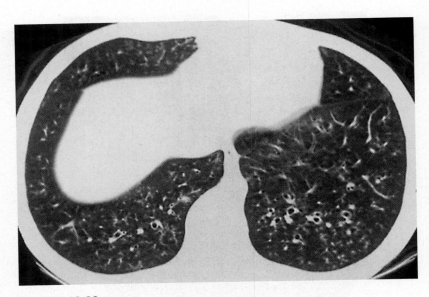

FIGURE 13-23

FIGURES 13-22 and 13-23 CT scans from two patients with AIDS again show the spectrum of pulmonary disease manifested by cytomegalovirus. Note the parenchymal consolidation (Fig. 13-22) and bronchiectasis (Fig. 13-23). Biopsy is essential in diagnosis.

Cytomegalovirus *(continued)*

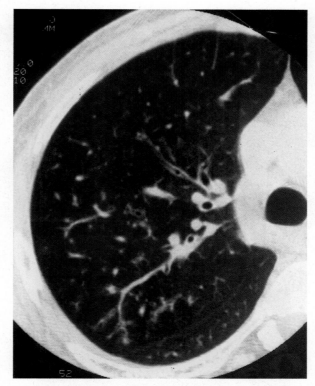

FIGURE 13-24 HRCT scan through the right upper lobe from a patient with AIDS and bronchitis and bronchiolitis secondary to cytomegalovirus infection shows dilatation and wall thickening of both bronchi and bronchioles. Indistinct interfaces with the lung parenchyma suggest peribronchiolar inflammation. Note the absence, however, of alveolar disease.

Varicella pneumonia

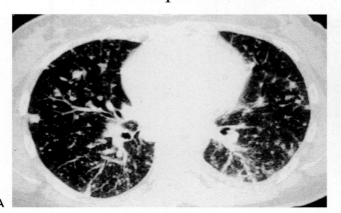 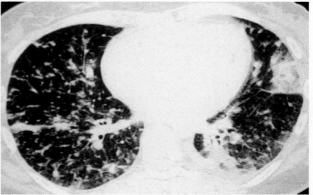

A   B

FIGURE 13-25 A,B: HRCT scans from a patient with AIDS and varicella pneumonia show multiple, fairly well-defined peripheral nodules of various sizes, the largest of which contains air bronchograms. These findings are nonspecific and may represent a number of pathogens or neoplasms.

Varicella zoster virus is one of the herpes viruses (the others are cytomegalovirus, Epstein-Barr virus, herpes simplex viruses, and herpes virus 6). Varicella zoster is an unusual infection in AIDS patients and may be a primary or copathogen.

Cryptococcosis

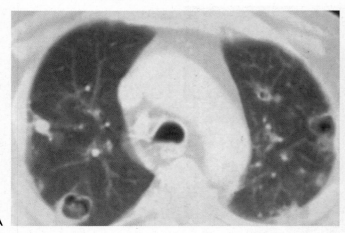
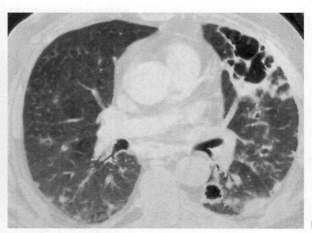

A   B

FIGURE 13-26

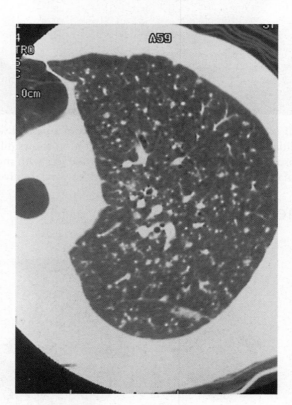

FIGURE 13-27

FIGURES 13-26 A,B and 13-27 CT scans from two patients with AIDS and pulmonary cryptococcosis show numerous, bilateral, cavitary thick and irregular-walled nodules and focal consolidation (Fig. 13-26A,B) and miliary nodules (Fig. 13-27).

Cryptococcus neoformans is a ubiquitous soil fungus that rarely causes lung disease in hosts with a normal immune system; the most common pulmonary fungal infection in patients with AIDS is caused by *C. neoformans*. As shown above, common CT findings of cryptococcal lung infection are poorly marginated nodules or masses and diffuse scattered miliary nodules. Associated lymphadenopathy, pleural effusions, and cavitation are uncommon.

Cryptococcosis *(continued)*

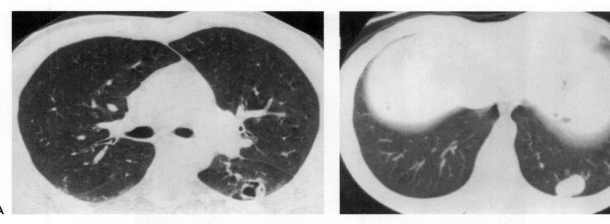

FIGURE 13-28 A,B: HRCT scans from a patient with AIDS and pulmonary cryptococcosis show both solid and cavitary masses. The HRCT pattern of cryptococcal pneumonia is usually nonspecific and may mimic other opportunistic infections or neoplasms. Diagnosis requires biopsy or culture.

Histoplasmosis

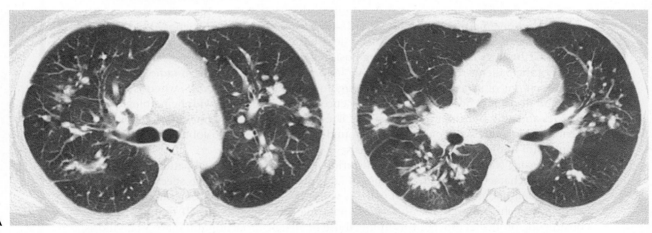

FIGURE 13-29 A,B: HRCT images from a patient with HIV infection and pulmonary histoplasmosis show multiple clusters of small lung nodules.

Obstructing bronchial aspergillois

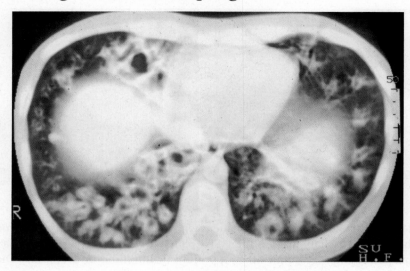

FIGURE 13-30 CT scan from a patient with AIDS shows multiple, rounded, and tubular densities in both lower lobes consistent with mucus-filled airways. At bronchoscopy, the lumens were packed with inflammatory material. Microscopic examination showed massive *Aspergillus* hyphae.

Whereas invasive aspergillosis is strongly associated with defects in granulocytic and phagocytic function, airways-invasive aspergillosis has been reported in nonneutropenic patients after bone marrow transplant. Airways-invasive aspergillosis is diagnosed histologically on the basis of identification of organisms deep to the basement membrane.

The CT findings in pulmonary aspergillosis are variable depending on the immunologic status of the patients. Thick-walled cavitary lesions are the most common radiologic manifestations of invasive pulmonary aspergillosis in patients with AIDS, whereas consolidation and ill-defined nodules are frequently encountered in patients with hematologic malignancies and after bone marrow transplant. The predominant CT manifestations are lobar or peribronchiolar areas of consolidation, ground-glass opacities, centrilobular nodules less than 5 mm in diameter, and bronchiectasis.

Obstructing bronchial aspergillosis is a descriptive term for the unusual pattern of airway involvement characterized by the presence of large quantities of *Aspergillus* species, usually *Aspergillus fumigatus*, in the airways of patients with AIDS. Patients may cough up fungal casts of their bronchi and present with severe hypoxemia. The characteristic CT findings in obstructing bronchial aspergillosis mimic those of allergic bronchopulmonary aspergillosis, consisting of bilateral bronchial and bronchiolar dilatations, mucoid impactions, and diffuse lower lobe consolidation caused by postobstructive atelectasis.

Invasive aspergillosis

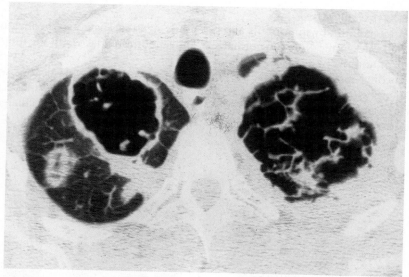

FIGURE 13-31 HRCT scan through the apices from this patient with AIDS and invasive aspergillosis shows a large right apical cyst, with nodular walls and internal material. Laterally the poorly marginated nodular density, a less advanced lesion, may represent either tissue invasion and abscess or angioinvasion and infarction. Internal lucencies suggest early cavitation. The left apical parenchyma is replaced by a complicated cavity with internal septations.

Kaposi sarcoma

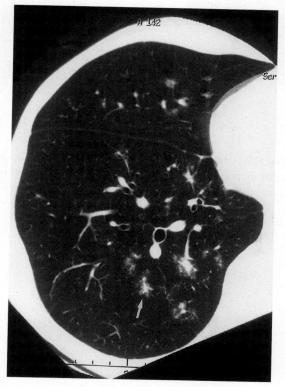

FIGURE 13-32 HRCT scan through the right lower lobe from a patient with AIDS and early Kaposi sarcoma shows many vessels of apparent increased size and ill-defined interfaces with the aerated lung (*arrow*), the "vascular interface" sign. This is due to infiltration of the

(continued)

Kaposi sarcoma *(continued)*

FIGURE 13-32 *(continued)*
perivascular interstitium by tumor cells and is a subtle sign that may precede obvious bronchial wall thickening. Note the normal size and smooth interface with the lung parenchyma of noninvolved vessels.

Kaposi sarcoma and lymphoma are the most common forms of neoplastic disease encountered in patients with AIDS. Pulmonary involvement is fairly common with Kaposi sarcoma, whereas lymphoma only rarely involves the lungs. HRCT can show borderline enlarged lymphyadenopathy, but true enlarged lymph nodes are unusual with Kaposi sarcoma.

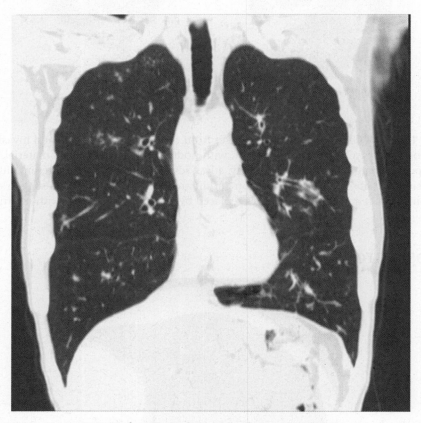

FIGURE 13-33 Coronal HRCT from a patient with AIDS and early Kaposi sarcoma shows many vessels of apparent increased size and ill-defined interfaces with the aerated lung. Note the normal size and smooth interface with the lung parenchyma of noninvolved vessels.

Kaposi sarcoma *(continued)*

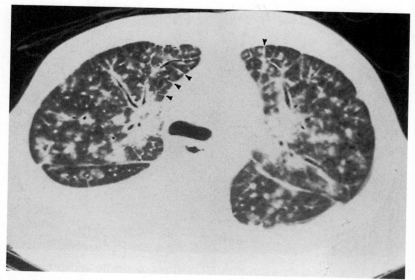

FIGURE 13-34

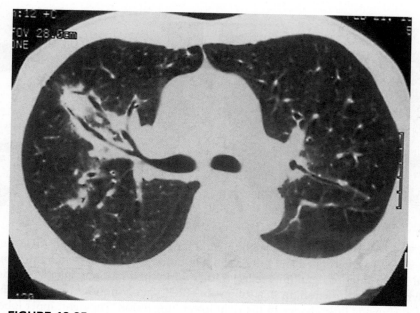

FIGURE 13-35

FIGURES 13-34 and 13-35 HRCT scans from two patients with AIDS show characteristic peribronchovascular consolidation of Kaposi sarcoma extending into the adjacent pulmonary parenchyma along the bronchovascular bundles. Figure 13-34 has an appearance similar to lymphangitic carcinomatosis note the interlobular septal thickening (*arrowheads*).

Kaposi sarcoma (continued)

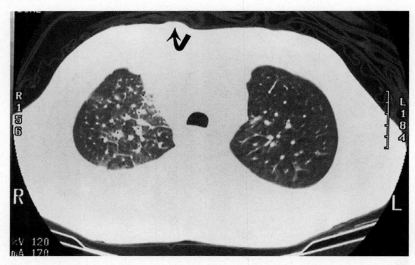

FIGURE 13-36 CT scan from a patient with AIDS shows moderate thickening of the right upper lobe bronchovascular structures and interlobular septa in this milder case of Kaposi sarcoma. Note the skin lesions on the anterior chest wall (*curved arrow*).

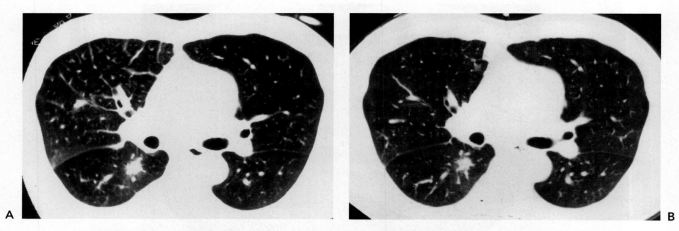

FIGURE 13-37 A,B: HRCT scan through the mid lungs from a patient with AIDS and Kaposi sarcoma shows **(A)** spiculated and lobular lung nodules. Interlobular septal thickening, appreciated in the anterior right lung, reflects either tumor infiltration or edema secondary to central lymphatic obstruction. In **B**, a follow-up HRCT scan 2 months after chemotherapy was started showing little change in the right lower lung lesion. The right upper lobe lesion was smaller. Note the interlobular septal thickening resolved with chemotherapy.

Kaposi sarcoma *(continued)*

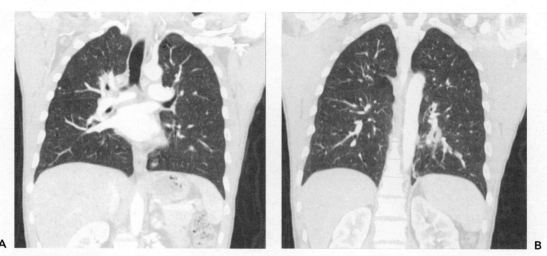

FIGURE 13-38 A,B: Coronal HRCT scans through the mid and posterior chest from a patient with AIDS and Kaposi sarcoma show extensive typical bronchovascular bundle thickening radiating out from both hila.

Lymphoid interstitial pneumonia

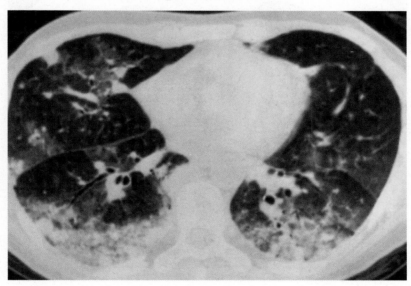

FIGURE 13-39

FIGURES 13-39, 13-40 A,B, and 13-41 HRCT scans from three patients with AIDS and lymphoid interstitial pneumonia (LIP) show both nonspecific, patchy parenchymal consolidation and ground glass opacities (Fig. 13-39) and nonspecific, diffuse, poorly marginated, 2- to 4-mm miliary nodules (Figs. 13-40 and 13-41) representing poorly formed granulomas in the lung interstitium in the absence of airspace disease. There is a predilection for the nodules to occur in centrilobular regions, best appreciated in the periphery; this suggests an association with bronchial-associated lymphoid tissue (see Figs. 11-19 and 11-20).

LIP is a chronic condition that primarily affects adults and is becoming more common in patients with AIDS. LIP is an AIDS-defining illness in children with human immunodeficiency virus infection. Histologically, mature polyclonal lymphocytes infiltrate and expand the interstitium of the lung. Amyloid can also be deposited in the lung.

(continued)

Lymphoid interstitial pneumonia *(continued)*

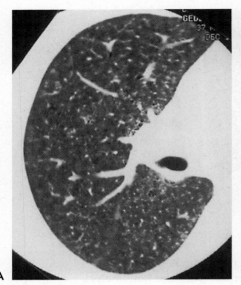

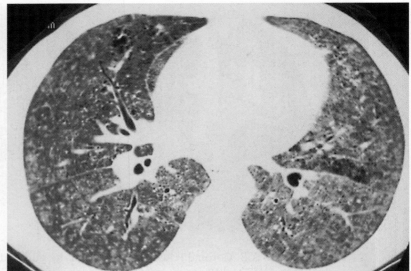

A

B

FIGURE 13-40

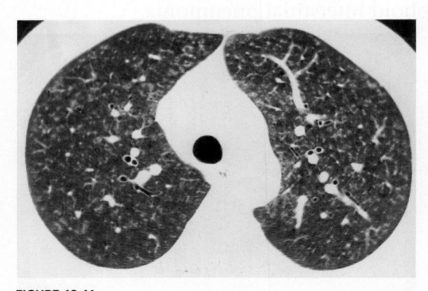

FIGURE 13-41

FIGURES 13-39, 13-40 A,B, and 13-41 *(continued)*

Lymphoproliferative disorder

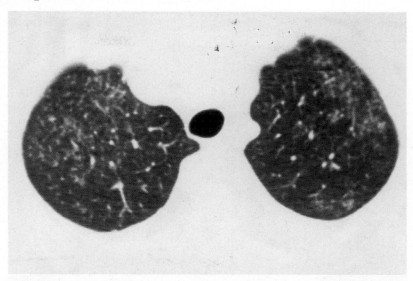

FIGURE 13-42 HRCT scan through the apices from a patient with AIDS shows a pattern radiographically similar to LIP. In this disease, however, the interstitial infiltration is polymorphous, atypical lymphocytes, including immature forms. There is a spectrum of lymphoproliferative interstitial diseases in AIDS, each pathologically distinct but with considerable radiographic overlap in appearances. They tend to occur in advanced AIDS but typically have an indolent clinical course.

Non-Hodgkin's lymphoma

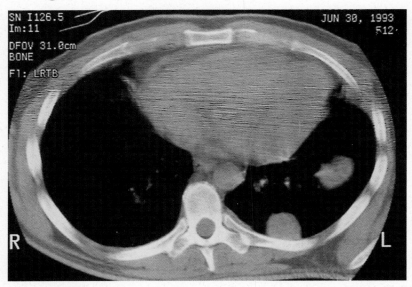

FIGURE 13-43

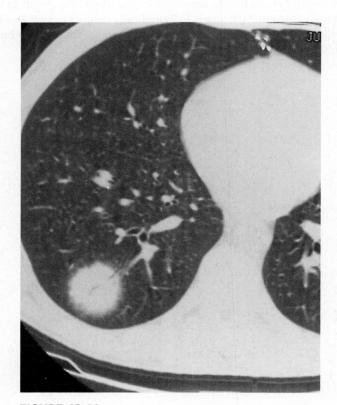

FIGURE 13-44

FIGURES 13-43 and 13-44 HRCT scans from two patients with AIDS and non-Hodgkin's lymphoma show multiple, nonspecific masses (Fig. 13-43) and a solitary, nonspecific mass with a central air bronchogram (Fig. 13-44).

Index